PUBLIC HEALTH IN THE 21ST CENTURY

OVERWEIGHTNESS AND WALKING

PUBLIC HEALTH IN THE 21ST CENTURY

OVERWEIGHTNESS AND WALKING

CALEB I. BLACK
EDITOR

Nova Science Publishers, Inc.
New York

NOTICE TO THE READER

The Publisher has taken reasonable care in the preparation of this book, but makes no expressed or implied warranty of any kind and assumes no responsibility for any errors or omissions. No liability is assumed for incidental or consequential damages in connection with or arising out of information contained in this book. The Publisher shall not be liable for any special, consequential, or exemplary damages resulting, in whole or in part, from the readers' use of, or reliance upon, this material.

Independent verification should be sought for any data, advice or recommendations contained in this book. In addition, no responsibility is assumed by the publisher for any injury and/or damage to persons or property arising from any methods, products, instructions, ideas or otherwise contained in this publication.

This publication is designed to provide accurate and authoritative information with regard to the subject matter covered herein. It is sold with the clear understanding that the Publisher is not engaged in rendering legal or any other professional services. If legal or any other expert assistance is required, the services of a competent person should be sought. FROM A DECLARATION OF PARTICIPANTS JOINTLY ADOPTED BY A COMMITTEE OF THE AMERICAN BAR ASSOCIATION AND A COMMITTEE OF PUBLISHERS.

LIBRARY OF CONGRESS CATALOGING-IN-PUBLICATION DATA

Overweightness and walking / Editor, Caleb I. Black.
   p. cm.
Includes index.
ISBN 978-1-60741-298-4 (hardcover)
1. Obesity. 2. Walking. I. Black, Caleb I.
RC628.O945 2009
616.3'98--dc22
          2010002301

Published by Nova Science Publishers, Inc. † New York

CONTENTS

PREFACE

This book presents and discusses current data on the topics of overweightness and walking. Angular momentum as a metric of human walking is discussed as well as the influence of visual, somatosensory and vestibular information and their interaction in relation to postural control and adaptive walking. The most recent evidence concerning the spinal and supraspinal control of human walking is examined as are stride-to-stride variability in patterns of lower extremity muscle activity after stroke. Also discussed in this publication is the effectiveness of school-based policies to reduce childhood obesity; and obesity as a complication of cancer or as a side-effect of a treatment of cancer in children, as well as obesity among community-dwelling older adults and their health-related issues and treatments. Traditionally human walking has been characterized by kinematic (position) and kinetic (force/acceleration) descriptors. However, recent work has suggested that angular momentum of body segments and that of the total body about a walker's center of mass (CoM) may provide additional insights into walking. Angular momenta are a way to characterize human walking using the velocity (linear and angular) of the segments.

Chapter 1 - However angular momentum in human walking has been little studied. In the past this may have been in part due to the fact that somewhat more extensive measurements and modeling that are required to compute angular momentum. Computation of the whole body angular momentum requires knowledge of the anthropometrics of the individual. Specifically one needs to know the location of both the center of mass (CoM) and the moments of inertia (I) of each segment. In addition, the motion, in three dimensions, of each segment is needed. Today's sophisticated motion capture systems combined with biomechanical models of human bodies allows computation of the angular momenta with some accuracy.

Naturally, merely having the technology to measure and compute a parameter provides no motivation to do so. The first modern work to look at angular momentum during walking is generally attributed to Elftman. Using the anthropometric data of Braun and Fischer and movement data from Fischer from the 19th century he reported that the angular momentum of the arms about the vertical axis countered that of rest of the body and that the arms did not act as pendulums but required muscular action.

For the next 60 years there was little research investigating the angular momenta of walking until two studies of angular momenta in the elderly were published. In 1998 Kaya et al. studied elderly subjects and found differences in the maximum HAT (head, arms and torso) angular momenta in the sagittal and lateral planes between healthy elders and elders with bilateral vestibular hypofunction. Simoneau and Krebs reported similar total body angular momenta about the center of mass (CoM) for an entire gait cycle between elderly fallers and non-fallers. Both studies found the whole body angular momentum normalized by body mass was small (<0.03 m^2 rad/s).

While angular momentum was of little interest to students of human walking, it was of interest to the researchers searching for control strategies for legged robots. Over a period of time, such as a gait cycle, the angular momentum on the total body of a walker must be zero or the individual or legged robot would rotate. As this is not the case, one strategy is to maintain zero angular momentum of the total body about its CoM throughout the gait cycle; referred to as zero angular momentum control. Thus when controlling the gait of a legged robot, the placement of a "foot" is planned so that the ground reaction force goes through the zero moment point (ZPM), the point where the force vector passes through the CoM of the walker and thus results in no moment on the CoM. Several control strategies employing some form of angular momentum control have been put forward. Of special interest is the work of Herr and coworkers, because as part of their work they investigated the gait of humans walking.

Culminating in a study of ten individuals walking at their comfortable walking speed (CWS) Herr and Popovic computed the angular momentum of total body about the total body CoM with a 16 segment model. They used principal component analysis (PCA) to show that most of the variation of the normalized angular momenta is contained in the first few principal components. They suggest that the regulation of angular momenta is part of the strategy to minimize work during walking.

Bennett et al. followed this work with an analysis exploring the effects of changing walking speed on angular momenta. Their results were in agreement with those of Herr and Popovic and showed how angular momenta changed with walking speed while the principal components of the whole body angular momenta remained constant. In a related article Robert, et al. examined the organization of the angular momenta from motor control perspective and showed that certain angular momenta act synergistically possibly representing a method for controlling walking.

This chapter presents data and analysis of angular momentum of healthy adults, typically developing children, and children with cerebral palsy (CP) walking. The author begin by reviewing the physics and mathematics of computing angular momenta. The author then present the angular momenta of the whole body and body segments of individuals walking at their comfortable walking speed. The author include descriptions of how the angular momenta of different body segments oscillate to maintain a low total angular momentum and the whole body data can be represented by a reduced data set. The author then discuss how angular momenta change with changes in walking speed. The author next present data of children with CP and typically developing children and use this data to describe the relationship of angular momentum to other gait parameters, including energy and work. Next there is a discussion of the implications of the angular momenta patterns for motor control of walking. Finally, the author conclude our analysis and discuss future directions for research into the angular momenta of walking.

Chapter 2 - Sensorimotor processing is necessary to perform motor actions according to environmental demands. The influence of visual, somatosensory and vestibular information, as well as their interaction, is largely studied in relation to postural control. Sensory integration is also crucial during adaptive locomotion and depends on both the task and the individual constraints. Several studies have been designed to observe the effects of the visual system on walking behavior, whereas the role of vestibular information, which is responsible for detecting linear and angular accelerations of the head in space, remains unclear. In this way, a series of three experiments was developed to investigate the contribution of the vestibular system on adaptive walking. In the first study, two different ways of disrupting vestibular system information in young adults were compared. Caloric and rotational stimulations were applied and subjects were asked to estimate the disturbance perceived. Rotational stimulation proved to disturb the vestibular system more intensively. In the second experiment, after rotational stimulation the author asked young adults to walk and step over an obstacle. The results revealed that subjects' walking pattern changed in the presence of vestibular perturbation when compared to the condition of no stimulation. In the third experiment the author used the same procedures and tasks of Experiment 2, but in older adults with no history of vestibular sickness. Older adults also showed spatial and temporal adjustments in their walking pattern. The results of these studies allowed us to conclude that vestibular information is not used to control limb elevation over an obstacle, but it is quite important in controlling locomotion direction. In addition, involvement in physical activity programs seems to minimize the effects of vestibular deficits.

Chapter 3 - Plantar pressure can contribute to the systematic measurement, description, and assessment of quantities that characterize human locomotion and its analysis may provide additional insight into the etiology of pain and lower extremities complaints allowing for injury prevention.

Plantar pressure measurements during walking or other activities can demonstrate the pathomechanics of the abnormal foot and yield objective measures for outcomes evaluation or to track disease progression. In order to reduce the risk of tissue damage and to prevent diabetic foot ulceration in the neuropathic foot, the reduction of plantar pressure shall be a goal. In looking forward to avoid or minimize foot pain discomfort in rheumatoid arthritis, the reduction of plantar pressure is also a therapeutic goal .

Walking represents an ideal physical activity to initiate a change in the behavior, which is needed to acquire health benefits, and which is accessible to all the community segments. It can be incorporated in the daily routine as a way of displacement in the surroundings of home, a way of exercise, to move from a place to another or for simple pleasure. Therefore, considering that the interest in physical fitness continues to grow in postmenopausal women, as a result of promoting health and wellness, the understanding of the dynamic characteristics of the symptom-free foot during the human locomotion provides the necessary basis for objective evaluation of movement dysfunction . This review includes relevant information for the assessment of the human locomotion based on plantar pressure in symptom-free postmenopausal women.

Our aim is to provide a selected review of information relevant to the assessment of the human locomotion based on plantar pressure, indicating several methodological concerns that must be taken into consideration, in order to achieve valid, reliable and accurate data. With this paper, the author hope to contribute to the improvement of gait analysis as an effective tool in the clinical decision, by making a process for improving treatment outcome in individuals.

Chapter 4 - This review will focus on both the most recent evidence concerning the spinal and supraspinal control of human walking, in both health and disease, as well as the new and emerging techniques for performing these studies. In recent years our understanding of how humans control walking has undergone a revolution. Animal studies indicated that the spinal cord plays a critical role in the control of locomotion. Even in the absence of sensory input the spinal cord of cats and rats are capable of generating a 'locomotor rhythm'. Sensory input, such as that arising from a moving treadmill belt, can alter this rhythm such that animals will adapt the speed of the rhythm to match the treadmill, and can even decouple the two sides of the body so that one leg steps faster than the other. More recent studies from individuals with spinal cord injuries have indicated that although the spinal cord, and the circuitry within the spinal cord are critically important to human walking, the cortical drive to the spinal cord appears to be of greater importance in humans than other species.

In large part our change in understanding of the control of human walking has come apart because of studies utilising new, neurophysiological techniques, as well as studies on individuals with damage to their nervous system. These new approaches to studying the neural control of walking have included such methods as transcranial magnetic stimulation and temporal and spectral analysis of muscle activity (EMG) as well as the more established reflex approaches, many of which have been refined in recent years. These new and refined neurophysiological approaches will be described and the evidence they have provided will be presented and evaluated and emerging techniques described.

Chapter 5 - This article brings the biomechanical analysis of sport – Nordic walking – for patients with osteoporotic fractured vertebrae and shows that it is suitable for them.

Based on the biomechanical model of skeletal load the author have developed a method of walking movement for patients, different from the method of walking movement for healthy people. And so came into being the "first sport"for patients with osteoporotic fractures. They can go for regular walks in easy terrains outdoors with friends and family, and so be liberated from social isolation. It requires only one-off financial costs of buying the poles and special footwear.

Chapter 6 - This chapter presents neurological and biomechanical principles of human bipedal walking and their potential application to humanoid walking robots by proposing two computational models. First, a computational model of cerebrocerebello-spinomuscular interaction during sagittal planar walking provides insight into each neural system's function based on neuro-anatomy and physiology. The neural systems substantially decouple gait cycle generation and postural stabilization, with a spinal pattern generator fulfilling the former function, and a cerebrocerebellar feedback system fulfilling the latter. A muscle synergy network facilitates control of redundant muscular actuators in descending pathways. Two control variables: horizontal position of the center of mass, and trunk pitch angle, are estimated from sensed information through the ascending neural pathways. Therefore, the space of the controller is simpler than the space of the actuators and plant. In this way, a simple control strategy is constructed.

The second computational model features a hierarchical task execution architecture that is suitable for control of a 3-D biped, for a variety of challenging walking tasks, including walking on difficult terrain with foot placement constraints. This approach supports exploration of performance limits based on biomechanical structure for such challenging tasks. The model uses an enhanced multivariable feedback linearizing controller, inspired by the muscle synergy approach used in the first computational model, to transform the biped into an abstracted plant that is easier to control. As with the first computational model, key control variables are the biped's center of mass, posture, and stepping foot position. The plant abstraction linearizes and decouples these variables, but the linearization has constraints based on actuation limits, and on limits of the biped's base of support. A reachability analysis is performed, in terms of the abstracted plant, in order to generate families of trajectories that satisfy task goals while observing constraints. Use of such trajectory sets supports high performance execution of difficult tasks such as kicking a soccer ball, or dynamic walking on a path of irregularly placed stones, while rejecting disturbances that may occur.

Chapter 7 - Overweight is defined as an excess accumulation of body fat. Overweight is a chronic multifactorial complex disease resulting from a long-term positive energy balance, in which both genetic and environmental factors are involved. It increases the risks of cardiovascular disease (CVD), type 2 diabetes, dyslipidemia, arthritis, and certain cancers and ultimately reduces the average life expectancy.

The purpose of the present review focuses on the current status of our knowledge concerning the genetic determinants of overweight related with CVD, including heart disease, vascular disease, atherosclerosis, stroke and hypertension. The review describes the anthropometric measurements of overweight, the sex steroid hormones involved in the distribution of adipose tissues and the occurrence of CVD, the pathogenesis of overweight, the relationship between overweight and CVD, and the environmental and genetic factors involved in regulating overweight development.

Simple anthropometric measurements of overweight that can be used to measure not only the total amount of fat but also the distribution of fat in the body include BMI, waist circumference, and fat mass, among others. Currently, adipose tissue is recognized not only as a storage deposit of excess energy but also as a major endocrine and secretory organ. Sex steroid hormones including the estrogen, progesterone and androgen receptors are involved in the metabolism, accumulation and distribution of adipose tissues. With a decrease in sex steroid hormones, there is a tendency to increase overweight, which is a major risk for CVD. Based on the current knowledge of the pathogenesis of overweight, genetic factor involvement in the development of overweight is estimated to be at the 30-70% level. There are several plausible mechanisms for a causative role for overweight in producing CVD. These include changes in blood pressure, lipids, glucose metabolism, and systemic inflammation. In addition, evidence is emerging that factors produced by adipose tissue in overweight can directly impact the atherogenic environment of the vessel wall through the regulation of gene expression and function in the endothelial cells, arterial smooth muscle, and macrophage cells. There is also substantial support in the literature that adipose tissue distribution plays an important role in atherosclerotic risk. The heredity of overweight is usually due to an interaction of more than 30 multiple candidate genes that are found at different locations on the gene map, and therefore, is considered to be polygenic in nature. At the present time, research is still attempting to determine the gene variants that cause most cases of overweight.

Chapter 8 - It is well known that the prevalence of obesity in the general population of children is increasing and that this is likely related to sedentary lifestyles and poor eating habits. Obesity is also being seen as a complication of treatments being used for cancer therapy in children as well as cancer itself. This can have a significant impact on a child's future health, especially since survival rates are being improved for many childhood cancers. When obesity results as a complication of a cancer or as a side effect of a treatment for cancer, children will be at risk for problems such as dyslipidemia, impaired glucose tolerance, hypertension, and cardiovascular disease.

Obesity as a complication of cancer in children can be either short-term or long-term. Treatment for cancer such as high dose steroids can result in transiently increased appetite, Cushing's syndrome and obesity during the treatment course. However, other forms of therapy such as radiation to the hypothalamus or surgical manipulation near the hypothalamic/pituitary region can result in permanent damage and cause hypothalamic obesity. In addition, tumors that invade or disrupt the hypothalamic/pituitary region can result in permanent hypothalamic dysregulation and cause obesity.

Trends in the prevalence of childhood cancer related obesity will be examined and a review of the etiology and pathogenesis behind these causes of obesity will be discussed. Current pharmacologic and surgical treatment options will also be reviewed.

Chapter 9 - The prevalence of childhood obesity has increased significantly over the past three decades. It is estimated that approximately 17% of all school-aged children are overweight or obese. Childhood obesity has a huge impact on the health of children as it is associated with an increased risk of hypertension, hypercholesterolemia, diabetes, and a wide range of additional physiological and psychosocial consequences.

Because school settings offer continuous, intensive contact with children during children's formative years, they have several advantages for implementation of interventions. For example, school educational programs can develop student attitudes, knowledge, and skills for a healthy lifestyle. In addition to education, schools can promote healthy dietary practices and regular physical activity by modifying school environments through offering healthier choices in cafeterias and vending machines and by providing physical activity curriculum. Overall, school infrastructure and physical environment, policies, curricula, and personnel have great potential to positively influence children's weight and health.

Based on prior review articles examining interventions implemented at school settings, strategies involving a combination of nutrition and physical activity interventions seem to be effective at achieving weight reduction in school settings. However, less attention has been paid to developing, implementing and evaluating school-based policy on childhood obesity prevention and management. This chapter intends to summarize evidence regarding the effectiveness of school-based policy interventions and to provide possible policy recommendations for researchers, practitioners and policy makers.

The author first provide the definition of overweight and obesity and describe the obesity trends in the US and the world. Physiological, psychosocial and economic consequences related to obesity are also presented. The author then discuss school-based policies and programs. Finally, policy recommendations for preventing obesity are provided.

Chapter 10 – Background: Good dictary habits are important for health enhancement, while inadequate nutrition may increase susceptibility to and delay recovery from illness. To meet the needs of frail older persons and to promote functional longevity, health education on proper nutrition and exercise is important. Obesity is a relatively serious problem in Hong Kong Chinese, as elsewhere in the developed world, owing to the associated increased risks for Type 2 diabetes mellitus, cardiovascular disease and cancer.

Project Aims & Preliminary Findings: In this study, the prevalence of overweight and obesity among community-dwelling older persons was explored, and health-related issues regarding obesity were discussed. The study also examined the effects of a nutrition education program.

A total of 61 older persons (12 males and 49 females, ages ranging from 60 to 89 years, with mean age 73 years) from two elderly community centers took part in the study.

Education level, self-reported health status, body mass index, dietary habits and physical exercise pattern were recorded.

Over 50% reported receiving no formal education. The majority were suffering from at least one chronic illness (hypertension, diabetes, hyperlipidemia or osteoporosis). None knew their BMI. The prevalence of overweight and obesity were very high, with 70% (n=38) overweight or obese.

Consumption of 'desirable' foods (fruits, vegetables, dairy and bean curd products) was low. Participants' intake of fruits and vegetables was inadequate, with 65% of the participants consuming ≤ 1 serving of fruit/day and 33% consuming < 3 servings of vegetables/day. The majority (80%) did not consume any dairy products.

Intervention: Nutrition Education Programme: A nutrition and lifestyle program (NLP) was provided to these elderly in the community centers, and a learning contract approach was used to encourage older people to adhere to the programe.

The NLP lasted for 8 weeks, and covered nutritional labeling, identifying healthy and unhealthy snacks and food (e.g. those high in cholesterol, saturated fat, salt), meal planning, and encouraging physical activity.

Evaluation & Conclusion: Participating elderly were followed up weekly regarding their learning contract on dietary modification and physical activity. Participation in the nutrition education program was high (nearly 95%); participants demonstrated increased knowledge and awareness of their health and nutritional status and were willing to follow the advice on dietary modification and lead a more active lifestyle.

Nutrition behavior is a complex process; a holistic health promotion approach seems to be essential for implementing healthy nutrition behavior.

In: Overweightness and Walking
Editor: Caleb I. Black, pp. 1-33

Chapter 1

ANGULAR MOMENTUM AS A METRIC OF WALKING

C. Bradford Bennett[1,2], Shawn Russell[1,2] and Thomas Robert[3]

[1]Department of Mechanical and Aerospace Engineering, University of Virginia
[2]Department of Orthopaedic Surgery, University of Virginia
[3]INRETS, Biomechanics and Impact Mechanics Laboratory (LBMC),
University of Virginia

INTRODUCTION

Traditionally human walking has been characterized by kinematic (position) and kinetic (force/acceleration) descriptors. However, recent work has suggested that angular momentum of body segments and that of the total body about a walker's center of mass (CoM) may provide additional insights into walking. Angular momenta are a way to characterize human walking using the velocity (linear and angular) of the segments.

However angular momentum in human walking has been little studied. In the past this may have been in part due to the fact that somewhat more extensive measurements and modeling that are required to compute angular momentum. Computation of the whole body angular momentum requires knowledge of the anthropometrics of the individual. Specifically one needs to know the location of both the center of mass (CoM) and the moments of inertia (I) of each segment. In addition, the motion, in three dimensions, of each segment is needed. Today's sophisticated motion capture systems combined with biomechanical models of human bodies allows computation of the angular momenta with some accuracy.

Naturally, merely having the technology to measure and compute a parameter provides no motivation to do so. The first modern work to look at angular momentum during walking is generally attributed to Elftman[1]. Using the anthropometric data of Braun and Fischer and movement data from Fischer from the 19th century he reported that the angular momentum of the arms about the vertical axis countered that of rest of the body and that the arms did not act as pendulums but required muscular action.

For the next 60 years there was little research investigating the angular momenta of walking until two studies of angular momenta in the elderly were published. In 1998 Kaya et al. studied elderly subjects and found differences in the maximum HAT (head, arms and torso) angular momenta in the sagittal and lateral planes between healthy elders and elders with bilateral vestibular hypofunction. Simoneau and Krebs[2] reported similar total body angular momenta about the center of mass (CoM) for an entire gait cycle between elderly fallers and non-fallers. Both studies found the whole body angular momentum normalized by body mass was small (<0.03 m^2 rad/s).

While angular momentum was of little interest to students of human walking, it was of interest to the researchers searching for control strategies for legged robots. Over a period of time, such as a gait cycle, the angular momentum on the total body of a walker must be zero or the individual or legged robot would rotate. As this is not the case, one strategy is to maintain zero angular momentum of the total body about its CoM throughout the gait cycle; referred to as zero angular momentum control. Thus when controlling the gait of a legged robot, the placement of a "foot" is planned so that the ground reaction force goes through the zero moment point (ZPM), the point where the force vector passes through the CoM of the walker and thus results in no moment on the CoM. Several control strategies employing some form of angular momentum control have been put forward. Of special interest is the work of Herr and coworkers[3-5], because as part of their work they investigated the gait of humans walking.

Culminating in a study of ten individuals walking at their comfortable walking speed (CWS) Herr and Popovic computed the angular momentum of total body about the total body CoM with a 16 segment model[3]. They used principal component analysis (PCA) to show that most of the variation of the normalized angular momenta is contained in the first few principal components. They suggest that the regulation of angular momenta is part of the strategy to minimize work during walking.

Bennett et al. followed this work with an analysis exploring the effects of changing walking speed on angular momenta[6]. Their results were in agreement with those of Herr and Popovic and showed how angular momenta changed with walking speed while the principal components of the whole body angular momenta remained constant. In a related article Robert, et al. examined the organization of the angular momenta from motor control perspective and showed that certain angular momenta act synergistically possibly representing a method for controlling walking[7].

This chapter presents data and analysis of angular momentum of healthy adults, typically developing children, and children with cerebral palsy (CP) walking. We begin by reviewing the physics and mathematics of computing angular momenta. We then present the angular momenta of the whole body and body segments of individuals walking at their comfortable walking speed. We include descriptions of how the angular momenta of different body segments oscillate to maintain a low total angular momentum and the whole body data can be represented by a reduced data set. We then discuss how angular momenta change with changes in walking speed. We next present data of children with CP and typically developing children and use this data to describe the relationship of angular momentum to other gait parameters, including energy and work. Next there is a discussion of the implications of the angular momenta patterns for motor control of walking. Finally, we conclude our analysis and discuss future directions for research into the angular momenta of walking.

ANGULAR MOMENTUM: THE PHYSICS AND MATHEMATICS

Angular momentum is the rotational counterpart of linear momentum. The fundamental nature of momentum seems often overlooked in physics. However, Sir Isaac Newton himself formulated his second law of motion laws of physics in terms of momentum writing his famous equation not in the familiar form of $F=ma$, but as the time rate of change of momentum $(d(mv)/dt)$. It is only when the mass remains constant does the equation degenerate into the familiar $F=ma$.

Momentum is a vector quantity in both its linear and angular forms. However the determination of angular momentum and its properties requires more sophisticated mathematics and more abstraction. The linear momentum vector points in the direction of the velocity vector. However the angular momentum vector, $L =m(rxv)$, is computed as the cross product of the velocity vector and the vector from the point about which the angular momentum is being computed to the "particle" that is moving. Thus angular momentum is computed relative to a specific point in space which itself may be stationary or in motion.

The fact that the angular momentum is computed as vector cross products creates a resultant that is orthogonal to the vectors in the product. Thus motions in the XY plane create an angular momentum in the Z direction, using the standard right hand coordinate system. Correspondingly, the angular momentum in the X direction is a result of motions in the YZ plane and angular momentum in the Y direction is the result of movements in the XZ plane. This property can cause confusion when comparing angular momentum results to velocity and position parameters.

Another important feature of momentum is that it is a conserved property, Newton's first law of motion. Thus, if no outside forces act upon a body, its velocity does not change and its momentum is unchanged. This is the principal at play when a skater spinning on the ice brings her arms closer to her center of rotation. As **r**, the distance from the arms to the center, decreases the angular velocity (ω) must increase to keep the total angular momentum constant.

While one can compute the angular momentum of a point mass about a position, in biomechanics we are usually more interested in the angular momentum of a body, usually assumed to be rigid. Using the property that momentum is that it is a linear quantity; that is to say the total angular momentum of a group of objects/segments is the sum of the angular momentums of each object/segment, it can be shown that the angular momentum about an arbitrary point in space can be computed as the sum of the local angular momentum, the segment revolving about its own CoM, and a transfer term, the result of the CoM of the segment moving relative to the body CoM. The terms are defined for the ith segment as:

$$\vec{L}_{i,local} = I_{CoM_i}\vec{\omega}_i$$

$$\vec{L}_{i,transfer} = \vec{r}_i \times \vec{p}_i = \vec{r}_i \times m_i\vec{v}_i$$

$$\vec{L}_{total} = \sum_{i=1}^{N} = \vec{L}_{i,local} + \vec{L}_{i,transfer}$$

where I_{CoM_i} is the moment of inertia tensor of the segment, $\vec{\omega}_i$ is the angular velocity vector, $\vec{r}_i$ and $\vec{v}_i$ are the relative position and velocity of the ith segment CoM to the whole body CoM respectively, $\vec{p}_i$ is the linear momentum of the ith segment, m_i is the mass of the segment, and N is the total number of segments, see Figure 1.

Computation of Angular Momentum from Experimental Data

The computation of the angular momenta of a subject walking requires the measured velocities of the walkers segments and the anthropometrics of the subject. The experimental data is collected using a motion capture system with the subject wearing a full body set of markers, so that each segments movement can be measured. A common full body model often includes 16 body segments consisting of the: head/neck, upper torso, central torso, lower torso, upper arms (2), lower arms (2), hands (2), upper legs (2), lower legs (2), and feet (2). However, we have found that the results using a simpler 12 segment model with a single torso segment, a combined head-neck segment, and combining the hands and forearms were not appreciably different from the 16 segment model. Another input into models to compute angular momentum are the subject specific anthropometric data (segments' physical properties (mass, length, CoM, and moment of inertia)) based upon subject age, weight, height, and gender. Again results were not significantly different using either the Generator of Body Data (GeBOD) database[8] or using the method validated by Eames [9]. Finally, it should be noted that for walking the transfer term dominates the total angular momentum.

The coordinate system used in this chapter has the positive X axis pointing in the direction of walking, the positive Y axis pointing up and the Z axis in the medial lateral direction formed by the right hand rule. Thus the angular momenta in the X-direction reflect movements in the frontal plane, while moments in the Y and Z-directions reflect movements in the transverse and sagittal planes, respectively.

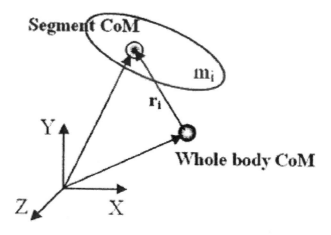

Figure 1. Whole body CoM and i^{th} segment represented in a global coordinate system

ANGULAR MOMENTUM OF ADULTS

In this section we present and interpret the angular momentum analysis of adults walking at their comfortable walking speed (CWS). We show that the angular momenta about all three axes are well organized and reproducible between individuals when normalized by the individual's height, mass, and walking speed. In addition to presenting data of both groupings (eg. upper body) and individual body segments, the cancellation coefficients (the fraction of the total momenta that are cancelled by opposing momenta) about each axis are presented. Finally, a principal component analysis (PCA) is presented revealing how a reduced set of orthogonal parameters can describe the angular momentum of the whole body.

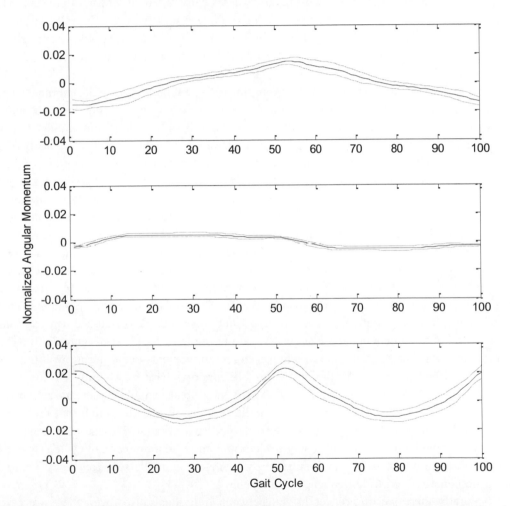

Figure 2. Mean ± standard deviation of the normalized (non-dimensional) angular momentum of walking at CWS. Angular momentum is normalized by subject walking speed, height, and mass. (a) Momentum about the X axis (frontal plane movements), (b) Momentum about the Y axis (transverse plane movements), (c) Momentum about the Z axis (sagittal plane movements).

Angular Momentum of Walking at CWS

Over a gait cycle the net angular momentum of the total body of the walking human must be zero. However, this does not rule out variations away from zero during the gait cycle. To determine the angular momentum of healthy adults walking at their comfortable walking speed (CWS) data were collected on 11 adult males. The subjects were free of any neurological or musculoskeletal conditions or injuries that would have affected their gait. Subject consent was approved by the University of Virginia's Human Investigation Committee and obtained for all subjects.

The subjects performed overground walking trials at their self-selected CWS. Three-dimensional kinematic data were collected using a six camera Vicon Motion Analysis System at 120 Hz. As is inherent in overground walking there was some variation in walking speed at each condition. The three strides that were closest to the desired speed with negligible acceleration and complete data were analyzed. This resulted in walking speeds within +/- 6.5% of the CWS..

Figure 2 shows the variation of the mean normalized total body angular momenta about the three principal axes for subjects at their CWS over a gait cycle. (For this plot and all subsequent plots in this chapter the gait cycle is defined as beginning and ending with left foot contact.) These results, where the angular momenta are normalized by subject height, mass, and walking speed, are typical of what has been reported in the literature[3;6;7;10]. Figure 2a shows the angular momentum about the X-axis, the direction of walking, the result of movements in the frontal plane. This momentum has its extrema during single support and is mostly due to lateral movement of the torso/CoM. Thus as an individual accepts weight onto the front foot at the start of double support, the CoM shifts from over the back foot to be more centered between the feet in the frontal plane. This results in a relative motion between the lower limbs and upper body and the CoM creating angular momentum. The angular momentum about the vertical, Y, axis behaves somewhat differently, see Figure 2b. The angular momentum of the transverse plane is the smallest of the whole body momenta. This is mostly a result of cancellation between the upper and lower body as discussed below. Finally, the angular momentum tends to be largest that about the lateral axis, see Figure 2c; the result of movements in the sagittal plane where the largest movements occur during walking. Here we see that the maxima occur during the double support phase of walking. During double support two legs are moving in a fashion where they create angular momenta in the same direction relative to the CoM and are thus additive. It is also worth noting that the angular momentum about the Z axis is has two maxima and two minima. This is in contrast to the other two momenta that have only a single maximum and minimum per gait cycle. Thus the Z angular momentum reveals it is dominated by phenomena at the step frequency while the other momenta reflect stride frequency phenomena.

Naturally there are differences in gait between individuals. However, there are certain gait parameters that consistent between individuals. Performance parameters such as joint angles and non-dimensionalized joint moments and CoM motion are subject independent. While the relatively small standard deviations of the normalized momenta shown in Figure 2 suggest there is little deviation between subjects further validation of this can be found by computing the correlation coefficients of the time dependent angular momentum curves between individuals. The traditional correlation formulas for comparing two curves were extended to simultaneously compare the waveforms from all 11 subjects following the method of Gerstenfeld, et al [11]:

$$\rho = \frac{\sum_{S=1}^{11}\left[\sum_{i=1}^{n}(X_i - \overline{X}) \times (Y_i - \overline{Y})\right]}{\sum_{S=1}^{11}\sqrt{\sum_{i=1}^{n}(X_i - \overline{X})^2 \times \sum_{i=1}^{n}(Y_i - \overline{Y})^2}}$$

where X and Y are vectors of length n representing the two waveforms to be compared. Using this technique the correlations between all 11 subjects were 0.94, 0.97, and 0.85 for the momenta about the X, Y, and Z axes, respectively, revealing the high coherence between the gaits of different individuals.

Additional insight into gait can be gained by looking at the angular momenta of groups of segments and individual segments. Although any arbitrary group of segments can be grouped there are certain groupings that make some intuitive sense. Here we will look at the groups of the upper and lower body segments as well as the arms and legs.

Figure 3 shows the angular momenta of the upper (head/neck, torso, and arms) and lower body (feet, shanks, and thighs). From this figure it can be seen that the contributions of the upper and lower body are comparable about the X axis and are additive, of the same sign. About the Y axis the lower body contribution is larger, and the curve is almost 180° out of phase with that of the upper body. This feature is a result of the human contralateral gait. The result is the small total body angular momentum about the vertical axis throughout the gait cycle. Thus as Elftman reported, the angular momenta of the swinging arms counters that of the swinging legs. Finally, the angular momentum in the sagittal plane is mostly due to the lower body, but the two momenta are additive (have the same sign) over most of the gait cycle.

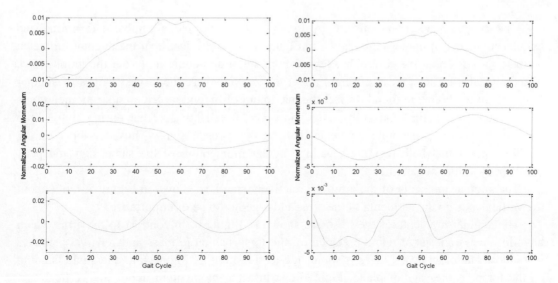

Figure 3. Normalized angular momenta of (a) the upper body (head-neck, torso, and arms) and (b) the lower body (feet, shanks, thighs) at CWS

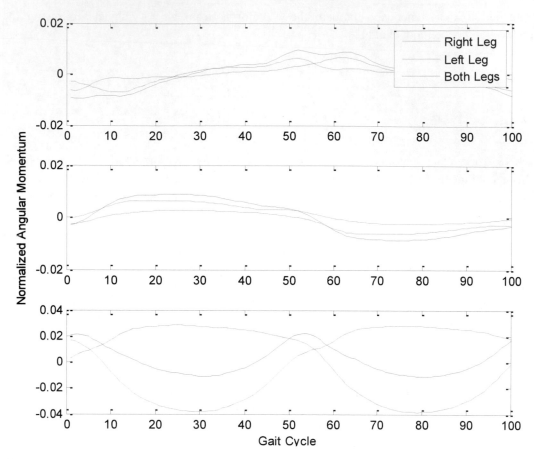

Figure 4. Normalized angular momenta of both legs and their sum about the (a) X axis, (b) Y axis, and (c) Z axis.

One can gain additional insight by looking at the individual limbs. The normalized angular momenta of the legs are shown in Figure 4. It can be seen that the angular momenta of the two legs about the X and Y axes are both small and additive. (Note the graphs have different scales.) The story is different about the Z axis where the largest values of angular momenta in the body are found. In fact the maximum of individual leg angular momentum is greater than that of the total body value. However, it can be seen that during single limb support the two legs generate momenta that are of opposite signs. Thus it is only during double support that both legs are creating angular momentum of the same sign and peak whole body values are attained.

The angular momenta of the arms are relatively small, as shown in Figure 5. Only about the vertical axis do the momenta of the arms add together to be of importance.

The angular momenta of the torso are shown in Figure 6. In contrast to the arms which have low mass and large relative velocities, the torso has large mass and relatively smaller velocities. The plots reveal there is some side-to-side motion, Figure 6-a, and some bending of the torso in the sagittal plane, Figure6-c, while the momentum about the vertical axis remains small during the entire gait cycle. The angular momentum of the head (not shown) is also small throughout the gait cycle about all three axes.

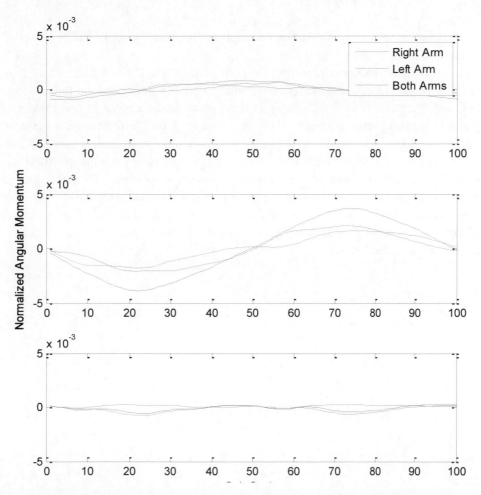

Figure 5. Normalized angular momenta of both arms and their sum about the (a) X axis, (b) Y axis, and (c) Z axis

Angular Momentum Cancellation

Since momentum is a vector quantity it can have opposite signs and thus the angular momentum of different segments can cancel each other when they are summed. As seen above when looking at different groups of segments there is significant cancellation of angular momenta. To examine the amount of cancellation Bennett and co-workers[6] defined a coefficient of cancellation, κ, to reflect the degree that the angular momenta of the body segments canceled each other. The Coefficient of Cancellation, κ, was defined as:

$$\kappa = \frac{\sum_{i=1}^{N} |L_i| - |\sum_{i=1}^{N} L_i|}{\sum_{i=1}^{N} |L_i|}$$

where L_i is the angular momentum in a plane of the ith body segment and N is the total number of segments. If there was no net angular momentum, all segments cancelled each other out perfectly, $\kappa=1$. If there were no cancelation, then the two terms in the numerator are equal and $\kappa=0$.

Plots of the cancellation coefficients for each plane at the CWS are shown in Figure 7. The X momentum had the least cancellation, mostly between the upper and lower body, with a mean coefficient value of 0.22. There is little cancellation except in the middle of the swing/single support phases. The cancellation coefficient of the Y momentum was larger with a mean value of 0.54, with peaks during double support. The most cancellation was found in the Z momentum with mean coefficient of 0.76. There was nearly complete cancellation of the sagittal plane movements during swing/single support phases, but much less during double support when both legs move in the same direction relative to the CoM. Also note that each plot has two peaks and two minima each stride, showing that cancellation phenomena are related to the step frequency, as opposed to the stride frequency. The cancellation is discussed in more detail below.

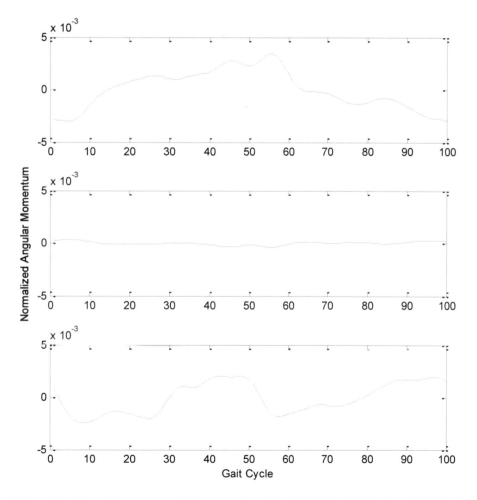

Figure 6. Normalized angular momenta of the torso about the (a) X axis, (b) Y axis, and (c) Z axis

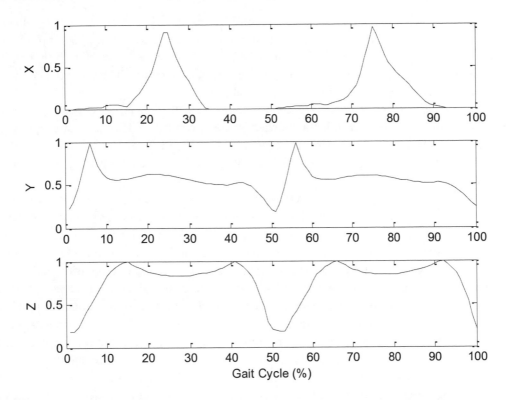

Figure 7. Mean values of the coefficient of cancellation for the angular momentum at CWS in the frontal plane (X), transverse plane (Y), and sagittal plane (Z). A value of 1 means there is no net angular momentum and a value of 0 means the angular momenta of all segments are in the same direction and there is no cancellation

Principal Component Analysis

Principal component analysis (PCA) can be viewed as a mathematical least squares statistical procedure that can transform a large data set of correlated variables into a smaller number of linear uncorrelated variables called principal components (PCs). Thus, PCA can reveal whether data can be described by a reduced set of primitives or basis vectors. The PCs are ordered so that the first principal component accounts for as much of the variability in the data set as possible, and each succeeding component accounts for the maximum amount of variance that is left while being orthogonal to all preceding PCs.

Principal component analysis (PCA) was used to explore whether the angular momentum data could be represented by a reduced data set. (An excellent tutorial on the use of PCA for biomechanical studies can be found in the article by Daffertshofer, et al.[12].) PCA was performed on the time dependent angular momentum of each segment for each principal axis to obtain the set of 12 angular momentum primitives (the body was modeled with 12 segments).

Since PCA basis vectors are data set dependent it is not guaranteed that the PCs computed for each individual are co-linear. The method of Krishnamoorthy et al.[13] was applied to determine the similarity of basis vector sets. In this analysis a central vector of each set of vectors is determined and the dot product of a vector with the PCs in each plane is computed. The closer the dot product is to 1.0 the smaller the "angle" between the two vectors in 12-dimensional space. The results confirm that the basis vectors, PCs, are similar between individuals, see Table 1. The mean dot products were greater than 0.96 and 0.87 for the first and second PCs, respectively. For the third PC the values were slightly lower, but these components account for only small variations in the momenta. Thus like the curves of angular momenta the PCs were similar between subjects.

Principal component analysis, see Figure 8, revealed that the time dependent angular momenta could be represented by a reduced set of primitives. The first three principal components of the average data account for more than 97% of the data variation in all three planes. Looking at just the first two PCs, 88%, 94%, and 96% of the variability of the data is accounted for.

Capturing this large percentage of the variability within a few PCs reflects a very well organized system. The data suggests that just two or three parameters are enough to describe or control the angular momentum during walking. The PC coefficients for the first three principal components and the percentage of the data variability they account for are plotted for each body segment in Figure 8. The coefficients reflect the relative contribution of each segment to the angular momentum about a particular axis for a particular principal component. Coefficients of opposite sign reveal segments whose angular momenta will tend to cancel each other. Examining the first PCs for each axis we see that for movements in the frontal plane the upper and lower body generate angular momenta in the same direction, as was seen above. In the transverse plane the upper and lower body generate angular momenta in opposite directions, which tend to cancel each other. In the sagittal plane, the right and left sides have opposite signs and we see most of the angular momentum is generated in the lower body. Thus the PC coefficients provide much of the information that was found in the plots of the angular momenta themselves.

Figure 9 shows the time dependent PC scores or weighting coefficients on the momenta data for each axis for the first 3 PCs. The first PC has a period that is coincident with a single stride. The second PCs about the Y and Z axes have two periods coincident with a single stride.

The coefficients of the PCs and their respective weighting coefficients provide insight into the generation and cancelation of angular momentum. As mentioned above only 22% of the X-direction total angular momentum was cancelled. This low value is suggested by the coefficients of the first PC all having the same sign. The second PC coefficients of the right and left sides of the body had opposite signs showing they tended to cancel each other, see Figure 3, but this PC explained less than 11% of the dataset variability. The normalized weighting coefficients reveal the time-dependent contributions of the PCs. The weighting coefficient for the first PC revealed the dominant contributions were from movements that repeat once each stride. We also see that at the points where the cancellation peaks, the weighting coefficient of the second PC was largest while the weighting coefficient of the first PC was near zero. The third PC explained only slightly less of the data, 10%, than the second PC and was almost 180° out of phase with that of the second PC2.

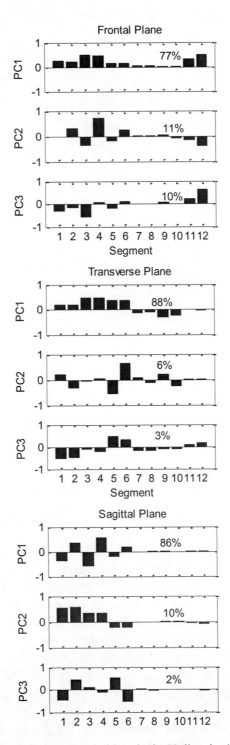

Figure 8. The first three angular momentum primitives in the X-direction/frontal plane (top), Y-direction/transverse plane (middle), and Z-direction/sagittal plane (lower) and their percent data explained. The abscissa numbers correspond to the following segments: Left (L) foot (1), Right (R) foot (2), L shank (3), R shank (4), L thigh (5), R thigh (6), L upper arm (7), R upper arm (8), L forearm/hand (9), R forearm/hand (10), head/neck (11), torso (12) Taken from Bennett, et al.[7]

Table 1. Mean dot product values of the first three PCs between individuals

	Frontal	Transverse	Sagittal
PC1	0.975	0.969	0.999
PC2	0.874	0.909	0.973
PC3	0.859	0.778	0.849

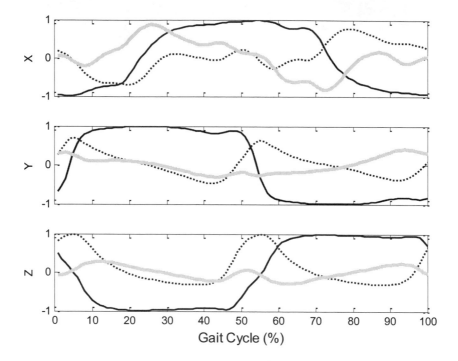

Figure 9. Normalized weighting coefficients for the X-direction/frontal plane (top), Y-direction/transverse plane (middle) and Z-direction/sagittal plane (lower). The black lines are the first PC, the dotted lines on the second PC and the thick grey lines are the third PC in each plot.

In the Y-direction the coefficients of the first PC of the upper and lower body had opposite signs, see Figure xx, reflecting our contralateral gait. They had their largest contributions during leg swing/single support. In the second PC the sides of the body opposed each other, see Figure 3, and were most dominant during double support, see Figure 4, creating the peaks in cancellation shown in Figure xx. For the third PC the main contributors were the feet opposing the thighs, but this accounted for only 3% of the data.

The first PC coefficients, see Figure 8, in the Z-direction revealed that most of the angular momentum was generated by the lower limbs and that the left and right sides opposed each other. This contribution was most dominant during swing phase where the legs create momenta that are of opposite sign. During double support there was very little cancellation because both legs were moving in the same direction relative to the CoM. The second PC had the feet and shanks opposed by the thighs and head and torso momenta. This component, 10%, had its strongest effect during stance when there was little contribution from the first PC, see Figure 4. The third PC was also dominated by the lower body with the two sides opposing each other, but explained only 2% of the data.

Summary

The angular momenta are well regulated and consistent between individuals when nondimensionalized by height, mass, and walking speed. There is an elegant organization of movement that keeps whole body angular momentum small by generating momenta of opposite directions with different parts of the body. Thus we see that the upper body and lower body generate opposing momenta in the transverse plane while the right and left side cancel each other in the sagittal plane. We can examine the dimensional values of angular momenta to better understand the magnitude of the momenta generated during walking. If we assume a 2m tall person with a mass of 75 kg walking at 1.3 m/s the maximum angular momentum on the person is less then 4 kg-m^2/s. This is approximately the angular momentum of a 10 speed bicycle wheel spinning at 5 rev/s. In other words the angular momentum of a the wheel at 4 mph (1.8 m/s), a fast walk. In addition the variability of the angular momenta can be accounted for by only two or three independent (orthogonal) primitives (PCs). The implications of this are discussed below in the section on angular momentum synergies.

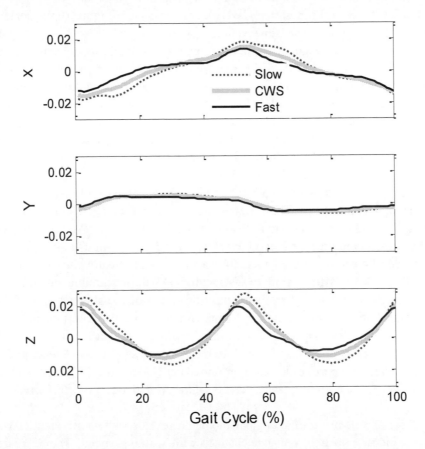

Figure 10. The average total body normalized angular momentum during a gait cycle. The gait cycle was defined as starting and ending with left heel contact (0% and 100%) with the right heel strike at 50%. Starting at the top the momentum in the frontal (X), transverse (Y), and sagittal planes (Z). The wide grey lines are at CWS, dotted lines are slow, and the solid black lines are fast walking. The standard deviations of the curves varied little with walking speed and averaged 0.0031 in the frontal plane, 0.0015 in the transverse plane, and 0.0042 in the sagittal plane.

EFFECTS OF WALKING SPEED ON ANGULAR MOMENTUM

The picture painted by the nondimensional angular momentum analysis becomes even more colorful when the effects of changing the speed of walking. It might be assumed that the angular momentum remains constant with changes in walking speed since it is normalized by the walking speed and is computed relative to the walker's CoM. However, this is not the case. As walking speed increases, the peaks of the normalized angular momenta decrease. This is a result of a more "coherent" gait and the changing of the timing of the gait phases. However, the PCs of the total body angular momenta are invariant with respect to walking speed suggesting this organization may be of importance in the control of walking.

Angular Momentum at Different Walking Speeds

The velocity dependence was investigated with the same subjects discussed above walking at 0.7, 1.0, and 1.3 times their CWS. As can be seen in Figure 10 the peaks in angular momentum were largest at the slow walking speed. In fact there was a negative linear correlation between the angular momentum peaks and walking speed with correlation coefficients of 0.55, 0.66, and 0.76 for momenta about the X, Y, and Z axes, respectively. (Without velocity normalization the peak values increase with walking speed.) There was tendency for the phase to shift with velocity, with the mean curves at the fast speed leading those at the slow speed by 26°, 22°, and 9° in the transverse, sagittal, and frontal planes, respectively, reflecting the shifting in relative timing of the gait phases with walking speed.

While qualitatively similar there was also variation in the cancellation of angular momentum with walking speed, see Figure 11. The total cancelations, areas under the curves, in the Y and Z directions were found to be velocity dependent with cancellation increasing with increasing walking speed. The X momentum had the least cancellation with tendency of mean coefficient values to increase from 0.21 to 0.27 from slow to fast. There was a phase shift in the X momentum cancellation curves with the fast leading the slow data by 36°. The cancellation coefficient of the Y momentum was larger with mean values that increased from 0.46 to 0.60 ($p < 0.0005$) from slow to fast, with peaks during double support. There was a tendency for the cancellation of fast walking to lead that of the slow trials by 11° ($p < 0.05$). The most cancellation remained in the Z momentum with mean coefficients that increased from 0.70 to 0.79 ($p < 0.0005$) from slow to fast. The fast trial cancellation data tended to lead the slow trial cancellation data by 8° ($p < 0.01$). The decrease in the momenta with increasing speed may reflect in part a decrease in movement variability[14] and increase in the coherence[15] between limbs that researchers have found occurs with increasing walking speed.

The effect of velocity on the angular momenta reveals a dynamic view of walking that provides a window into how our gait changes with walking speed. The decrease in the X momentum extrema at higher walking speeds reflects the lower side to side relative velocities at higher walking speeds. The decrease in the Y momentum with increasing speed may reflect in part a decrease in movement variability[14] and increase in the coherence[15] between limbs. The increased coherence is reflected in the increase in momentum cancellation (from 46% to 62% from slow to fast walking) between the upper and lower body in the Y-direction.

While the above argument can also be applied to the momenta in the Z-direction, we also see that the decrease in normalized angular momentum paralleled the decreasing amount of the gait cycle spent in double support. (This was likely impacting the data in the Y and X-directions as well.) The less time spent in double support the longer relative time for the leg to swing and thus a slower leg velocity relative to the CoM. The longer relative swing time also increased the percentage of the gait cycle when cancellation of momenta was high, i.e. the two legs are generating opposing momenta. The changing time in double support was also reflected in the phase shifts of the momenta and cancellation curves with changing speed.

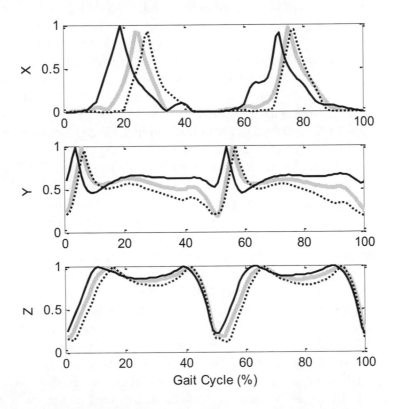

Figure 11. Mean curves of the coefficient of cancellation for the angular momentum at different walking speeds in the frontal plane (X), transverse plane (Y), and sagittal plane (Z). The wide grey lines are CWS, dotted lines are slow, and the solid black lines are fast walking. The peaks of cancellation occur earlier at faster speeds and the total cancellation (area under the curve) increases with walking speed. A value of 1 means there is no net angular momentum and a value of 0 means the angular momenta of all segments are in the same direction. The gait cycle was defined as starting and ending with left heel contact (0% and 100%) with the right heel strike at 50%.

Table 2. Mean dot product values of the first three PCs at different walking speeds

Between Speeds			
	Frontal	Transverse	Sagittal
PC1	0.999	0.995	1.000
PC2	0.950	0.974	0.990
PC3	0.952	0.858	0.994

Principal Component Analysis

The principal components of the angular momenta are independent of walking speed[5;6]. This can be demonstrated by using the method of central vector analysis described above. This analysis was performed on the mean data at each walking speed and is shown in Table 2 the dot products were greater than 0.95 for the first and second PCs in all planes. Thus the PCs are very co-linear between walking speeds.

However, there were aspects of the analyses that were velocity dependent. In the frontal plane the percentage of data variance explained by each PC was independent of velocity, but this was not the case in the transverse and sagittal planes. In both planes the degree to which the data is explained by the first PC increased with increasing speed. In the transverse plane the percentage increased from 83.3% (slow) to 89.5% (fast) (p<0.0001), while in the sagittal plane the percentage increased from 82.0% (slow) to 88.1% (fast) (p<0.0001). The second PCs reduced from 7.6% to 6.1% (p<0.05) and 12.5% to 8.4% (p<0.0001) from slow to fast in the transverse and sagittal plane data, respectively. The third PCs went from 4.9% to 2.4% (p<0.0001) and 3.3 to 2.0% (p<0.0005) from slow to fast in the Y and Z data, respectively.

The invariance of the PC vectors means that the *directions* (in the 12 dimensional segment angular momentum space) that had the most angular momentum variation were independent of walking speed. In other words the organization of the PCs did not change. However the percentage of the data variation that was explained by each PC did change with velocity reflecting changes in the gait structure, such as the changing relative time spent in stance with changing walking speed, as noted above.

The effect of shorter stance times can be seen in the structure of the PCs and their weighting coefficients. As shown in Figure 9, the weighting coefficients of the first PCs about the Y and Z axes were minimal (near zero) during double support (approximately 0% - 20% and 50% - 70% of the gait cycle) while the coefficients of the second PCs reach their maximums. During single support the situation reversed and the weighting coefficients of the first PCs about the Y and Z axes achieve their extremas while the second and third PCs reach their minimums (zero). Thus a shorter double support period increases the 'influence' of the first PC and decreases the contributions of the second and third PCs. In addition, the first PCs the momenta about the Z and Y axes are responsible for most of the cancellation, both because they are the major contributors to the momentum and have components (coefficients) that generate momenta in different directions (are of opposite signs) as shown in Figure 8 Thus while the structure of the PCs (the coefficients) did not change with velocity, the changes in the structure of the gait with increasing velocity resulted in a decrease in the total normalized angular momenta from the increased cancelation without any change in the structure of the PCs.

Summary

The normalized angular momenta extrema are inversely proportional to walking speed. This seems to be a result of increased cancellation caused by both a more coherent walking structure and a decrease in time spent in double support with increasing speed. This change is also seen in the increasing percentage of variability accounted for by the first PCs about the Y and Z axes with a corresponding decrease in the percent variance explained by the second and third PCs. However, it is of importance that the PC vectors (coefficients) remained invariant. The invariance of the PC vectors means that the *directions* (in the 12 dimensional segment angular momentum space) that had the most angular momentum variation were independent of walking speed. The analysis of angular momentum with changing gait speed further suggests that angular momentum may be an organizing factor in walking.

CHILDREN WITH CP AND THE RELATIONSHIP TO ENERGIES AND WORK

In the present section we examine the work, both internal and external, energy, and angular momenta of TD children and children with CP at preferred walking speeds. We relate the angular momenta to traditional gait parameters and compare it between the two groups. We demonstrate that angular momenta are greater in children with CP compared to TD children. However, because of overall gait similarities the shape of the angular momenta over the gait cycle the principal components are not be different between the two groups. Also due to the relation of momenta and internal work/energy we also show that the angular momentum of the body can be used as an indicator to quantify the contribution of individual limbs and segments to the total internal work done over a gait cycle.

The relationship between momenta and work are presented in an effort to quantify the contribution of gait kinematics to internal work, much as the determinants of gait[16-19] have been used to quantify kinematic effect on external work. Momentum is a convenient method of quantification of work and it represents dynamic motion over the entire gait cycle as opposed to the determinants, which represent a static snapshot of one instant in the gait cycle [16]. A cursory review of the equations for energy and momentum reveal that momentum equations are the derivative of the energy equations, though in reality this is not a direct relation since energy is a scalar while momentum is a vector quantity. However, the energy due to relative motion about the CoM can be broken up into orthogonal components for comparison to directional momentum in place of work as discussed previously.

Kinematic data on a convenience sample of 24 children were collected and analyzed. This group of children consisted of two populations. The first group of age-matched controls was comprised of 8 children without known musculoskeletal, neurological, cardiac, or pulmonary pathology, and included 2 females and 6 males averaging 10.3 ± 1.9 years of age, 141.8 ± 12.9 cm in height, and 39.8 ± 14.7 kg in mass. The second group consisted of 16 children diagnosed with spastic diplegic CP. These subjects were community ambulators, with a mean score of $92 \pm 7\%$ on the Gross Motor Function Measure[20] and walked without aids. They included 7 females and 9 males averaging 10.1 ± 4.1 years of age, 135.5 ± 29.4 cm in height, and 34.4 ± 16.9 kg in mass. None of the subjects had undergone surgery or other significant treatments within the 12 months prior to being tested and all subjects with CP walked with some degree of equinus gait, i.e. they had no true heel strike.

Work/Energy Computation

The total energy of a system can be described via the following method developed by Willems[21]:

$$E_{Total} = MgH + \frac{1}{2}MV_g^2 + \sum_{i=1}^{n}\left(\frac{1}{2}m_i v_{i,g}^2 + \frac{1}{2}I_i\varpi_i^2\right)$$

for segments $i = 1 \to n$

The first two terms represent the "external energy" or the energy state of the CoM as it moves through space and is based only on the motion of the composite CoM. It is this energy and the work associated with its change that is used in current energy evaluation methods such as determinants of gait[16-18] and others[22;23] based on CoM movement. The two other terms represent "internal energy" or the energy of the limbs as they move about the CoM and are based on the rotational motion of each segment about its own CoM and the velocity of the segments CoM relative to the composite CoM. Similar to the momentum calculations it is this relative velocity component that dominated the internal energy, as seen in the results section. It is these terms which relate with angular momentum.

Work is the total change in energy, and were calculated following the method of Willems[21], allowing energy transfer between the segments of a limb only, i.e. the thigh, shank, and foot of a leg, with no transfer between limbs.

$$W_{wo/trans} = |\Delta PE| + |\Delta KE|$$
$$W_{w/trans} = |\Delta PE + \Delta KE|$$

Unlike momentum, work/energy is a scalar and typically cannot be split it up into components in different directions. This holds for internal energy due to the rotational motion of each segment, because it is the product of two tensors, I and ω : $E_{int/rot} = \varpi^T I\varpi$. Because mass is a scalar as apposed to a tensor like inertia, the relative energy can be reported as the sum of the energy due to the motion in three orthogonal planes resulting in easier comparison with the directional momentum.

Angular Momenta

The average normalized angular momenta were small for the entire gait cycle as it was in the adults, see Figure 12. In fact the momenta for the children with TD are almost identical to that found for the adult walkers. Overall the angular momenta of the total body about the CoM have the same general pattern for children with CP and the controls as shown in Figure 12. However, there were some noteworthy differences. For the Z axis, the absolute area under the curve, momentum area, was 73% larger in the group with CP, $P < 0.01$, Figure 12. In addition the momenta curve of the children with CP lagged that of the TD children by 31°, $p < 0.01$. The momentum area about the X axis reflect the side to side leaning motions of the body and is larger in the group with CP by 50%, $p = 0.058$, (Figure 12). The extrema occurred just before the swing foot left the ground and were about twice as large in the children with CP. The momenta about the vertical, Y, axis were small and similar for the two groups.

The cancellation of angular momenta curves in the typically developing children, Figure 13 was very similar in both shape and total amount of cancellation per gait cycle to that of adults, Figure 7. However the curves are somewhat different for the children with CP, Figure 13. While retaining the overall shapes of the typically developing children and adults, the children with CP had increased cancellation in the transverse plane motions. (The slight increase in the frontal plane was not significantly different.) The 30% increase in the cancellation about the Y axis reflects the larger angular momenta generated by both the lower and upper body in the children with CP. However, the upper and lower bodies remain nearly 180° out of phase. The end result is there is no difference in the total body angular momentum in the transverse plane.

The story is very different in the sagittal plane. There we see a 15% decrease in cancellation over the whole gait cycle, with a corresponding increase in total body angular momentum. It is important to recall the most of the cancellation in the sagittal plane is from the legs generating opposing moments during the single limb support. However, children with CP, including this group, have longer double support phases. This decreases the percent of the gait cycle that is available for the swing leg to move forward, requiring a greater velocity relative to the CoM. This same phenomena was seen in the adult data at slower walking speeds. The longer double support times also contribute to the phase shifts seen in the cancellation curves.

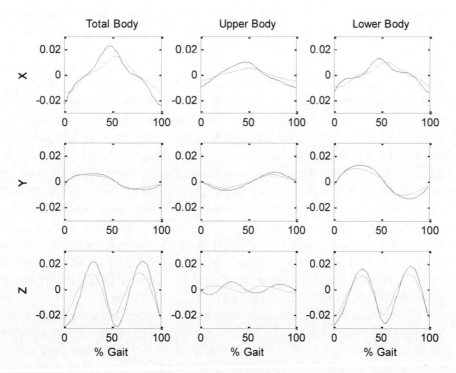

Figure 12. The angular momentum of the total body, the upper body, and the lower body for both TD children (solid line) and children with CP (dashed line) about the three principle axis, X frontal, Y transverse, and Z sagittal plane. Non-dimensional momentum was normalized by height, mass, average velocity, and is reported with respect to gait cycle.

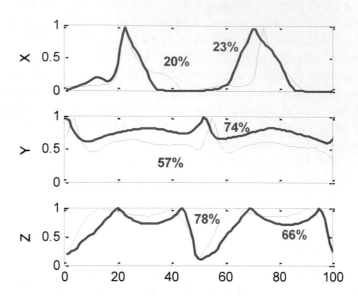

Figure 13 Mean values of the coefficient of cancellation for the angular momentum at CWS in the frontal plane (X), transverse plane (Y), and sagittal plane (Z) for children with TD (blue) and children with CP (red_. A value of 1 means there is no net angular momentum and a value of 0 means the angular momenta of all segments are in the same direction and there is no cancellation.

Other differences between the CP and TD groups occur when comparing properties of the upper and lower body (Figure 12). **In the upper body the CP group's momenta area** are larger about both the X and Z axes, P=0.025 and P<0.01 respectively. The increased side-to-side motion represented by the angular momentum about the X axis reveals an accommodation for equinus gait where the subject leans to one side in order to lift the hip of the swing leg to increase foot clearance during swing. Also of note is the phase difference about Z axes, where the CP group led the TD group by 75°, P=0.01. Thus children with CP are moving their upper bodies at very different times than the children with TD, most likely related to the circumduction of the foot during swing.

Comparisons of the lower body data revealed that the subjects with CP had a greater momenta area about the Y and Z axis than the TD group, P<0.01 about both axes. Unlike the upper body, the lower body momentum phase was different in all three axis, X, Y, and Z, with the CP population, lagging 18° in the X axis, P=0.01, and leading 7° in the Y axis, P=0.03, and leading 18° about the Z axis, P=0.04. For both groups the angular momenta *area* was larger for the lower body about both the Y and Z axis, P<0.001 for all cases, while there was no difference for the CP group about the X axis, the momenta was slightly larger about the X axis for the TD group, P=0.043 (Figure 12).

Narrowing the focus of the analysis to individual limbs and limb segments offers more insight into individual movements. The swing leg of children with CP had larger angular momentum about all three axes (X P<0.01, Y P<0.01, and Z P<0.05) but particularly about the X and Y axis during swing, i.e. 10-55% gait (Figure 15). This represent circumduction of the leg/foot during swing, a common adaptation employed to increase foot clearance in equinus gait. The angular momenta and internal work of the arms were similar for both groups.

Work/Energy

When walking at their comfortable walking speed, children with CP did 59% more total work per unit mass and distance traveled than the typically developed group, 1.64 J/kg-m and 1.03 J/kg-m respectively, P<0.01. For subjects with CP 60% of this total work is attributed to external work or movement of the body center of mass, while external work accounted for 47% of total work for typically developed, or 0.99J/kg-m and 0.49 J/kg-m respectively, P<0.01. This means that the body center of mass motion of children with CP results in 102% more work being done per kg-m than for typically developing children. The balance of the total work is the internal work or the work associated with the motion of body segments about the body center of mass. While walking, children with CP did 21% more internal work than typically developing children, P=0.053. For children with CP this results in 0.66 J/kg-m of internal work being done vs. 0.54 J/kg-m for typically developing children, 40% and 53% of the total work respectively. Looking at the upper and lower body internal work revealed a trend of increased work for the children with CP. For the upper body the CP group had 0.0986 J/kg-m compared to the TD group, 0.0646 J/kg-m, P=0.18, while for the lower body the CP group had 0.562 J/kg-m compared to the TD mean of 0.481 J/kg-m, P=0.06. The associated internal work of the swing leg over an entire gait cycle shows little overall difference between groups (CP 0.263 J/kg-m, TD 0.234 J/kg-m, P=0.15).

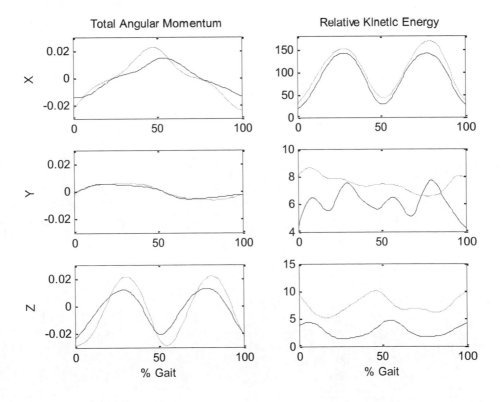

Figure 14. Non-dimensional total body angular momentum about the X frontal, Y transverse, and Z sagittal axis over a gait cycle for both TD children (solid) and children with CP (dashed). And the relative energy component of internal energy along the three orthogonal axis, presented as mJ/kg-m.

Multiple regression analyses were conducted to relate the momenta and energy of the total body (Figure 14), and the swing leg in gait (Figure 15). For the total body analysis the relative energy in the X and Z directions correlated with the associated momentum for both groups, TD: $R^2=0.75$ and 0.95 respectively, $P<0.0001$, and CP: $R^2=0.88$ and 0.72 respectively, $P<0.0001$. There was a poor correlation of the relative energy in the Y direction, TD: $R^2=0.33$ $P<0.0001$ and CP: $R^2=0.09$ $P<0.0035$.

Results for the swing leg were similar to the whole body results. The relative energy in the X and Z axis correlated to the associated momentum for both groups, TD $R^2=0.91$ and 0.82 respectively, $P<0.0001$, and CP $R^2=0.95$ and 0.78 respectively, $P<0.0001$ with a poor correlation for the relative energy in the Y direction, TD: $R^2=0.33$ $P<0.0001$ and CP: $R^2=0.01$ $P<0.024$. A cross correlation was also conducted to relate the time dependent momentum of the swing leg in the X and Y directions with energy in the Z and X directions respectively for TD and CP subjects. For TD children the momentum about the X axis and energy in the Z direction had a correlation coefficient of $C=0.8334$ and $C=0.7943$ for momenta about the Y axis and energy in the X direction. Children with CP showed similar correlations $C=0.7871$ for momenta about X and energy in Z direction and $C=0.9196$ for momenta about the Y axis and energy in the X direction.

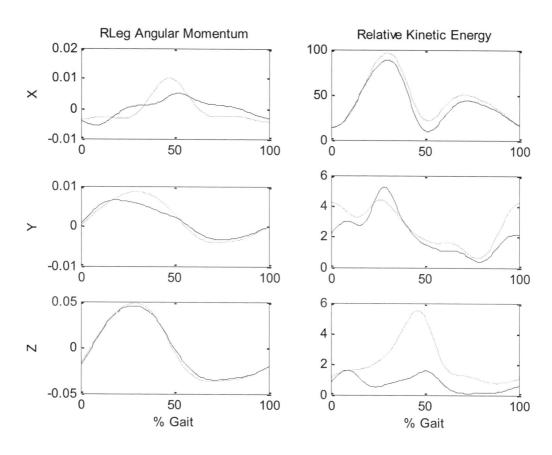

Figure 15. Non-dimensional angular momentum of the right (swing) leg about the X frontal, Y transverse, and Z sagittal axis over a gait cycle for both TD children (solid) and children with CP (dashed). And the relative energy component of internal energy along the three orthogonal axis, presented as mJ/kg-m.

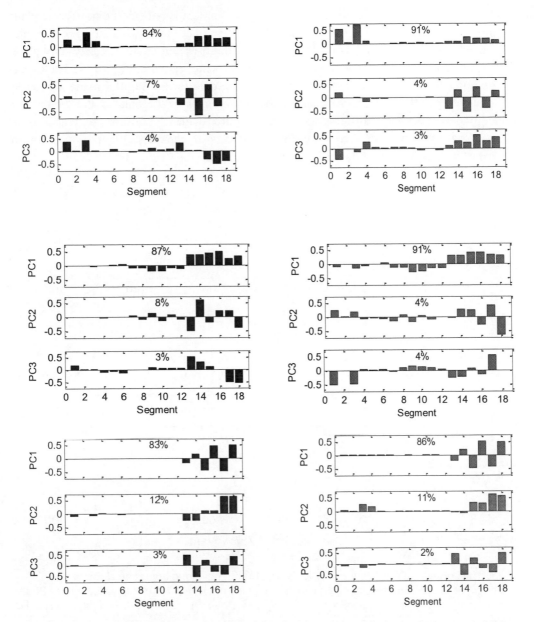

Figure 16. the first three principal components for typically developing children (blue) and children with CP (red) about the X (top), Y (middle), and Z (bottom) axes. The numbers represent the percentage of variabilty accounted for by the individual PC. The segments correspond to the following: 1) Head, 2) Neck, 3) UpperChest, 4) UpperTorso, 5) CentralTorso, 6) LowerTorso, 7) RUpperArm, 8) LUpperArm, 9) RLowerArm, 10) LLowerArm, 11) RHand, 12) LHand, 13) RUpperLeg, 14) LUpperLeg, 15) RLowerLeg,16) LLowerLeg, 17) RFoot, 18) LFoot

A principal component analysis was performed on an 18 segment model. The results, shown in Figure 16, show that overall the organization of the PCs of the two groups is quite similar to each other and similar to that of the adults presented above. To quantify this similarity we used the dot product of the principal component vectors of the two groups to computer the co-linearity of the vectors, see Table 3. For the first PCs there is excellent alignment in all three planes. For the second PCs the alignment is poor in the transverse plane where the asymmetries of the gaits of children with CP affect the coefficients. For the third PC, which accounts for 4% or less of the variability, there was good co linearity only about the Z axis. The weighting coefficients of the first two PCs are shown in Figure 17. The curves are very similar for the first PC. For the second PC the data for the sagittal plane are nearly for the two groups. However, there a substantial differences in the data of the frontal and transverse planes. The frontal differences suggest children with CP are more regular in these movements that children with TD, while the coefficients of transverse plane movement are suggestive of the asymmetry of the gait of children with CP.

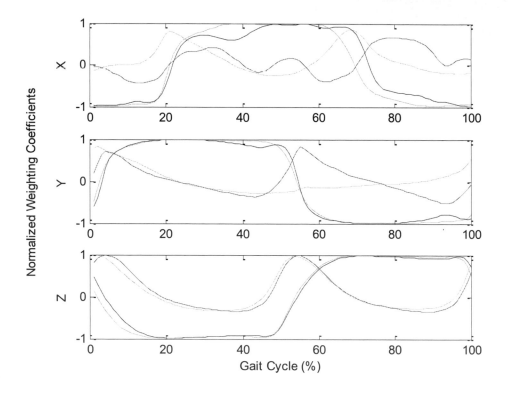

Figure 17. The normalized weighting coefficients for TD children (solid lines) and children with CP (dashed lines) of the first and second PCs. (The third PCs are not shown for clarity and the third PCs accounted for 4% or less of the variability in all three axes. However they were dissimilar between the two groups.)

Table 3. Mean dot product values of the first three PCs between children with TD and children with CP

Between Groups			
Plane	Frontal	Transverse	Sagittal
Axis	X	Y	Z
PC1	0.88	0.97	1.00
PC2	0.90	0.06	0.86
PC3	-0.67	0.29	0.97

Summary

Overall the angular momenta of both TD children and those with CP were similar both on a global scale, looking at the total, upper, or lower body, and at a more segmental scale looking at individual limbs, or individual segments. The momenta of children with CP did tend to exhibit greater excursion and also tended to be larger, i.e. larger moment area that is representative of the exaggerated motions associated with CP gait.

As the momenta analysis was refined to look at smaller groupings its representation of specific kinematics became more obvious. The cancelation of the momenta about the Y axis between the upper and lower body for both groups revealed contralateral gait. The higher amplitude of negative momenta of the lower body about the Z axis represented double support, where both legs are traveling in the same direction, is another example.

Regression analysis of the momenta and energy associated with the whole body demonstrate that the momenta can be effectively used to explain the relative energy in the X and Z directions during gait. Momentum does little to explain the energy in the Y direction because of cancellation, however energy due to vertical motion represents little of the total internal energy. This work/momenta relation, while valid, does little to increase our understanding of the relation of specific kinematics to increased work due to the transfer of energy between segments and the cancelation of momenta between body segments i.e. the cancelation of momenta about the Y axis between the upper and lower body. The usefulness of angular momentum analysis becomes more obvious as it is applied to smaller groupings of body segments such as the legs, arms, or torso.

The relation between momenta and work/energy is convoluted due in part to the nature of the quantities compared i.e. scalar vs. vector quantities, the nature of energy transfer between body segments, and the cancelation of momentum between segments as they move together. Comparison of quantities is complicated by the planer rotational properties acting in both linear directions within the plane of rotation resulting in non-linear in-determinant relationships, due the relative energy in any direction being a function of motion in two orthogonal rotational planes. Yet despite these complications we were still able to use momenta to relate the kinematics of leg circumduction to increased internal work/energy. This raises the need to continue work on relating momenta to gait kinematics. As a better understanding of the relation of momenta and gait kinematics is developed, the ability to use momenta to correlate increased internal work with specific kinematics will also increase.

It appears the angular momenta, as was the case for adults, are both highly controlled and well organized. The angular momenta peaks and the cancellation were group dependent. However, the organization of the angular momenta of the body segments, the PC coefficients, was independent of group. In addition, this organization can be represented by only two independent parameters. This organization and that found in the adults is highly suggestive of a neuromuscular synergy that can in part be scaled by velocity. Below the uncontrolled manifold hypothesis (UCM) of Sholz and Schöner[24] is used to explore whether angular momenta conforms to this definition of synergy.

REGULATION OF THE WHOLE BODY ANGULAR MOMENTUM DURING THE GAIT CYCLE

The previous sections have highlighted the particular features of the angular momenta during the gait cycle. More particularly, they showed that the whole body angular momentum (WBAM) follows a very reproducible pattern from stride to stride. In addition these studies showed that the angular momenta of the individual segments (SAM) are organized in a specific way: they co-varied such that can they can be grouped into a small number of primitives, whose composition is invariant of the walking speed. Moreover, the composition of these primitives tended to keep the WBAM small (high coefficients of cancellation). Taking together, these facts seem to indicate that the WBAM is an important variable that is made reproducible by the Central Nervous System (CNS) from stride to stride. However this point is not clearly demonstrated in these studies. More particularly they do not focus on how the controller acts on these groups of individual variables.

An interesting way to study this question is the notion of multi-segmental synergies[24;25] These authors define a synergy as *a particular organization of individual variables that allows producing a better Performance Variable (PV) as compared to if these variables were acting independently from each others*. More particularly, by studying human motions these authors showed that these synergies were an interesting way for the controller to deal with the mechanical redundancy of the human body. Not only it allows the controller to solve the redundancy problem, i.e. to find a way to share the task among the different individual variables in order to produce the desired PV, but it also allows it to take advantage of the redundancy in order to be stable against perturbations.

The quantification of the multi-segmental synergies has been done within the so called uncontrolled manifold framework (UCM). Within this framework, the control is viewed as a two-level hierarchy: at the lower level, the individual variables are grouped into Elemental Variables (EV) based on their co-variation. Although the origin of such grouping is still debated (does it originate from the CNS or is it a consequence of biomechanical constraints?), the result is that the controller can act at the upper level on a fewer number of independent EV. At this upper level, the neural controller forms in the space of EV a subspace, named UCM, corresponding to a desired value (time profile) of an important performance variable (PV). By confining the EV to that subspace, the controller guarantees a constant value of the PV. In other terms, the controller defines not only a unique solution among the EV but a set of solutions (the UCM) that will result in the desired PV. For a given task, successfully performed by a subject many times, this will result in a large amount of trial-to-trial variability of the EV along the UCM subspace. If this phenomenon is observed, a conclusion can be drawn on a synergy among the EV "stabilizing", i.e. decreasing its variability across trials.

By using this framework, Robert et al.[7] addressed the question of the control of the WBAM during the gait cycle. They studied the possible synergies among the SAM (being the individual variable in this study) that would lead to a stable time profile value of the WBAM (the performance variable).

Seven male subjects walked on a treadmill at their comfortable walking speed. A 17-segment model, fitted to the subject's anthropometry, was used to reconstruct their kinematics and to compute SAM and WBAM around the whole body COM in three dimensions (normalized by the mass, height and CWS of the subject). For each subject 40 strides were identified using the kinematics of the left heel markers[26], time normalized and resampled over a 100 time windows. The following analyses were performed independently for each of the three direction of the space.

A principal component analysis was used to represent the 17 SAM by the magnitudes of the first five principal components.

$$\mathbf{L} = \mathbf{PC} \cdot \mathbf{M} \qquad \qquad (Eq.\ 1)$$

Where **L** the vector of segmental angular momenta Li (17 by 1); **PC** the matrix made of the five principal components orthonormal vectors (17 by 5), constant across frames and trials; **M** the vector of the magnitudes of each of the 5 PCs (5 by 1).

These first five principal components, independent by property of the principal component analysis, were later used as EV. Within the UCM framework we need to investigate how the stride to stride variations of the EV affected the PV. In this case, the relation between EV and PV can be deducted from the linear relation between the WBAM (L_{WB}) and the SAM (L_i):

$$\overrightarrow{L_{WB}} = \sum_{i=1}^{17} \overrightarrow{L_i} \qquad \qquad (Eq.\ 2)$$

Considering Eq. 1 and Eq. 2, the relation between EV and PV can be written using a Jacobian matrix **J** as followed:

$$L_{WB} = \mathbf{J} \bullet \mathbf{M} \qquad \qquad (Eq.\ 3)$$

where **J** is a Jacobian matrix, here degenerated to a 5 by 1 vector.

The component of **J** can be computed as:

$$J_j = \sum_{i=1}^{17} PC_{ij} \ , \mathrm{j} = 1 \rightarrow 5; \qquad \qquad (Eq.\ 4)$$

The UCM being the subspace where any change in EV does not affect the PV, it is by definition the null space of this Jacobian matrix. For each time window, the trial-to-trial variance of the EV was computed and projected onto this null-space and its orthogonal complement. The variances projected were then normalized by the dimension of the subspaces (4 and 1 for the UCM and its orthogonal complement, respectively). An index ΔV was used to compare these two normalized components of variance:

$$\Delta V = \frac{V_{UCM} - V_{ORT}}{V_{TOT}} \qquad \qquad (Eq.\ 5)$$

Where V_{UCM} and V_{ORT} are the normalized component of variance projected on the UCM and its orthogonal complement respectively; V_{TOT} is the total variance of the EV, normalize by the dimension of the space of the EV (here 5).

Strongly positive values of ΔV indicate that there is more variance within the UCM than orthogonal to it. By definition of the synergies, one can thus claim that there is a synergy among the EV stabilizing the PV. Negative values of the index of synergy, less classically discussed, are more complex to handle (see Robert et al.[7] for a discussion). Nevertheless, ΔV different from zero indicates that the motor abundance is organized in a non-trivial way with regard to its effect on the PV (remember that for a random process, the variance would be spread randomly between the two subspaces resulting in a ΔV statistically not different from zero).

In this study, non-zero values of ΔV were observed in two of the three planes (see Figure 18): the frontal plane during the double support phase and the sagittal plane for both double support and swing phases. This is a clear indication that, during walking activities, the WBAM is a particular variable that the CNS tends to regulate via the individual SAM. This result constitutes a support to the numerous studies about humanoid gait control which considered the WBAM as a controlled variable[27].

However, results showed that the value of ΔV changed significantly between double support and swing phase, for at least two of the three planes (from negative values to zero and from negative values to positive values for the frontal and sagittal plane respectively, see Figure 18). It implies a modification of the nature and goal of the control between double support and swing phase. Interestingly, the mechanical state of the body also changes between two phases: from a complex chain with kinematical loop to a less stable open chain between these two phases. A possible interpretation consists of linking the change in control to the difference of stability during the gait phases. The relation between mechanical stability and the use of synergies has already been proposed in the literature, by Black and colleagues[28] for example. They showed that children with Down syndrome take more profit of their motor abundance than typically developed children, and interpreted it as a way to compensate the fact that they are inherently less stable than their typically developed peers.

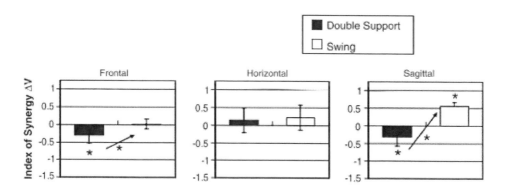

Figure 18. Index of synergy ΔV for the double support phase (black bars) and swing phase (white bars), averaged across subject (± one standard deviation) for the 3 planes. The stars over the bars indicate that ΔV is significantly different from zero (p<0.05). The stars over the arrows indicate a statistically significant change of ΔV (p<0.05) between the double support and swing phases. See text for details. Note the change of sign for ΔV in the sagittal plane.

In this study, higher values of ΔV during the swing phase, during which the body is in a less stable state, was understood as way to take profit of the motor abundance of the segments, i.e. to produce reproducible patterns of an important whole body parameter (the WBAM) with an increased robustness against perturbations. On the opposite, during the more stable double support phase, smaller or negative values or ΔV indicate that the segmental redundancy was used to adjust the value of the whole body parameters from stride to stride.

Summary

In this section we show that the Whole Body Angular Momentum (WBAM) is a particular variable for the CNS, who tends to regulate its value along the gait cycle by exploiting the human body motor abundance. We also show that this motor abundance was used in different ways during the different phases of the gait cycle. During the swing phase, in which the body is in a less stable state, the CNS tends to take profit of the segments redundancy in order to produce reproducible patterns of whole body angular momentum with an increased robustness against perturbations. This was interpreted as synergies among the individual segmental angular momenta stabilizing the whole body angular momentum. On the opposite, during the more stable double support phase, the segmental redundancy was used to adjust the value of the whole body angular momentum from stride to stride. This was interpreted as "anti-synergies" among the individual segmental angular momenta used to adjust the whole body angular momentum. Results could be extended by studying these synergies in walking with various situations of constraints.

CONCLUSION

Research has shown that the angular momentum of the body about its center of mass (CoM) during walking is highly regulated. In addition, if the angular momentum is normalized by a walker's height, mass, and walking speed it is similar between walkers at their preferred walking speed. Methods such as principal component analysis (PCA) reveal that the angular momenta of the body segments are not independent and that a reduced set of orthogonal components can account for very high percentage of the angular momentum variation. Lastly it is shown that the organization of particular whole body angular momenta fit the strict definition of a synergy that is regulated by the CNS.

The use of angular momentum analysis of bipedal gait is in its infancy. We expect that additional research in this area will bring additional insight into walking and how it is controlled. These results could be used in the field of human walking, including impaired gait and rehabilitation, and has direct implications in gait control of bipedal robot.

REFERENCE

Elftman, H. The Function of the Arms in Walking. *Human Biology*, 1939, 11 IS - 4, 529.

Simoneau, GG; Krebs, DE. Whole-body momentum during gait: A preliminary study of non-fallers and frequent fallers. *Journal of Applied Biomechanics*, 2000, 16, 1-13.

Herr, H; Popovic, M. Angular momentum in human walking. *Journal of Experimental Biology*, 2008, 211, 467-81.

Popovic, M; Englehart, A. Angular momentum primitives for human walking: *biomechanics and control*. 2004, 1685-1691.

Popovic, M, Englehart, A; Herr, H. Angular momentum primitives for human walking: biomechanics and control. Proceedings 2004 IEEE/RSJ International Conference on Intelligent Robots and Systems 2004, 2, 1685-91.

Bennett, BC; Russell, SD; Sheth, P; Abel, MF. The Effect of Walking Speed on Whole Body Angular Momentum. *Human Movement Science*, 2009.

Robert, T; Bennett, B; Russell, S; Zirker, C; Abel, M. Angular momentum synergies during walking. *Experimental Brain Research*, 2009, 197, 185-97.

Cheng, H; Obergefell, L; Rizer, A. Generator of Body Data (GEBOD) *Manual*. 1994. Dayton, OH, Systems Research Labs, Inc.

Eames, MHA; Cosgrove, A; Baker, R. Comparing methods of estimating the total body centre of mass in three-dimensions in normal and pathological gaits. *Human Movement Science*, 1999, 18, 637-46.

Russell, S; Bennett, BC; Ledoux, A; Sheth, PN; Abel, MF. The Gait of Children with and without Cerebral Palsy: *Work, Energy, and Angular Momentum. In: Gait & Posture*. (In Press).

Gerstenfeld, EP; Dixit, S; Callans, DJ; Rajawat, Y; Rho, R; Marchlinski, FE. Quantitative comparison of spontaneous and paced 12-lead electrocardiogram during right ventricular outflow tract ventricular tachycardia. *J Am Coll Cardiol*, 2003, 41, 2046-53.

Daffertshofer, A; Lamoth, CJC; Meijer, OG; Beek, PJ. PCA in studying coordination and variability: a tutorial. *Clinical Biomechanics*, 2004, 19, 415-28.

Krishnamoorthy, V; Goodman, S; Zatsiorsky, V; Latash, ML. Muscle synergies during shifts of the center of pressure by standing persons: identification of muscle modes. *Biological Cybernetics*, 2003, 89, 152-61.

Jordan, K; Challis, JH; Newell, KM. Walking speed influences on gait cycle variability. *Gait & Posture*, 2007, 26, 128-34.

Donker, SF; Daffertshofer, A; Beek, PJ. Effects of velocity and limb loading on the coordination between limb movements during walking. *Journal of Motor Behavior*, 2005, 37, 217-30.

Russell, SD; Bennett, BC; Kerrigan, DC; Abel, MF. Determinants of gait as applied to children with cerebral palsy. *Gait & Posture*, 2007, 26, 295-300.

Kerrigan, DC; Della Croce, U; Marciello, M; Riley, PO. A refined view of the determinants of gait: Significance of heel rise. *Arch Phys Med Rehabil*, 2000, 81, 1077-80.

Saunders, J; Inman, VT; Eberhart, HD. The major determinants in norma and pathological gait. *J Bone Jnt. Surg.*, 1953, 35A, 543-58.

Della Croce, U; Riley, PO; Lelas, JL; Kerrigan, DC. A refined view of the determinants of gait. *Gait & Posture*, 2001, 14, 79-84.

Russell, D; Gowland, C; Hardy, S; et al. *Gross Motor Function Measure Manual Intrathecal baclofen for generalized dystonia*. 2 ed. Hamilton, ON: Neurodevelopmental Clinical Research Unit, McMaster University, 1993.

Willems, PA; Cavagna, GA; Heglund, NC. External, Internal and Total Work in Human Locomotion. *Journal of Experimental Biology*, 1995, 198, 379-93.

Unnithan, VB; Dowling, JJ; Frost, G; Bar-Or O. Role of mechanical power estimates in the O2 cost of walking in children with cerebral palsy. *Medicine & Science in Sports & Exercise*, 1999, 31, 1703-8.

Bennett, BC; Abel, MF; Wolovick, A; Franklin, T; Allaire, PE; Kerrigan, DC. Center of Mass Movement and Energy Transfer During Walking in Children With Cerebral Palsy. *Archives of Physical Medicine & Rehabilitation*, 2005, 86, 2189-94.

Scholz, JP; Sch+|ner, G. The uncontrolled manifold concept: identifying control variables for a functional task. *Experimental Brain Research*, 1999, 126, 289-306.

Latash, ML; Scholz, JP; Schoner, G. Toward a new theory of motor synergies. *Motor Control*, 2007, 11, 276-308.

Zeni, J; Richards, JG; Higginson, JS. Two simple methods for determining gait events during treadmill and overground walking using kinematic data. *Gait & Posture*, 2008, 27, 710-4.

Goswami, A; Kallem, V. *Rate of change of angular momentum and balance maintenance of biped robots*. 2004, 3785-3790.

Black, DP; Smith, BA; Wu, JH; Ulrich, BD. Uncontrolled manifold analysis of segmental angle variability during walking: preadolescents with and without Down syndrome. *Experimental Brain Research*, 2007, 183, 511-21.

In: Overweightness and Walking
Editor: Caleb I. Black, pp. 35-57

ISBN: 978-1-60741-298-4
© 2010 Nova Science Publishers, Inc.

Chapter 2

THE CONTRIBUTION OF VESTIBULAR INFORMATION TO ADAPTIVE LOCOMOTION IN YOUNG AND OLDER INDIVIDUALS

T. B. Lilian Gobbi[1]*, Renato Moraes[2], C. Taís Gonçalves[1],
H. P. Marins Francisco [1], O. Camila Ricciardi[1], A. Fabio Barbieri[1],
P. Marcelo Pereira[1] and Veronica Miyasike-daSilva[1,3]

[1]UNESP – São Paulo State University at Rio Claro,
Posture and Gait Studies Lab, São Paulo, Brazil
[2]USP – University of São Paulo at Ribeirão Preto, São Paulo, Brazil
[3]UW – University of Waterloo at Waterloo, Ontario, Canada

ABSTRACT

Sensorimotor processing is necessary to perform motor actions according to environmental demands. The influence of visual, somatosensory and vestibular information, as well as their interaction, is largely studied in relation to postural control. Sensory integration is also crucial during adaptive locomotion and depends on both the task and the individual constraints. Several studies have been designed to observe the effects of the visual system on walking behavior, whereas the role of vestibular information, which is responsible for detecting linear and angular accelerations of the head in space, remains unclear. In this way, a series of three experiments was developed to investigate the contribution of the vestibular system on adaptive walking. In the first study, two different ways of disrupting vestibular system information in young adults were compared. Caloric and rotational stimulations were applied and subjects were asked to estimate the disturbance perceived. Rotational stimulation proved to disturb the vestibular system more intensively. In the second experiment, after rotational stimulation we asked young adults to walk and step over an obstacle. The results revealed that subjects' walking pattern changed in the presence of vestibular perturbation when compared to the condition of no stimulation. In the third experiment we used the same

---

* Corresponding author: Phone/Facsimile + 55 19 3534-6436; E-mail ltbgobbi@rc.unesp.br

procedures and tasks of Experiment 2, but in older adults with no history of vestibular sickness. Older adults also showed spatial and temporal adjustments in their walking pattern. The results of these studies allowed us to conclude that vestibular information is not used to control limb elevation over an obstacle, but it is quite important in controlling locomotion direction. In addition, involvement in physical activity programs seems to minimize the effects of vestibular deficits.

Key words: human, aging, vestibular system, locomotion, obstacles

INTRODUCTION

Sensorimotor processing is necessary to perform motor actions, including body balance and walking. The influence of visual, somatosensory and vestibular information, as well as their interaction, is largely studied in relation to postural control (Horak & Macpherson, 1996). Sensory information and integration is also crucial during adaptive locomotion and depends on the task and the individual constraints. Several studies have been designed to observe the effects of the visual system of gait control on even and uneven terrains (Mohagheghi et al., 2004; Patla & Greig, 2006; Rietdyk & Rhea, 2006; Graci et al., 2009), whereas the role of the vestibular system has only recently been investigated and it remains to be fully clarified.

In the past, the sensation of motion sickness and disorientation reported during space flights motivated studies about the role of the vestibular system on motor actions (Lackner & DiZio, 2009). The vestibular organ comprehends the otoliths (utricle and saccule) and semicircular canals, which are responsible for detecting linear and angular accelerations of the head in space, respectively (Kelly, 1991a; Angelaki & Cullen, 2008). The vestibular system is related to the control of motor actions, and function disruption affects the performance of locomotion, sport, dance and other skills (Brooks, 1986; Kelly, 1991b; Horak & Macpherson, 1996; Horak, 2009). The specific contributions of the vestibular system to motor actions have been investigated with regard to postural control (Ghez, 1991; Daniel & Redfern, 2000; Fitzpatrick & Day, 2004; Rama-López & Pérez-Fernández, 2004; Lenggenhager et al., 2008), locomotor control (Bent et al., 2000; Gonçalves et al., 2000; Yamamoto et al., 2002; Kennedy et al., 2003; Bent et al., 2004; Bent et al., 2005; Marques et al., 2007), or both (Iles et al., 2007). Some studies with animals have shown that dynamic tasks such as locomotion are impaired when there is lack of bilateral vestibular information (Igarashi et al., 1970; Goldberg et al., 1982).

Vestibular system perturbation can be elicited by simple tasks such as a subtle head rotation. In the experimental settings, vestibular disturbance has been induced by a variety of invasive and noninvasive methods. Galvanic vestibular stimulation (GVS) and caloric stimulation are among these invasive methods. GVS is typically delivered through a small current (~1 mA) on anodal and cathodal electrodes placed on the mastoid process behind each ear (Fitzpatrick & Day, 2004). This configuration causes a person to sway to the side of the anodal electrode. Caloric stimulation consists of the excitation of a larger cortex area on the ipsilateral side and inhibition of the contralateral side by water irrigation on the external ear (Bottini et al., 2001). The temperature change produces an endolymph flux either towards the ampullae of the excited side (warm test) or away from it (cool test). Self-rotations and rotational stimulations (rotary chair) are among the noninvasive methods (Clarke, 2001). For the vestibular stimulation using a motorized rotary chair, individuals are seated on a chair that rotates at a constant frequency.

Just recently, studies have used GVS during human locomotion (Bent et al., 2000; Deshpande & Patla, 2005; Iles et al., 2007). Also recently, the motorized rotary chair has been used for studying the contribution of the vestibular system to locomotion control (Gonçalves et al., 2000). In both cases, a medium-lateral deviation of walking was observed due to vestibular system stimulation. For the GVS the deviation is to the side of the anode, whereas for the rotary chair the deviation is to the side of rotation.

Structural changes occur in the vestibular system during the aging process. Individuals over the age of 70 have a loss of 40% of the vestibular system's sensorial cells (Spirduso, 1995). This morphological loss may lead to functional changes. One of the characteristics attributed to this decrease in the vestibular system's sensorial capacity is denominated vertigo. In an otolaryngology study conducted to verify the dizziness caused in patients over 60 years of age, it was observed that 18% of the 50 patients evaluated had vertigo attributed to peripheral vestibular disorder (Lawson et al., 1999). The vertigo attributed to peripheral vestibular disorder is directly related to fall occurrence, which is one of the most dangerous and common factors of body injuries, such as hip fractures, in elderly people (Mcauley et al., 1997). It has also been showed that vertigo in older adults persists for a long time; it is caused by a great number of factors and causes a higher incapacity in comparison with vertigo in young adults, since its recovery is slower in older adults in comparison with young adults (Davis, 1994).

A difference in recovery time after unilateral labyrinthectomy was noted between older and young squirrel monkeys. The older animals needed more time than the young ones to compensate for the loss of one of the labyrinths (Igarashi et al., 1970). Hence, we can infer that older adults with vestibular loss attributed to the aging process perform daily tasks such as walking in cluttered environments with more difficulty, which can contribute to tripping, sliding and falling.

Although there were studies that investigated the contribution of vestibular information to locomotor control, most of them were conducted on even terrains with young adults. The influence of vestibular inputs to locomotion on uneven terrains (i.e., adaptive locomotion) and on older adults remains unclear. Therefore, the main question driving the studies presented in this chapter was related to the effects of vestibular inputs on adaptive locomotion, using the motorized rotary chair to perturb the vestibular system. In order to answer this question a series of three experiments was designed and conducted. Since there is a lack of knowledge about the effect of the motorized rotary chair in perturbing the vestibular system, in the first experiment we compared both caloric and rotational stimulations to perturb the vestibular system in young adults, who estimated perceptually the magnitude of the disturbance. In the second experiment, after the rotational stimulation, we asked young adults to walk and step over an obstacle placed a few steps in front of the chair. In the third experiment we perturbed the vestibular system of older adults by means of the same stimulation and asked them to perform the same task given in Experiment 2.

EXPERIMENT 1: SUBJECTIVE PERCEPTION OF VESTIBULAR PERTURBATION BY ROTATIONAL AND CALORIC STIMULATIONS

Introduction

The vestibular receptors detect head motion. These afferent signs inform the central nervous system about head angular and linear accelerations and orientation related to gravity. The vestibular information is processed by the central nervous system to adjust body motion as needed (Brooks, 1986; Kelly, 1991b; Horak & Macpherson, 1996).

For clinical and experimental purposes, a variety of methods have been applied to induce vestibular perturbation such as galvanic stimulation, caloric stimulation and rotational stimulation (rotary chair). All these methods induce the afferent activity but the rotational stimulation is a noninvasive method (Lysakowski & Goldberg, 2004). However, since the rotary chair used by our group was self-built it was necessary to validate it. We used as gold standard the disturbance to the vestibular system caused by caloric stimulation. The stimulation of the horizontal semicircular canals by the caloric test allows the clinician to assess the integrity of the peripheral vestibular system while for researchers it is used to control the perturbation only on the semicircular canals. The caloric testing can be done with water or air. The classic test of Fitzgerald-Hallpike is the most common and it uses water on 44°C (warm test) and 30°C (cool test), both with 40 s of irrigation time and a volume of 250 ml. The individual should be lying supine with the head elevated to 30° in order to verticalize the lateral canals. The caloric stimulation produces an endolymph flux towards the ampullae of the excited side (warm test) or away from it (cool test). Caloric vestibular stimulation, with water, has been applied to verify its effects on the cardiorespiratoy system (Jauregui-Renaud et al., 2000), the clinic symptoms and the recovery of labyrinthine function in patients with *vestibular neuronitis* (Taborelli et al., 2000), and on the motor actions (Yamamoto et al., 2002).

Rotational forces are able to elicit responses from the semicircular canals' afferents endings. In order to achieve that, it is necessary to keep the head stationary or move it at a constant velocity (Lysakowski & Goldberg, 2004). Rotational stimulation by rotary chair was first introduced by Bárány, in 1907, for vestibular-ocular reflex testing. At that time, the patient's head was restrained and the chair was manually rotate in 10 times over 20 seconds followed by a sudden stop of the chair. In the past few years, motorized rotary chair is used and it stimulates the vestibular system at frequencies in a range of 0.01–1.28 Hz. In this procedure, the patient's head is tilted forward at 30°, which place the horizontal canals perpendicularly to the plane of gravity. Rotational stimulation is based on angular head acceleration. During this procedure, the semicircular canals follow the head movement while the endolymph rotates in the opposite direction exciting the hair cells. With the sudden stop of the rotational stimulation, the semicircular canals stop while the endolymph moves in the opposite direction, inhibiting the hair cells (Guyton, 1993). This perturbation is kept only for 20s, when the hair cells stop firing and return to their resting discharge level. Rotational stimulation of the vestibular system has been applied by means of the flight simulator to verify the inclination perception from the vertical position in patients with unilateral vestibular deficits (Aoki et al., 1999) and by self-rotation to assess patients' vertigo (Belafsky et al., 2000).

We considered using a motorized rotary chair to transitorily disturb the vestibular system to reveal its role on adaptive locomotion. However, little is known about the perceived intensity of the disturbance elicited by both an invasive and a noninvasive method. In order to apply a noninvasive method and observe the adaptive locomotion of young and older adults, we must first know if the perceived intensity of the perturbation applied by both methods is similar. The caloric and the rotational stimulations were chosen because both affect primarily the horizontal semicircular canal (Brandt & Strupp, 2005) and a constant sensation of rotation can be induced by caloric stimulation (Fasold et al., 2002). Therefore, the caloric test of Fitzgerald-Hallpike was adapted to induce a transitory, caloric stimulation, with water, not only because it is a classic method but also because it is largely used for research and clinical purposes. On the other hand, a motorized rotary chair was used in this study to induce a transitory vestibular perturbation. Our motorized rotary chair has a control mechanism that allows us to adjust the rotation velocity and to guarantee the same rotation frequency for all participants, independently of their body mass. With the control of these parameters, we can verify how many rotations per minute are necessary to perturb the vestibular system. In this way, the aim of this experiment was to verify the relationship between the subjective perception generated by both caloric and rotational stimulations in young adults using a psychophysical tool. We expected to observe a high and positive relationship of the subjective perception of the perturbation between the two methods.

Methods

Twenty-four undergraduate young adults (8 males and 16 females) with mean age equal to 22 ± 2 years old volunteered to participate in the present study. All participants were healthy and without any known motor or sensory deficit, especially in the vestibular system. Initially, participants were interviewed about the occurrences of dizziness, nausea or difficulty of balance control. They were informed about the procedures and signed a consent form to participate in the study, which was approved by the University Ethic Committee.

In two visits to the laboratory, a week apart, each participant was assigned to the rotational and caloric stimulations. The presentation order of the stimulations was counterbalanced among the participants. Participants were instructed to avoid eating at least 6 hours before each visit.

The rotational stimulation was applied on a motorized rotary chair (Figure 1). An engine was fixed under the chair seat by means of an iron frame to prevent the contact of the participant feet with the engine. The engine was controlled by a digital frequency converter (Toshiba VF-SX) to monitor the chair rotation frequency. A circuit breaker was placed beside the frequency converter to allow the firing of the chair. The participant was instructed to sit on the chair, with the back resting against the backrest, supporting arms comfortably on chair arms, resting the feet on the footrest, and keeping head tilted at approximately 30° back and closing their eyes to avoid any visual fixation. After the chair stopped rotating, the participant opened their eyes, stood up as quickly as possible and verbalized the intensity of disturbance that they perceived at that moment. For this purpose a psychophysical scale containing five levels was used. The scale ranged from 1, not disturbed; 2, little disturbed; 3, disturbed; 4, very upset; 5, overly disturbed. The scale was attached on a panel and each level was explained to the participant to guarantee higher level of the accuracy in the subjective perception.

The chair was rotated at a frequency of 30 rotations per minute and completed three turns. Four trials were performed in this experimental condition. A one minute-rest period was used between attempts to avoid a possible trial effect, dissipating the disturbance occurred in the previous attempt.

The warm caloric stimulation was applied according to the classical technique of Fitzgerald-Hallpike. In order to give similar conditions in the two procedures, participants were asked to sit on a chair with the head tilted at approximately 30° back and slightly tilted to the opposite side of the irrigated ear with eyes closed. A quarter of warm water (44°C) irrigates each ear for about 60s.

A physiologic solution (NaCl 0.9%) was used for the irrigations to avoid possible changes in ion concentrations and dehydration of the tissue cells of the ear. The solution was warmed on propane fire. The 250 ml were graduated by a beaker and the temperature was controlled by a thermometer (Incoterm®, graded from −10 to 110°C, with 1°C degree, reading of metallic mercury). The irrigation was applied by means of a latex tube and an eppendorf. The eppendorf had the tip cut and it was introduced in the external ear. Two irrigations in each ear were applied in each participant. The interval between irrigations was kept constant (at least 5 minutes). Towels and a plastic sheet covered the participants' shoulders to prevent the contact with the solution.

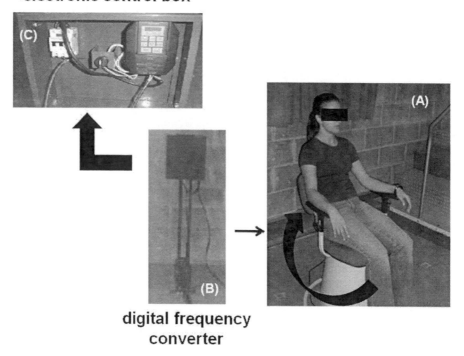

Figure 1. Illustration of the motorized rotary chair showing the participant position (A), as well as the electronic tool box (B) and the digital frequency converter that control the chair rotation frequency (C)

After each irrigation, participants were asked to open the eyes, to stand up as quick as possible and to subjectively judge the intensity of the perturbation at that moment using the same 5-level psychophysical scale presented above. The comparison of the subjective judgments in each of the procedures (medians) was statistically treated by the Wilcoxon test and the Kendall's correlation with a significance level of 0.05, which employed SPSS 15.0 (SPSS, Inc.) software.

Results

All participants responded positively to both procedures. The presentation order of the rotational and caloric stimulations did not affect the participants' subjective perception of the perturbation ($F_{1,22} = 1.226$; $p > 0.05$). The subjective perception of the intensity generated by the rotational stimulation (median = 3, ranging from 1 to 4) was higher than one generated by the caloric stimulation (median = 1, ranging from 1 to 3). The Wilcoxon test confirmed this observation ($Z_{23} = -4.266$; $p < 0.001$). The Kendall's correlation analyses revealed a moderate, positive and significant relationship between the subjective perception of the rotational and caloric perturbations ($\tau = 0.352$; $p = 0.05$; Figure 2).

Discussion

The aim of this experiment was to verify the relationship between the subjective perception of vestibular perturbation generated by caloric and rotational stimulations in young adults. We were expecting to observe a high and positive relationship of the subjective perception of the perturbation imposed by the two methods. Our results confirmed our hypothesis, although the relationship was moderate. In this way, we can affirm that the rotational stimulation applied by a motorized rotary chair is as efficient in perturbing the vestibular system as the caloric stimulation.

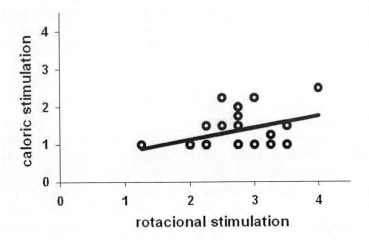

Figure 2. Relationship between the subjective perception of the perturbation intensity generated by both rotational and caloric stimulations

The rotational stimulation disturbs the vestibular system at two different moments: at the beginning and at the end of the perturbation. At the beginning, the endolymph tends to stay stationary, but since the head is moving the endolymph will move the cilia of the hair cells. At the end, the endolymph keeps moving inside the semicircular canals after the sudden stop (Guyton, 1993). The head position, tilted backwards also generates the afferent activity of the hair cells, but this position was kept the same in both procedures. Differently, on caloric stimulation the vestibular system of the excited side is disturbed, in a continuous way (Bottini et al., 2001; Fasold et al., 2002). Our data confirm that young adults reported more intense perturbation under the rotational stimulation than the caloric stimulation.

In addition, the caloric stimulation was applied unilaterally, disturbing only the ipsilateral side of the irrigation. On the other way, the rotational stimulation disturbed the vestibular system bilaterally. In the caloric stimulation, the conflict can be characterized by the difference in signs from the irrigated side and the non irrigated side. Differently, in the rotational stimulation, there was no sensory conflict, since it was applied in the clockwise direction for all participants, with the same intensity in both sides.

The structural and functional features of the vestibular system can also explain the increased subjective perception of the rotational stimulation. More specifically, the endolymph motion and the activation of the hair cells must to be considered. In movements in the horizontal plan, head angular accelerations move the endolymph in the opposite direction of the rotation. The endolymphatic flow moves toward the ampullae in the lateral canal of the same side of the rotation, flexing the cupula in the direction of the utricule. The cupula motion moves the stereocilias toward the kinocillium, depolarizing the hair cells. In the contralateral side, the endolymphatic flow moves against the ampullae of the lateral canal, moving the stereocilias away from the kinocillium, hiperpolarizing the hair cells. These endolymphatic flows act in a cooperative manner in both body-sides and do not induce any conflict between sides. Differently, the caloric stimulation is not a physiological procedure and induces the endolymphatic flow towards (warm test) or away (cool test) from the ampullae of the horizontal semicircular canal by means of creating a temperature gradient between the lateral and the medial portions of the canal. This flow creates an activation of hair cells only in the stimulated side (Ganança et al., 1999).

The spatial distribution of the semicircular canals could contribute to the lower subjective perception of the perturbation intensity generated by the caloric than the rotational stimulation. The semicircular canals in each side of the head are perpendicularly oriented in a way to constitute three synergic pairs. Each pair is sensible to head rotation in one plan (Guyton, 1993; Kelly, 1991b). However, the head position was imposed in this experiment (tilted backwards) to isolate the lateral canals which can be more sensitive to rotational than to caloric stimulation.

The present experiment attested that the rotational stimulation is a noninvasive procedure that fit same objectives that invasive methods and it can be used for clinical, rehabilitation and research purposes. This test was useful to disturb the vestibular system and therefore, to verify the contribution of the vestibular inputs to the control of motor actions. The results of this experiment motivated us to observe the role of the vestibular information in the control of adaptive locomotion in young (Experiment 2) and older (Experiment 3) adults.

EXPERIMENT 2: EFFECTS OF VESTIBULAR PERTURBATION ON ADAPTIVE LOCOMOTION IN YOUNG ADULTS

Introduction

Environmental stimuli provide information that allows individuals to guide themselves during locomotion. The individual uses sensory and perceptual mechanisms to receive and process environmental information. Uneven surfaces require the integration of intrinsic (organism) and extrinsic (environment) information to finely tune the effector system accordingly. Adaptive locomotion requires accurate visual information. Head and eye movements were observed during the approach to obstacle crossing driving the attention to the environmental information (Patla & Vickers, 1997). Sensory information provided by the visual, vestibular and somatosensory systems must be integrated in order to perform complex actions (Stein & Meredith, 1993) such as adaptive locomotion (Gobbi & Patla, 1997). Adaptive locomotor strategies indicate different modulations of the effector system according to the integration of the sensory signs. However, gait adaptations are not only simple variations of the basic gait pattern but also reveal a complex and functional reorganization of the normal walking (Patla, 1991).

This reorganization can occur under a feedforward control mechanism. By definition, proactive strategies are related to the resources used to maintain stability and progression. The anticipatory postural control adaptations to a voluntary arm motion during walking characterize a feedforward response (Nashner & Forssberg, 1986; Patla, 1986). The adaptive strategies involve all changes in the gait pattern to accommodate it to different surfaces that the individual cannot avoid and wish to overcome. It also includes the necessary changes to avoid obstacles in the pathway, such as a curb, a hole, and others. Adaptive strategies to obstacle crossing can be implemented within one stride cycle (Patla et al., 1991; Patla, 2003).

The obstacle avoidance paradigm has been used to test this integration between sensory and effector systems (Patla, 2003). Several studies showed adaptive locomotor strategies during obstacle crossing (Chen et al., 1991), revealing the role of vision (Mohagheghi et al., 2004; Patla & Greig, 2006; Patla & Vickers, 2003; Patla et al., 2002), the influence of spatial and temporal constraints (Moraes et al., 2004) and describing the motion of the center of mass (Chou et al., 2003). However, little is known about the contribution of the vestibular signs to adaptive locomotion. Deshpande and Patla (2005) investigated the integration of visual and vestibular signs in the locomotion direction, using GVS. Gonçalves et al. (2000) applied a manual rotary chair to stimulate the vestibular system in young adults before crossing obstacles. Their results revealed that toe clearance was not affected by the vestibular stimulation. Toe clearance is a robust variable that integrate the motor plan and it is affected neither by the obstacle height nor the vestibular stimulation. Differently, the take-off distances were modulated according to the obstacle height and the vestibular stimulation.

However, the use of a manual rotary chair was an important limitation of Gonçalves et al.'s study, since it was not possible to guarantee a constant rotation of the chair within and between subjects. Then, to improve the control over the vestibular perturbation to study the contribution of the vestibular system to adaptive locomotion, we used a motorized rotary chair and analyzed the medial-lateral deviations and maximum horizontal velocity among the crossing variables. In this context, we asked if the same adaptive strategies used on normal conditions, were used after transitory rotational vestibular stimulation. The purpose of this experiment was, therefore, to analyze the effects of the transitory rotational vestibular stimulation delivered by a motorized rotary chair on adaptive locomotor strategies in young adults. We expected to observe an increased medial-lateral deviation under low obstacle (less challenging condition) associated with the vestibular stimulation.

Methods

Six young adults, undergraduate students 18 to 30 years of age, 3 male and 3 female, volunteered to participate in this study. All participants had either normal or corrected-to-normal vision and no known neurological or musculoskeletal impairment or sensory-motor disorders that could incapacitate them to perform the proposed activities or increase task difficulty. The individuals signed a consent form approved by the local University Ethics Committee.

Initially, the following anthropometric characteristics were measured: thigh, shank and foot lengths, ankle height and total body mass and height. Then, participants were invited to sit on the chair with the head in a pitch position and with eyes closed (to avoid possible visual targets during the rotations and before standing up). After the rotational perturbation, the participant was instructed to extend the head, open the eyes, stand up and walk towards the obstacle. The distance from the chair to the obstacle was about three steps.

The magnitude of the transitory vestibular perturbation was established by a pilot study. Ten young adults (from 18 to 27 years old) were asked to report the perceived intensity of the transitory vestibular perturbation using a scale ranging from 1 to 5 (1, not disturbed; 2, little disturbed; 3, disturbed; 4, very upset; 5, overly disturbed). The combination of five rotation frequencies (from 20 to 40 rpm) and three rotation magnitudes (from 2 to 4 rotations) totalized 15 conditions. Two attempts of each condition were randomly applied for each participant. The results showed that the perceived intensity of the vestibular perturbation increased linearly with the increased rotational frequencies and magnitudes. As no vertigo episodes were reported at the high frequencies and magnitudes conditions, the rotational frequency was set at 40 rpm and the rotational magnitude at 4 consecutive rotations.

The obstacle heights were individually established according to the participant knee height. Patla (1997) showed that the knee height is the threshold for the adaptive locomotor behavior in young adults. The high obstacle corresponded to 10 cm above the knee height and the low obstacle was set 10 cm below the knee height. Our aim was to challenge the locomotor control system for both the obstacle height and the vestibular perturbation.

The combination of the temporary vestibular perturbation and the obstacle heights generated six experimental conditions: no vestibular perturbation and no obstacle (control for both factors), with vestibular perturbation and no obstacle (control for vestibular perturbation), no vestibular perturbation and high obstacle, no vestibular perturbation and low obstacle, with vestibular perturbation and high obstacle and with vestibular perturbation and low obstacle. Five attempts for each experimental condition were set, totalizing thirty fully randomized trials. Participants had a rest period of twenty seconds between each trial in order to guarantee the temporary vestibular perturbation dissipation and a 1-minute interval every 10 trials to adjust the experimental environment.

Infrared emitting diodes (IREDs) were attached on the following body landmarks on right (head of the fifth metatarsal, lateral side of calcaneus and lateral maleolous) and left (head of the first metatarsal, medial side of calcaneus and medial maleolous) lower limbs. The IREDs trajectories in tri-dimensional space were tracked by the OPTOTRAK system (Northern Digital Inc., Canada) at 60 Hz. The raw kinematic data were initially interpolated by the OPTOFIX 1.6 software (Mishac Kinectics, Ontario, Canada) using a cubic spline function for missing data. The following dependent variables were calculated in Matlab 5.3 (Maths Works Inc): leading toe clearance (vertical distance between the head of the fifth metatarsal and top of the obstacle), leading take-off distance normalized by the leg length (horizontal distance between head of the fifth metatarsal and the base of the obstacle), right and left medial-lateral deviation and maximum horizontal velocity in anterior-posterior direction. The differences within these dependent variables can show the locomotor adjustments, allowing us to infer the adaptive locomotor strategies utilized by young adults under different challenging conditions.

All dependent variables were statistically treated by the descriptive statistic using means and standard deviations. The comparisons among conditions were performed by trial using two way repeated measures ANOVAs (2 perturbation X 2 obstacle). The significance level was set at 0.05.

Results

Toe clearance was affected only by the obstacle height ($F_{1,106}$ = 20.923; p < 0.001). Participants elevated less the toe over the high obstacle (12.8 ± 8.2 cm) than over the low obstacle (22.3 ± 12.5 cm). The normalized take-off distance, the left medial-lateral deviation and the maximum horizontal velocity were affected neither by the obstacle height nor by the vestibular perturbation (p>0.05). There were no interactions between the factors for toe clearance, take-off distance, left medial-lateral deviation and maximum horizontal velocity (p>0.05). Differently, the right medial-lateral deviation was affected by the rotational vestibular perturbation ($F_{1,270}$=5.263, p < 0.024; Figure 3).

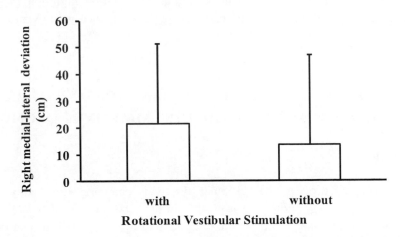

Figure 3. Means and standard deviations for right medial-lateral deviation according to the rotational vestibular perturbation

Discussion

The purpose of this experiment was to analyze the effects of the motorized rotational vestibular stimulation on adaptive locomotor strategies of young adults. Obstacle height and vestibular stimulation affected the studied gait parameters in different ways.

Obstacle height affected toe clearance. Even with the obstacle height normalized for each subject's anthropometric feature, the safety margin on top of the obstacle was modulated by obstacle height independently of the vestibular stimulation. This result did not confirm the findings of Patla and colleagues (Patla & Reitdyk, 1993; Patla et al., 1996a; Patla et al., 1996b; Patla et al., 2004), which highlight that the mean values for the safety margin presented by young adults is about 10 cm independently of the obstacle height. The subjects of this experiment showed an average of about 20 cm on top of the low obstacle and 12 cm for the high obstacle. However, our finding about toe clearance is in agreement with another study that manipulated the obstacle height and vestibular stimulation in young adults (Gonçalves et al., 2000). These results suggest that although vestibular perturbation did not affect directly toe clearance, it seems reasonable to assume that the simple presence of the vestibular perturbation generated an overall increase in the safety margin over the obstacle in order to avoid an obstacle contact.

In another way, vestibular stimulation affected the right medial-lateral deviation. GVS produces an increased response to the opposite side of the stimulation (Kubo et al., 1997; Fitzpatrick et al., 1999; Bent et al., 2000). The rotational stimulation applied by the motorized rotary chair, which rotated in the clockwise direction, influenced the right medial-lateral deviation. One could expect that this effect would occur in the left medial-lateral deviation. However, the endolymph in the semicircular canals rotates in the inverse direction with the subtle stop of the rotary chair (Guyton, 1993), affecting gait in the same rotational direction. This result was previously described in young adults by Gonçalves et al. (2000).

The results of this experiments revealed that young adults adapt their locomotion strategies under the experimental manipulations of the obstacle height and the vestibular stimulation. The toe clearance modulation according to the obstacle height and the right medial-lateral deviation according to the vestibular stimulation highlight these strategies, which can be considered as conservative strategies. The balance maintenance must be the base of the observed behavior.

EXPERIMENT 3: EFFECTS OF TRANSITORY VESTIBULAR DISTURBANCE ON OLDER ADULTS' ADAPTIVE LOCOMOTION

Introduction

During the aging process, the vestibular system is changing structurally. Older adults over 70 years of age have a notable loss of 40% in the total number of sensorial cells of the vestibular system (Spirduso, 1995). This morphological loss may lead to functional changes. One of the characteristics attributed to this decrease in sensorial capacity of the vestibular system is denominated by vertigo. In an otolaryngology study conducted to verify the causes of dizziness in patients older than 60 years of age, it was observed that 18% of the 50 patients that were evaluated had the vertigo, mainly attributed with the peripheral vestibular disorder (Lawson et al., 1999).

Then we can infer that older adults with vestibular loss attributed to aging process perform the daily tasks, as walking in cluttered environments, with more difficulties, which can lead to tripping, sliding and falls. On the other hand, the enrollment of older individuals in physical activity programs has been shown to retard the structural and functional decline generated by the aging process. Active elders fall less and present higher mobility (Brach et al., 2004; Gobbi et al., 2005; Silsupadol et al., 2006; Verghese, 2006). Therefore, the purpose of this study was to verify the contribution of the vestibular information while stepping over obstacles in active and sedentary older adults. A motorized rotary chair was used to apply the transitory vestibular perturbation, mainly because it is less aggressive to older individuals than other invasive methods, such GVS.

Methods

Thirty individuals (55 to 75 years old) participated in this study after provided written informed consent. The local Ethic Committee approved the protocol and it is in accordance with the Declaration of Helsinki. Two groups were evaluated: fifteen participants were physically active and fifteen were sedentary. The Modified Baecke Questionnarie for Older Adults (Pereira et al., 1997; Voorrips et al., 1997) was used to classify individuals to both groups. In addition, the active participants should be enrolled in physical activities at least for 1 year. The participants were distributed in groups accordingly to their age: middle-age (55–60 years old), young-old (61–65 years old) and old-age (66–75 years old). After all, six groups were defined accordingly with their age and physical activity status: active and middle-age (n = 5), active and young-old (n = 5), active and old-age (n = 5), sedentary and middle-age (n = 5), sedentary and young-old (n = 5) and sedentary and old-age (n = 5). Table 1 presents the subjects' characteristics of age, height, body mass and physical activity level by group. Active and sedentary individuals within the age group were similar for age, height and body mass (p>0.05).

Table 1. Means and standard deviations of the subjects' characteristics by group

Groups		Age (years)	Height (cm)	Body mass (kg)	Physical activity level (points)
active	middle-age	56.40±1.67	160.80±5.02	61.60±7.27	16.28±6.93
	young-old	62.00±1.22	158.20±3.63	70.60±7.44	9.64±2.49
	old-age	69.00±1.58	157.80±12.11	67.80±17.89	10.93±5.43
sedentary	middle-age	57.60±1.82	160.80±6.83	77.44±19.11	2.19±1.15
	young-old	62.80±2.05	152.40±5.08	60.56±11.88	2.76±0.76
	old-age	70.60±2.70	165.40±6.91	71.90±11.61	2.25±0.71

Participants sat comfortably on a motorized rotary chair. This equipment allowed inducing a temporary vestibular perturbation. Based on a pilot study and considering the older individuals enrolled in this study, we decreased the rotational magnitude and frequencies by two rotations of 20 rpm. The designed system allowed the rotation at same frequency and velocity for all participants, independently of their anthropometrics features. The task performed consisted in walking in a 3 m length and 1.5 m width pathway and stepping over one of two obstacles personalized by lower limb anthropometric parameters of the participants. The high obstacle was defined as leg length minus 10 cm and the low was obtained as the ankle height.

Participants were instructed to seat on the chair with the head in a pitch position and with eyes closed (to avoid possibly visual targets during the rotations and before standing up). After the chair stopped participants should open their eyes, stand up as fast as possibly, initiate gait (in their preferred velocity) toward the obstacle and step over it. The obstacle was distant one stride from the chair. The combination of transitory vestibular perturbation and the obstacles created six experimental conditions: (1) without perturbation and without obstacle, (2) with perturbation and without obstacle, (3) without perturbation and low obstacle, (4) without perturbation and high obstacle, (5) with perturbation and low obstacle and (6) with perturbation and high obstacle. Each participant performed five trials in each experimental condition totalling thirty trials completely randomized. A 20-second rest interval was allowed after each trial for recovering from the transitory vestibular perturbation (Guyton, 1993). The interval was standardized for all participants; however it was given more time if necessary.

Displacements of six active markers (fifth metatarsi, heel, and ankle in both feet) were tracked by the OPTOTRAK system (Northern Digital, Canada) placed on the left side of the participant. The active markers were placed on the lateral side of the left foot and on the medial side of the right foot. The data was sampled at a frequency of 60 Hz. Kinematic data was filtered using a fourth-order Butterworth filter with cut-off frequency of 5 Hz. Five dependent variables were analyzed: toe clearance, take-off horizontal distance of the lead limb, maximum horizontal speed of toe marker and medial-lateral deviation. All dependent variables were statistically analyzed using a four-way ANOVA for repeated measures in the last two factors (3 age groups X 2 physical activity levels X 2 perturbation levels X 2 obstacles heights). Scheffé post-hoc test was used to identify the differences when main effects were present. The significance level was set at 0.05. Due to the great variability in the elderly behaviour it was considered $p < 0.08$ as a marginal result.

Results and Discussion

As shown in previous studies (Gonçalves et al., 2000; Bent et al., 2000; Fitzpatrick et al., 1999; Kubo et al., 1997), the vestibular perturbation produced a significant lateral deviation. The ANOVA for medial-lateral deviation identified a main effect of transitory vestibular perturbation ($F_{1,24} = 17.688$, $p = 0.0001$) (perturbation = 15.24±12.16cm; no perturbation = 11.01±11.53cm). Therefore, the use of the motorized rotary chair was successful to produce the transitory vestibular perturbation desired.

Sedentary participants presented higher medial-lateral deviation (16.52±11.78cm) in comparison to active ones (9.73± 11.31cm) ($F_{1,24} = 4.609$, $p = 0.042$). This result indicates that regular physical activity is helpful in the adaptive process followed by the vestibular perturbation. Some studies shown that the impaired vestibular system can be rehabilitated thought physical activities (Cass et al., 1996).

The significant interaction between perturbation and obstacle height ($F_{2,48}$ = 3.136, p = 0.05) showed that the participants increase the medial-lateral deviation without perturbation, whereas the medial-lateral deviation decreases with transitory vestibular perturbation when the obstacle height increases, although the medial-lateral deviation was always larger for the conditions with transitory vestibular perturbation than for the conditions without it (Figure 4).

It is possible that the visual target (obstacle) may help subjects to adapt their behaviour due to vestibular perturbation and, therefore, they were able to modulate the medial-lateral deviation. The increase in obstacle height represents a more dangerous situation, especially when associated to a transitory vestibular perturbation. Hence, the organism needs to increase the attention demand, what might be potentially provided by the visual system. Horak et al. (1990) showed that the organism needs at least one sensory system intact to recover successfully from a perturbation, through a sensory organization test with six experimental conditions with mixed vision and support perturbation during quiet standing. As both visual and somatosensory systems were not manipulated in the present study it would result in a suppression of the vestibular system information that could decreased the medial-lateral deviation under this condition. Since the low obstacle and absence of obstacle did not represent a real problem during walking, the central nervous system does not need to be alert in those conditions. Nevertheless, the medial-lateral deviation was increased for all obstacle heights during temporary vestibular perturbation condition showing that even a visual target was not able to minimize the medial-lateral deviation.

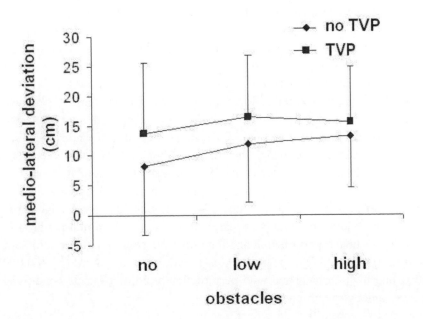

Figure 4. Interaction between transitory vestibular perturbation (TVP) and obstacle height in medial-lateral deviation (MLD)

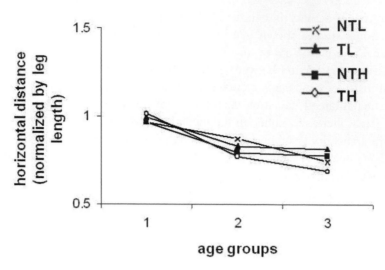

Figure 5. Interaction between transitory vestibular perturbation (TVP), obstacle height and age group for the take-off horizontal distance of the lead limb (HD); (conditions: NTL= no transitory vestibular perturbation and low obstacle; TL= with transitory vestibular perturbation and low obstacle; NTH= no transitory vestibular perturbation and high obstacle; and TH= with transitory vestibular perturbation and high obstacle)

For the take-off horizontal distance of the lead limb, it was verified that the transitory vestibular perturbation interfered in where participants landed their foot before stepping over the obstacle. This was seen in the interaction between transitory vestibular perturbation, obstacle height and age group ($F_{2,24}$ = 3.471, p = 0.047). Independently of physical activity, the older tend to decrease their take-off horizontal distance of the lead limb (Figure 5), what may be related to the aging process. The old-age group decreased its take-off horizontal distance when they needed to cross over the highest obstacle and more when the obstacle height was associated with transitory vestibular perturbation. Many factors may explain why elderly prefer to place the foot closer to the obstacle before crossing it. First, the aging is accompanied by many morph-physiologic changes, as joint stiffness and muscle weakness that constraints the movement performance. Therefore, stepping longer while cross-over the obstacle could imply in a slip, trip or even a non successful attempt. Second, it might be explained by the fact that older people decrease the dynamics of the whole event (e.g., short step length, low velocity) (Ferrandez et al., 1990) to achieve a more stable movement and to do not compromise their safety. This is especially performed by increasing their single support phase before step over the obstacle. Without transitory vestibular perturbation and low obstacle, the middle-age group was marginally different from old-age group (p = 0.054). With transitory vestibular perturbation and high obstacle condition, the middle-age group was different from young-old group (p = 0.034) and old-age group (p = 0.004). Without perturbation and high obstacle and with perturbation and low obstacle conditions there were no differences among age groups.

The results showed that transitory vestibular perturbation did not affect toe clearance. In this case it can be inferred that toe clearance is a variable that suffer less or no interference from temporary vestibular perturbation differently from take-off horizontal distance of the lead limb. Since toe clearance is a not dispensable variable to successfully step over an obstacle, the participants may have chosen to keep toe clearance, despite the lateral deviation, constant as a safe strategy. It seems that in this specific case, toe clearance is more important than take-off horizontal distance of the lead limb. Another factor that should be considered is the intensity of rotation used by the motorized rotary chair. Perhaps a higher intensity than that used (2 rotations at 20 rpm) is necessary to cause interference with toe clearance.

Independently of age and obstacle height, the active participants presented a higher maximum horizontal speed than the sedentary participants in both conditions: with and without perturbation. The interaction between perturbation and physical activity level was also significant ($F_{1,24}$ = 5.383, p = 0.029). Inactive participants have the same maximum horizontal speed in both conditions (Figure 6).

According to Brandt (2003), it is possible to suppress the vestibular system information when the speed of gait is increased. He affirmed that during slow walk or run with closed eyes patients with acute vestibular neuritis show a deviation of gait towards the affected ear. However, during running they maintained their direction much better than during walking. Hence, this result may explain the interaction showed in Figure 6. Sedentary participants showed a particular behaviour when walking under transitory vestibular perturbation. Differently from the actives, they did not change their velocity when walking under vestibular perturbation conditions. It is possible that the sedentary individuals chose to maintain the velocity, since during vestibular information suppression balance became easier to control on its condition. Although the active individuals changed the velocity, the safety was preserved and the medial-lateral deviation was much lower than sedentary as showed.

In addition, a marginal significant interaction between transitory vestibular perturbation and obstacle height was observed ($F_{2,48}$ = 2.953, p = 0.062; Figure 7). It is interesting to observe that, when the transitory vestibular perturbation was absent, the participants, independent of age and physical activity, performed the task quicker during the low obstacle and no obstacle conditions than in the high obstacle condition. When facing the high obstacle, the participants exhibited the same speed in both with and without perturbation.

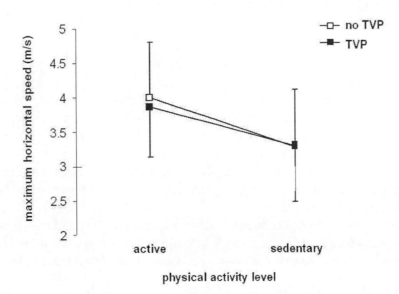

Figure 6. Interaction between temporary vestibular perturbation (TVP) and physical activity level for maximum horizontal speed

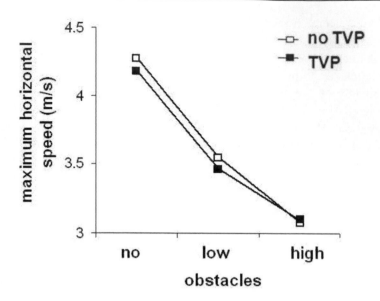

Figure 7. Interaction between temporary vestibular perturbation (TVP) and obstacle height for maximum horizontal speed (MHS)

The results showed that the integrity of the vestibular system appears to play an important role in the modulation of velocity during locomotion over obstacles. They showed that when the perturbation was absent the participants perform the task faster than when the perturbation was present. It was also noted that, independently of transitory vestibular perturbation, when the obstacle was higher the participants performed the task with the same velocity and it was slower than the other obstacle heights. There is no doubt that obstacle height is a restriction that has a direct influence on the locomotor pattern of the elderly and it seems to be more challenging when associated with transitory vestibular perturbation.

CONCLUSION

Young and old adults were able to plan and execute their motor actions according to the environmental (obstacle height) constraint. The presence of transitory vestibular perturbation did not affect limb elevation over the obstacle, suggesting that vestibular information is not used to control limb elevation during obstacle crossing in both young and old adults. On the other hand, the presence of transitory vestibular perturbation affected walking direction in both young and old adults. Therefore, vestibular information seems quite important for keeping straight ahead locomotion.

The medial-lateral deviation of the walking trajectory on even terrain under vestibular perturbation was previously documented (Bent et al., 2000). The results of Experiments 2 and 3 showed that this is also observed in adaptive locomotion for both young and old adults. The presence of a visual target (i.e., obstacle) was not able to minimize the medial-lateral deviation. For young adults, horizontal velocity was not affected by transitory vestibular perturbation and medial-lateral deviation could not be reduced by increasing gait speed as observed by Brant (2003). Older individuals, on the other hand, showed increased difficulties in adaptive locomotion. When compared to young adults, the results of Experiment 3 revealed that older adults produced some additional modifications of their gait pattern due to transitory vestibular perturbation. In particular, older adults exhibited reduced maximum horizontal speed and decreased take-off horizontal distance. These two adaptations can be related to the maintenance of dynamic stability and reveal a conservative strategy.

The observed differences and interactions related to physical activity level (medial-lateral deviation and maximum horizontal speed) highlight the benefits of enrollment in physical activity programs. Exercise can help in slowing morpho-physiological decline related to the aging process. In addition, more active elders have preserved the capacity to reweigh sensory information. As a consequence, active older persons show higher levels of mobility and fall less frequently (Brach et al., 2004; Gobbi et al., 2005; Silsupadol et al., 2006; Verghese, 2006).

The results of these experiments can also have an impact on the healthy population, which is related to the early detection of vestibular deficits and the subsequent development of preventive actions. The motorized rotary chair can be implemented on a large scale for early detection of vestibular deficits. This early detection of vestibular deficits can be used to generate actions to improve dynamic task performance and prevent falls. One such action can be engagement in exercise activities, since the present data supports intervention with physical activities to minimize vestibular deficits.

In summary, the motorized rotary chair can be used in research settings to disturb the vestibular system input, as shown in Experiment 1. The results of Experiment 2 showed that young adults could better compensate for the disturbance of the vestibular system than old adults (Experiment 3), even though the magnitude of the perturbation was higher for the young than for the old adults. Also, involvement in physical activity programs by older adults seems to help compensate for disturbance of the vestibular system.

REFERENCES

Aoki, M., Ito, Y., Burchill, P., Brookes, G. B. & Gresty, M. A. (1999). Tilted perception of the subjective 'upright' in unilateral loss of vestibular function. *American Journal of Otology, 20,* 741-747.

Angelaki, D. E. & Cullen, K. E. (2008). Vestibular system: the many facets of a multimodal sense. *Annual Review of Neuroscience, 31,* 125-150.

Belafsky, P., Gianoli, G., Soileau, J., More, D. & Davidowitz, S. (2000). Vestibular autorotation testing in patients with benign paroxysmal positional vertigo. *Otolaryngology-Head and Neck Surgery, 122,* 163-167.

Bent, L. R., Inglis, J. T. & McFadyen, B. J. (2004). When is vestibular information important during walking? *Neurophysiology, 92,* 1269-1275.

Bent, L. R., McFadyen, B. J. & Inglis, J. T. (2005). Vestibular contributions during human locomotor tasks. *Exercise Sport Science Review, 33,* 107-113.

Bent, L. R., McFadyen, B. J., Merkley, V. F., Kennedy, P. M. & Inglis, J. T. (2000). Magnitude effects of galvanic vestibular stimulation on the trajectory of human gait, *Neuroscience Letters, 279,* 157-160.

Bottini, G., Karnath, H. O., Vallar, G., Sterzi, R., Frith, C. D., Frackowiak, R. S. J. & Paulesu, E. (2001). Cerebral representations for egocentric space: Functional–anatomical evidence from caloric vestibular stimulation and neck vibration. *Brain, 124*, 1182-1196.

Brach, J. S., Simonsick, E. M., Kritchevsky, S., Yaffe, K. & Newman, A. B. (2004). The association between physical function and lifestyle activity and exercise in the health, aging and body composition study. *Journal of the American Geriatric Society, 52,* 502-509.

Brandt, T. (2003). *Vertigo: Its Multisensory Syndromes.* (2 ed). London: Springer-Verlag.

Brandt, T. & Strupp, M. (2005). General vestibular testing. *Clinical Neurophysiology, 116,* 406–426.

Brooks, V. B. (1986). *The Neural Basis of Motor Control.* (1 ed). New York, New York: Oxford University Press.

Cass, S. P., Borello-France, D. & Furman, J. M. (1996). Functional outcome of vestibular rehabilitation in patients with abnormal sensory-organization testing. *The American Journal of Otology, 17*, 581-594.

Chen, H. C., Ashton-Miller, J. A., Alexander, N. B. & Schultz, A. B. (1991). Stepping over obstacles: gait patterns of healthy adults. *Journal of Gerontology and Medicine Science, 46*, M196–203.

Chou, L. S., Kaufman, K. R., Hahn, M. E. & Brey, R. H. (2003). Medio-lateral motion of the center of mass during obstacle crossing distinguishes elderly individuals with imbalance. *Gait and Posture, 18*, 125-133.

Clarke, A. H. (2001). Perspectives for the comprehensive examination of semicircular canal and otolith function. *Biological Sciences in Space, 15*, 393-400.

Daniel, L. L. & Redfern, M. S. (2000). The role of initial conditions in the postural sway response to galvanic vestibular stimulation [online]. Available from: www.abs-biomech.org/onlineabs/abstracts2000/pdf/132.pdf.

Davis, L. E. (1994). Dizziness in elderly men. *Journal of the American Geriatrics Society, 42*, 1184-1188.

Deshpande, N. & Patla, A. E. (2005). Dynamic visual-vestibular integration during goal directed human locomotion. *Experimental Brain Research, 166*, 237–247.

Fasold, O., von Brevern, M., Kuhberg, M., Ploner, C. J., Villringer, A., Lempert, T. & Wenzel, R. (2002). Human vestibular cortex as identified with caloric stimulation in functional magnetic resonance imaging. *Neuroimage, 17,* 1384-93.

Ferrandez, A. M., Pailhois, J. & Durup, M. (1990). Slowness in elderly gait. *Experimental Aging Research, 16*, 79-89.

Fitzpatrick, R. C. & Day, B. L. (2004) Probing the human vestibular system with galvanic stimulation. *Journal of Applied Physiology, 96*, 2301-2316.

Fitzpatrick, R. C., Wardman, D. L. & Taylor, J. L. (1999). Effects of galvanic vestibular stimulation during human walking. *Journal of Physiology, 517*, 931-939.

Gananca, M. M., Caovilla, H. H., Munhoz, M. L. S., Silva, M. L. G., Gananca, F. F. & Gananca, C. F. (1999). As etapas da equilibriometria [The phases of the equilibriumetry]. In M. M. Gananca, H. H. Caovilla, M. S. L. Munhoz & M. L. G. Silva (Eds.), *Equilibriometria Clínica* [Clinical Equilibriumetry] (1 ed., pp.41-114). São Paulo, SP: Atheneu.

Ghez, C. (1991). Posture. In E. R. Kandel, J. H. Schwartz & T. M. Jessell (Eds.), *Principles of Neural Science.* (3 ed., pp. 598-607). Norwalk, CT: Appleton & Lange.

Gobbi, L. T. B., Gonçalves, C. T., Miyasike-da-Silva, V., Marins, F. H. P. & Gobbi, S. (2005). Elderly estimation and locomotor behavior after transitory vestibular perturbation. In: *Scientific Proceedings from the 6th World Congress on Aging and Physical Activity*. London, Ontario: Canadian Center for Activity and Aging, 28-32.

Gobbi, L. T. B. & Patla, A. E. (1997). Desenvolvimento da locomoção em terrenos irregulares: proposta de um modelo teórico [The development of locomotion over uneven terrain: the purpose of a theoretical model]. In A. M. Pellegrini (Ed.), *Coletânea de Estudos: Comportamento Motor I. [Studies Collection: Motor Behavior I]* (1 ed., pp. 29-44). São Paulo, SP: Movimento.

Goldberg, J. M., Ferrandez, C. & Smith, C. E. (1982). Responses of vestibular afferents in the squirrel monkey to externally applied galvanic currents. *Brain Research, 252*, 156-160.

Gonçalves, C. T., Moraes, R. & Gobbi, L. T. B. (2000). Efeito da perturbação vestibular transitória na transposição de obstáculos [Effect of transitory vestibular perturbation on obstacle crossing]. *Motriz, 6*, 57-63.

Graci, V., Elliott, D. B. & Buckley, J. G. (2009) Peripheral visual cues affect minimum-foot-clearance during overground locomotion. *Gait & Posture, 30*, 370-374.

Guyton, A. C. (1993). *Neurociência Básica: anatomia e fisiologia [Basic Neuroscience, Anatomy & Physiology]* (2 ed.). Rio de Janeiro, RJ: Guanabara Koogan.

Horak, F. B. (2009). Postural compensation for vestibular loss. *Annals of the New York Academy of Sciences, 1164*, 76–81.

Horak, F. B. & Macpherson, J. M. (1996). Postural orientation and equilibrium. In L. B. Rowell & J. T. Shepherd (Eds.), *Handbook of Physiology Section 12: Exercise: Regulation and Integration of Multiple Systems* (1 ed., pp.255-292). New York, NJ: Oxford University Press.

Horak, F. B., Nashner, L. M. & Diener, H. C. (1990). Postural strategies associated with somatosensory and vestibular loss. *Experimental Brain Research, 82,* 167-77.

Igarashi, M., Watanabe, T. & Maxian, P. M. (1970). Dynamic equilibrium in squirrel monkeys after unilateral and bilateral labyrinthectomy. *Acta Oto-Laryngologica, 69*, 247-253.

Iles, J. F., Baderin, R., Tanner, R. & Simon, A. (2007). Human standing and walking: comparison of the effects of stimulation of the vestibular system. *Experimental Brain Research, 178*, 151–166.

Jauregui-Renaud, K., Yarrow, K., Oliver, R., Gresty, M. A. & Bronstein, A.M. (2000). Effects of caloric stimulation on respiratory frequency and heart rate and blood pressure variability. *Brain Research Bulletin, 53*, 17 – 23.

Kelly, J. P. (1991a). Hearing. In E. R. Kandel, J. H. Schwartz & T. M. Jessell (Eds.), *Principles of Neural Science* (3 ed., pp. 481-499). Norwalk, CT: Appleton & Lange.

Kelly, J. P. (1991b). The sense of balance. In E. R. Kandel, J. H. Schwartz & T. M. Jessell (Eds.), *Principles of Neural Science* (3 ed., pp. 500-511). Norwalk, CT: Appleton & Lange.

Kennedy, P. M., Carlsen, A. N., Inglis, J. T., Chow, R., Franks, I. M. & Chua, R. (2003). Relative contributions of visual and vestibular information on the trajectory of human gait. *Experimental Brain Research, 153*, 113–117.

Kubo, T., Kumakura, H., Hihokawa, Y., Yamamoto, K., Imai, T. & Hirasaki, E. (1997). 3D analysis of human locomotion before and after caloric stimulation. *Acta Oto-Laryngologica, 117*, 143-148.

Lackner, J. R. & Dizio, P. (2009). Angular displacement perception modulated by force background. *Experimental Brain Research*, *195*, 335–343.

Lawson, J., Fitzgerald, J., Birchall, J., Aldren, C. P. & Kenny, R. A. (1999). Diagnosis of geriatric patients with severe dizziness. *Journal of the American Geriatrics Society, 47*, 12-17.

Lenggenhager, B., Lopez, C. & Blanke, O. (2008). Influence of galvanic vestibular stimulation on egocentric and object-based mental transformations. *Experimental Brain Research*, *184*, 211–221.

Lysakowski, A. & Goldberg, J. M. (2004). Morphophysiology of the vestibular periphery. In S. M. Highstein, R. R. Fay & A. N. Popper (Eds.), *The Vestibular System* (1 ed., pp. 57-152). Berlin, GE: Springer.

Marques, B., Colombo, G., Müller, R., Dürsteler, M. R., Dietz, V. & Straumann D. (2007). Influence of vestibular and visual stimulation on split-belt walking. *Experimental Brain Research*, *183*, 457–463.

Mcauley, E., Mihalko, S. L. & Rosengren, K. (1997). Self efficacy and balance correlates of fear of falling in elderly. *Journal of Ageing and Physical Activity*, *5*, 329-340.

Mohagheghi, A. A., Moraes, R. & Patla, A. E. (2004). The effects of distant and on-line visual information on the control of approach phase and step over an obstacle during locomotion. *Experimental Brain Research*, *155*, 459-468.

Moraes, R., Lewis, M. A. & Patla, A. E. (2004). Strategies and determinants for selection of alternate foot placement during human locomotion: influence of spatial and temporal constraints. *Experimental Brain Research*, *159*, 1–13.

Nashner, L. M. & Forssberg, H. (1986). Phase dependent organization of postural adjustments associated with arm movements while walking. *Journal of Neurophysiology*, *55*, 1382-1394.

Patla, A. E. (1986). Adaptation of postural responses to voluntary arm rises during locomotion in humans. *Neuroscience Letters*, *68*, 334-338.

Patla, A. E. (2003). Strategies for dynamic stability during human locomotion: Contribution of visual, vestibular and kinesthetic inputs to maintaining balance in complex environments. *IEEE Engineering in Medicine and Biology Magazine, 22*, 48-52.

Patla, A. E. (1997). Understanding the roles of vision in the control of human locomotion. *Gait and Posture*, *5*, 54-69.

Patla, A. E. (1991). Visual control of human locomotion. In A. E. Patla (Ed.), *Adaptability of Human Gait: Implications for the Control of Locomotion* (1st ed., pp. 55-97). Amsterdam: Elscvicr.

Patla, A. E., Davies, T. C. & Niechwiej, E. (2004). Obstacle avoidance during locomotion using haptic information in normally sighted humans. *Experimental Brain Research, 155*, 173 - 185.

Patla, A.E. & Greig, M. (2006). Any way you look at it, successful obstacle negotiation needs visually guided on-line foot placement regulation during the approach phase. *Neuroscience Letters*, *397*, 110-114.

Patla, A. E., Niechwiej, E., Racco, V. & Goodale, M. A. (2002) Understanding the contribution of binocular vision to the control of adaptive locomotion. *Experimental Brain Research*, *142*, 551-561.

Patla, A. E., Prentice, S. D. & Gobbi, L. T. B. (1996a). Visual control of obstacle avoidance during locomotion: strategies in young children, young and older adults. In A. Ferrandez

& N. Teasdale (Eds.), *Changes in Sensori-motor Behavior in Aging* (1 ed., pp. 257-277). Amsterdam: Elsevier.

Patla, A. E., Prentice, S., Robinson, C. & Neufeld, J. (1991). Visual control of locomotion: strategies for changing direction and for going over obstacles. *Journal of Experimental Psychology: Human Perception of Performance, 17*, 603-634.

Patla, A. E. & Riedtyk, S. (1993). Visual control of limb trajectory over obstacles: effect of obstacle height and width. *Gait and Posture, 1*, 45-60.

Patla, A. E., Rietdyk, S., Martin, C. & Prentice, S. (1996b). Locomotor patterns of the leading and trailing limb while going over solid and fragile obstacles: some insights into the role of vision during locomotion. *Journal of Motor Behavior, 28*, 35-47.

Patla, A. E. & Vickers, J. N. (2003). How far ahead do we look when required to step on specific locations in the travel path during locomotion? *Experimental Brain Research, 148*, 133-138.

Patla, A. E. & Vickers, J. N. (1997). Where and when do we look as we approach and step over an obstacle in the travel path? *NeuroReport, 8*, 3661-3665.

Pereira, M. A., Fitzgerald, S. J., Gregg, E. W., Joswiak, M. L., Ryan, W. J., Suminski, R. R., Utter, A. C. & Zmuda, J. M. (1997). Modified Baecke questionnaire for older adults. In A. M. Kriska & C. J. Caspersen (Eds.), A collection of physical activity questionnaires for health-related research. *Medicine and Science in Sports and Exercise, 29*, S117-S121.

Rama-López, J. & Pérez-Fernández, N. (2004). Characterization of the influence exerted by the visual factor in patients with balance disorders. *Revista de Neurología, 39*, 513-516.

Rietdyk, S. & Rhea, C. K. (2006). Control of adaptive locomotion: effect of visual obstruction and visual cues in the environment. *Experimental Brain Research, 169*, 272-278.

Silsupadol, P., Siu, K. C., Shumway-Cook, A. & Woollacott, M. H. (2006). Training of balance under single and dual-task conditions in older adults with balance impairment. *Physical Therapy, 86*, 269-281.

Spirduso, W. W. (1995). *Physical Dimensions of Aging*. Champaign, IL: Human Kinetics.

Stein, B. E. & Meredith, A. (1993). *The Merging of the Senses* (1 ed.), Boston, MA: A Bradford Book, The MIT Press.

Taborelli, G., Melagrana, A., D'Agostino, R., Tarantino, V. & Calevo, M.G. (2000). Vestibular neuronitis in children: study of medium and long-term follow-up. *International Journal of Pediatric Otorhinolaryngology, 54*, 117-121.

Verghese, J. (2006). Cognitive and mobility profile of older social dancers. *Journal of the American Geriatric Society, 54*, 1241–1244.

Voorrips, L. E., Ravelli, A. C. J., Dongelmans, P. C. A., Deurenberg, P. & Van Staveren, W. A. (1997). A physical activity questionnaire for the elderly. *Medicine Science Sports & Exercise, 29*, S117-21.

Yamamoto, K., Momoto, Y., Imai, T., Hirasaki, E. & Kubo, T. (2002). Effects of caloric vestibular stimulation on head and trunk movements during walking. *Gait and Posture, 15*, 274-281.

In: Overweightness and Walking
Editor: Caleb I. Black, pp. 59-73

ISBN: 978-1-60741-298-4
© 2010 Nova Science Publishers, Inc.

Chapter 3

ASSESSMENTS BASED ON PLANTAR PRESSURE: EMPHASIS ON ITS USE IN SYMPTOM-FREE POSTMENOPAUSAL WOMEN

Ronaldo Gabriel[1], Marco Monteiro[2], Helena Moreira[2], Aurélio Faria[3] and João Abrantes[4]

[1]Department of Sport Science, Exercise and Health – CITAB, University of Trás-os-Montes and Alto Douro, Vila Real, Portugal
[2]Department of Sport Science, Exercise and Health – CIDESD, University of Trás-os-Montes and Alto Douro, Vila Real, Portugal
[3]Department of Sport Science – CIDESD, University of Beira Interior, Covilhã, Portugal
[4]MovLab - CICANT, Universidade Lusófona de Humanidades e Tecnologias, Lisbon, Portugal

ABSTRACT

Plantar pressure can contribute to the systematic measurement, description, and assessment of quantities that characterize human locomotion and its analysis may provide additional insight into the etiology of pain and lower extremities complaints allowing for injury prevention [1, 2].

Plantar pressure measurements during walking or other activities can demonstrate the pathomechanics of the abnormal foot and yield objective measures for outcomes evaluation or to track disease progression [3]. In order to reduce the risk of tissue damage and to prevent diabetic foot ulceration in the neuropathic foot, the reduction of plantar pressure shall be a goal [4]. In looking forward to avoid or minimize foot pain discomfort in rheumatoid arthritis, the reduction of plantar pressure is also a therapeutic goal [5].

Walking represents an ideal physical activity to initiate a change in the behavior, which is needed to acquire health benefits, and which is accessible to all the community segments. It can be incorporated in the daily routine as a way of displacement in the surroundings of home, a way of exercise, to move from a place to another or for simple pleasure. Therefore, considering that the interest in physical fitness continues to grow in postmenopausal women, as a result of promoting health and wellness, the understanding of the dynamic characteristics of the symptom-free foot during the human locomotion provides the necessary basis for objective evaluation of movement dysfunction [6]. This review includes relevant information for the assessment of the human locomotion based on plantar pressure in symptom-free postmenopausal women.

Our aim is to provide a selected review of information relevant to the assessment of the human locomotion based on plantar pressure, indicating several methodological concerns that must be taken into consideration, in order to achieve valid, reliable and accurate data. With this paper, we hope to contribute to the improvement of gait analysis as an effective tool in the clinical decision, by making a process for improving treatment outcome in individuals.

INTRODUCTION

Pressure (p) is defined as force perpendicular to the surface (f) per unit area of this surface (a), specifically, $p = f/a$ [7] The magnitude of plantar pressure is then determined by dividing the measured force perpendicular by the known area of the foot in contact with the supporting surface. In the IS nomenclature the pressure values should be reported in units of Pascal (Pa) which equals a force of 1 Newton per 1 square meter (Nm^{-2}). For foot pressures, the values usually reach the kilopascal (kPa) or megapascal (MPa) range. Several research teams use units like Newton per square centimetre ($Ncm^{-2} = 10$ kPa).

In the biped locomotion, the foot has three fundamental biomechanical functions [8]: (1) body adaptation to the unevenness of the ground; (2) support and weakening of body mass and; (3) transmission of propulsory forces. As a result of its location and its associated locomotors functions, the foot becomes an essential study object in the control of this way of locomotion [9] and in the comprehension of gait adaptations during the act of walking, as well as the difficulties felt during its execution (ex. discomfort or pain in the inferior extremities). This may be a major factor in the predisposition to participate in habitual physical activity such as walking [10]. For instance, an unsuitable force distribution, may lead to an irregular movement, especially during the stance phase, which will cause an excessive stress and originate injuries in the soft tissues [11].

Messier et al [12] refer that changes in gait default due to attempts to avoid or minimize eventual discomfort, may be the cause for why pain appears in the lower limb. However, the regular practice of walking promotes an improvement in walking biomechanics and a reduction of pain sensation in the knee, during the performance of several daily routine tasks of biped locomotion [13]. Therefore, plantar pressure can contribute to the systematic measurement, description, and assessment of quantities that characterize human locomotion and provide additional insight into the etiology of pain and lower extremities` complaints, permitting injury prevention [1].

Concerning special population, plantar pressure measurements during walking or other activities can demonstrate the pathomechanics of the abnormal foot and yield objective measures for outcomes evaluation or to track disease progression [3]. Its evaluation may reduce the risk of tissue damage to prevent diabetic foot ulceration in the neuropathic foot [4] and minimize foot pain discomfort in rheumatoid arthritis [5].

Walking has been growing in the health and well-being promotion and in accordance to Myers et al [14], it is the kind of physical activity that tends to remain as most frequent in several age groups. Walking represents an ideal physical activity to commence a change in the behaviour, which is needed to acquire health benefits, and is accessible to all the community segments. It can be incorporated in the daily routine as a way of displacement in the surroundings of home, a way of exercise, to move from a place to another or by simple pleasure. This activity is sought by many individuals older than 60 years old, with the purpose of reducing the disease risk factors associated to the aging process [15].

In postmenopausal women, walking may constitute as an excellent cardiovascular stimulus, permitting the reduction of adiposity excess and improving the components of metabolic syndrome commonly exhibited by this population [16]. The active support of body weight confers an evident osteogenic stimulus, preserving the bone mineral density of the femur [17] and reducing approximately 55% of facture risk to the hip, in comparison to sedentary women in the same climateric phase [18].

The main objective of this lecture is to provide a selected review of information relevant to the assessment of the human locomotion based on plantar pressure, indicating several methodological concerns that must be taken into consideration, in order to achieve, valid, reliable and accurate data.

METHODOLOGICAL CONCERNS

The evaluation of plantar pressure is based in pressure transducers that measure the force of a known surface, providing in this context the necessary information to determine the pressure, through the division of the force by the area. When the aim of the study is the description of normal gait patterns, some methodological concerns must be taken into account to ensure the validity and reliability of data. Namely, factors related to subject, to motor task and to the equipment, must be taken and controlled during data collection.

Factors Related to the Subject

Foot structure and function - According to [19], foot structure and function predicted only approximately 50% of the variance in peak pressure, although the relative contributions in different anatomical regions varied dramatically. However, structure was dominant in predicting peak pressure under the midfoot and first metatarsal head, while both structure and function were important at the heel and hallux. This study developed some predictive models that seem useful to find potential etiological factors associated with elevated plantar pressure. When looking for the eventual effect of the foot type on in-shoe plantar pressure during walking and running [20], it was identified that individuals with low arches may be at decreased risk for the development of fifth metatarsal stress fractures.

Anthropometrical variables - Some studies analysed the gait characteristics of the obese adults [10, 21-23], describing increases in the plantar pressure values with obesity. The plantar pressure measures seem to have an important role in the treatment of obese subjects, having noticed a distinct relation, from those registered in control groups, between the pathological ponderal overload and the plantar surface contact area [23]. Subjective references are accomplished many times to the physical limitations, including the body mass motion difficulties of the obese. The problems normally referred, include general discomfort in general activities of daily living, such as walking and climbing stairs, pain in the lower limb joints, reduced circulation (including edema), ulceration, foot torpidity and predisposition to pathological gait patterns, particularly after periods in biped orthostatic support of the body. The study of Hills et al [10] was the first to expose peak pressure data under adult foot with evident ponderal overload. The subjects performed an evaluation protocol that included the basic locomotor tasks of walking and standing in biped orthostatic support of the body and the study gives important information concerning the specific functional limitations of the foot biomechanics in static position (biped orthostatic support of the body) and dynamic position (gait).

The obese subjects demonstrate an increase in the forefoot width and higher plantar pressure during the protocol of walking and standing in biped orthostatic support of the body. The higher increases of the plantar pressure in the obese were observed under the longitudinal foot arch and in the metatarsal heads [10].

Age – Specialty literature documents reductions in the magnitude of forces and pressures and greater relative duration of contact in older participants [24]. These findings confirm that there are significant changes in the structure and function of the foot with advancing age that have influence in plantar pressure behaviour, namely significant reductions in the magnitude of forces and pressures under the heel, lateral forefoot and hallux, but greater relative duration of contact under the heel, and midfoot of older participants. These age-related differences could be largely explained by differences in step length and selected foot characteristics.

Consequently, before plantar pressure assessments are made, all subjects should visit a physician for a comprehensive injury history [25], in order to validate the inclusion criteria, or to register some variables that must be controlled by the investigator, namely the absence of [10, 22, 25]: (1) foot pain and deformities; (2) acute lower extremity trauma; (3) lower extremity surgery like prosthesis operations of the hip, knee, ankle or foot; (4) leg length discrepancies; (5) eye, ear or cognitive disorders which interfere in conducting the motor task needed for the evaluation; (6) diabetes or related peripheral neuropathy and; (7) walking aids.

Factors Related to the Motor Task

Floor Surfaces - Floor surfaces have an important influence on gait and are likely to affect walking stability [26].

Obstacle crossing – When an obstacle appears, the centre of pressure velocity during stance phase prior to obstacle crossing appears to be regulated for the presence of different obstacle heights [27]. On the other hand, peak pressure and pressure-time integral during level walking correlated strongly with pressures during other activities like ramp climbing, stair climbing, and turning [28]. Therefore, and according to Maluf et al. [28], these results support the clinical evaluation of peak pressure during level walking as an efficient method in screening for maximum levels of stress on the foot, while patients with diabetes mellitus and peripheral neuropathy perform their daily activities.

Gait protocol – In the assessment of the plantar pressure, different gait protocols are used. One of them is the traditional and 'gold standard'' midgait protocol, in which pressure is measured during steady-state in the middle of a relatively long walkway. This protocol requires significant laboratory space and time to complete due to the relatively large number of barefoot steps [29]. The large number of barefoot steps required by this method can not allow the assessment of the people with painful pathologies and increase the risk of injury in the plantar surface of the weak foot. For these reasons, the 1-step and 2-step approach protocols are commonly used in alternative. In these protocols, pressure platform contact is made on the first step (1-step protocol) or on the second step (2-step protocol), after the gait initiation, and the subjects must be also instructed to walk until the end of the walkway, after the pressure platform contact (3-4 steps) [30]. For instance, the 1-step and 2-step protocols require the least amount of repeated trials for obtaining valid and reliable pressure data and may be recommended for assessment of patients with diabetic neuropathic foot [30].

Number of Trials – Typically, in assessments based on pressure platforms, barefoot pressure data from several repeated trials are collected in order to obtain the plantar pressures in a given subject. An important feature in the assessment of the plantar pressure pattern is the number of trials required to minimize the intra-individual variability in an experimental session and therefore to obtain reliable representation of the subject behaviour [31]. Using the EMED F system and based on the realization of 25 trials (three different velocities) in 10 volunteers, Hughes et al. [31] identified a reliability coefficient elevated by the use of three or more trials for most force/pressure.

Speed - Faster walking resulted in higher pressures [32] and variations in walking speed from slow to fast significantly influence the timing and magnitude of plantar pressure values, using the two-step gait initiation protocol [33]. The negative correlation observed in the midfoot implies a reduction to the collapse of the foot's longitudinal arch, with the increase of walking speed [34]. A prescribed walking speed will help to compare the pressure patterns of different subjects, but will most likely prevent the generation of a natural walking pattern for all subjects and the use of a metronome may cause an unnatural stride [35]. However, the obligation to record the speed and to try to keep it constant between repeated trials of one subject is suggested, in order to reduce the intra-subject variability. For instance, a trial must be discarded if the stance duration is higher than ±5% of that participant average stance duration, so as to minimize the effect of the walking speed on the data and to ensure that the participant cadence and velocity are consistent throughout the trials [36, 37].

Factors Related to the Equipment

Sampling frequency - Sampling frequency is the number of samples measured by each sensor per second and it is recorded in cycles (samples) per second or hertz (Hz). Sampling frequency determines the temporal resolution of the system. The minimum sampling frequency for the subsequent plantar pressures calculations was calculated as two times the highest measurable biological frequency, according to the Nyquist Theorem [38]. In this context, 100 Hz were considered adequate for walking [39], however, depending on the aim of the study, sampling frequencies smaller than 100 Hz could also be enough.

Spatial Resolution – The presence of a higher number of sensors confers a better spatial resolution, having observed the foot anatomy and function in measurement of the plantar pressure. The spatial resolution will be necessary to permit the obtainment of specific data concerning the behaviour of plantar pressure in certain restricted areas of the plantar support, as it is appropriate to the objectives of the investigation.

In-shoe device and pressure platform – Comparing to In-Shoe device, a pressure platform usually includes a greater number of sensors, thus a higher spatial resolution. In the pressure platform, sensors are always positioned parallel to the supporting surface to provide a perpendicular force measurement. However, the bigger number of steps required to collect data and the targeting of the pressure platform surface by the sample subject, arc the typical problems associated with this system for data collection. The use of In-shoe pressure measurement is thought to eliminate the problem of targeting and also permits the researcher to study other bipedal locomotion tasks, because it is located within the shoe. It is particularly important to assess the effect of specially designed and built footwear or foot orthoses with the aim to modify the plantar pressures to maximize their comfort and effectiveness.

Calibration – A plantar pressure system shall not only be valid but also reliable and calibration is critical to respect those characteristics of the plantar pressure system. There are several valid methods to calibrate the sensors, depending on the location (*in-shoe* or *pressure platform*) and the system. All of them have the same principle, compressing the sensors at several known levels of pressure to permit the generation of a calibration curve for each sensor or group of sensors in a matrix. With the help of specific software that takes into account that some sensors may not be loaded at all, the calibration can be achieved having a subject stand on the insole or platform generating calibration data for those sensors.

DATA PROCESSING AND ANALYSIS

Areas of interest – Every plantar pressure parameter can be obtained for the whole plantar surface or certain areas based on the foot anatomy and function, although, there is no general pattern for the foot subdivision in interest areas. A careful observation of the literature [10, 23, 25, 32], allows the identification of different footprint divisions, once they are obtained from the total plantar surface. Thus, such decisions must depend on the study objectives [35]. The foot subdivisions have to be small enough to avoid confusion with the neighbouring area, but large enough to include all useful information about that particular area. Ideally, divisions should correspond to foot anatomy and function, and should therefore take into consideration joint position in the foot [40]. For instance, in plantar pressure analysis resorting to the plantar pressure platform RsScan International (1m x 0.4 m, 8192 sensors, 253 Hz) a footprint is obtained from the pressure platform (Figure 1) being divided according to the predefined geometric criteria in ten anatomical pressure areas, with the scalable mask automatically provided (Footscan Software 7.1, RsScan International,

Belgium) under supervision of the researcher and based on the peak pressure footprint. These areas can be defined as medial heel (HM), lateral heel (HL), metatarsal I–V (M1, M2, M3, M4 and M5), the midfoot (MF), the hallux (T1) and the toes (T2-5) [41].

When the method that based on the predefined geometric criteria lose accuracy in the presence of foot deformity, an alternative method involves visual examination of the footprint, and selection of sub-areas based on a subjective assessment and identification of areas corresponding to anatomical landmarks [40]. The spatial resolution of the pressure platform, the anatomical knowledge of the researcher, and the clarity with which each landmark may be identified, influence the accuracy of that method [42]. To solve this problem [43] proposed an innovative method integrating pressure, force and kinematics measurements. The position of each reflective marker placed on appropriate anatomical landmarks on the foot is projected vertically onto the footprint at a point corresponding to mid-stance. Subdivisions of the foot may then be automatically defined based on the position of the reflective markers, making it possible to link the loading distribution under the foot and the position of the overlying anatomical structure. With this innovative method every foot joint can be reliably identified over the footprint, and local loads can be accurately associated with the specific joint. However, when is not possible to combine pressure and kinematics measurements, a new method to normalize plantar pressure measurements for foot size and foot progression angle are proposed in order to study the plantar pressure in more detail, even in the presence of foot deformity [44].

According to Keijsers et al. [44], to calculate the normalized foot, the plantar pressure pattern was rotated over the foot progression angle and normalized for foot size. The foot progression angle was defined as the average angle of the tangent lines to the medial and lateral side of the foot. Foot length was defined as the distance between the back of the heel and the forefoot line. Foot width was defined as the medio-lateral distance between the most medial and most lateral point of the contour line of the forefoot. This study gives us hopeful results concluding that the method allows the use of principal component analysis, clustering techniques, or other classification techniques to analyse plantar pressure or to discriminate between patient groups.

Plantar pressure parameters - After the data assessment from previous identification of different footprint divisions, the biomechanical analysis must be done according to the investigation purposes. Usually, several kinds of data are considered relevant in the biomechanical analysis of plantar pressure.

Absolute and relative temporal data – This allows the analysis of the foot support, the gait characteristics and interactions with functional limitations referred in the specialty literature [2]. They include the instants the regions make contact and instants on which the regions end foot contact, namely, total *foot contact time* (TCT), *first metatarsal contact* (FMC, instant when one of the metatarsal heads contacted the pressure plate), *forefoot flat* (FFF, the first instant all metatarsal heads made contact with the pressure plate), *first foot contact* (FFC, defined as the instant the foot made first contact with the pressure plate), *heel off* (HO, instant the heel region lost contact with the pressure plate) and *last foot contact* (LFC, defined as the last contact of the foot on the plate).

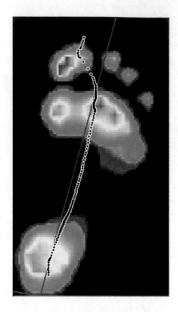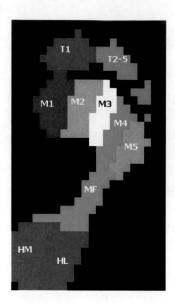

Figure 1. Footprint obtained from the pressure platform, being divided according to the predefined geometric criteria in ten anatomical pressure areas

Peak pressure and absolute impulses - This variable is associated with pain during barefoot walking [4, 5]. The shape of the peak pressure curve along the whole stance phase of gait, might contain more information than instantaneous peak values. A screening test based on peak pressure curve might be an effective tool in the early detection of patients at risk of ulceration [45].

Relative impulses - This parameter resorts from the product of the absolute impulses multiplied by 100 and divided by the sum of all the impulses, determined to the ten foot areas. Their calculation allows for the establishing of the foot areas that contribute mostly to the total vertical impulse and define with clearness in what sense the locomotor pattern efficiency is affected by the presence of certain conditions, namely those related to the subject body composition [46].

Two medio-lateral impulse ratios - The identification of the lateralization of the impulses distribution under the foot, particularly in the metatarsus areas, have consequences in the subject balance [41]. These ratios (*Ratio 1* = [(HM + M1 + M2) − (HL + M4 + M5)]/sum of absolute impulse underneath all areas; *Ratio 2* = (M1−M5)/sum of absolute impulse underneath all metatarsal heads), are calculated to each subject. *Ratio 1* describes the impulse distribution in the whole foot and *Ratio 2* the impulse distribution in the forefoot.

Forefoot-to-rearfoot plantar pressure ratio - The maximum peak pressures under the forefoot (F) and the rearfoot (R) were separately measured for each foot, and the forefoot-to-rearfoot plantar pressure ratio was calculated (F/R). It may play an important role in the etiology of diabetic foot ulceration [47].

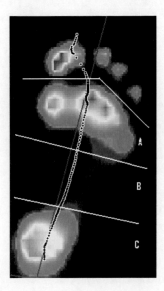

Figure 2. The summed footprint without the toes is divided into three equal parts. Dynamic arch index is calculated as a ratio of the midfoot area (B) to the total foot contact area (A+B+C).

Centre of pressure trajectory - The characteristics concerning the centre of pressure trajectory could serve as reference for future research, in which to study the dynamics of the foot rollover process and foot function. However, a distinction between different foot anatomy types should be made since they influence the centre of pressure path [48].

Dynamic arch index - After the data collection, some aspects must be taken into consideration, in attempt to assure their validity. Thus, if a subject exhibits an extreme flattening or accentuated plantar arch, this condition must be considered in treatment and in the discussion of the results [35]. The plantar pressure evaluation has the potential to reveal the relations between the foot multisegmented structure and function [41]. The arch index gives a simple quantitative way to access the medial longitudinal arch height [49]. However, the dynamic foot biomechanical evaluations, during the support phase, may provide a better starting point to a functional classification system [50]. Dynamic arch index can be calculated as the ratio of the midfoot contact area to the total contact area without the toes (Figure 2) calculated [41].

PLANTAR PRESSURE ASSESSMENTS IN POSTMENOPAUSAL WOMEN

Because the interest in physical fitness continues to grow in the postmenopausal women in order to promote health and wellness, this review includes information relevant to the assessment of the human locomotion based on plantar pressure in symptom-free postmenopausal women. According to the investigation purposes and concerning the general methodological cares to collect data in this population, once the selection of valid, reliable and precise equipment is done, certain attention should also be made in the sample selection, as well as in the experimental task to be conducted.

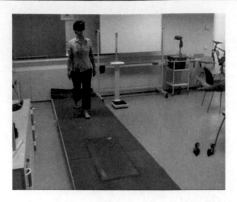 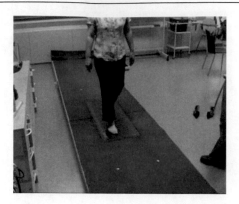

Figure 3. Set up for the walking plantar pressure evaluation

Explicitly, before testing, all subjects should visit a physician for a comprehensive injury history, in order to validate the inclusion criteria, or to register some variables that must be under control by the investigator, depending on the study. After sample selection and considering the methodological concerns related to the data assessment procedures, it is suggested a methodology and experimental protocols for data collection on the approach of the biomechanical parameters of plantar pressure in postmenopausal women. An experimental set up for the walking plantar pressure evaluation should consist of a 9 meter passage (Figure 3) in a 9 m route, above wood platforms, strict and removable, placed in series, with the plantar pressure platform positioned in the middle of the passage [41].

Subjects should be allowed a period of 10 min to practice walking, at a self selected speed, over the pressure platform, to help them become familiar with the test procedure. Simultaneously, the subjects must be instructed not to look at the ground while walking. Each subject must be tested using the 2-step protocol in which platform contact is made on the second step, after the gait initiation. In each protocol, subjects must be instructed to walk until the end of the walkway, after the platform contact (3-4 steps).

The two-step protocol is suggested (contact with the pressure platform at the second step) once, according to [30], because it allows the acquisition of reliable pressure data, with a small amount of trials.

The subjects should make three to five trial repetitions walking barefoot at a natural cadence. The control of gait velocity is not suggested because regardless of discussion it remains a matter of personal choice.

A trial must be discarded if the stance duration is higher than ±5% of that participant average stance duration, in order to minimize the effect of the walking speed on the data and to ensure that the participant's cadence and velocity are consistent across trials or if the foot contact with the pressure platform is incomplete or if the participant targets the platform.)

THE CHARACTERIZATION OF PLANTAR PRESSURE IN POSTMENOPAUSAL WOMEN

As far we know, few studies were made concerning the analysis of the foot biomechanics in postmenopausal women through plantar pressure parameters. The analysis of the influence of fat mass in the plantar pressure turns out to be important given that the persistent overload in the musculoskeletal system endangers the individual's mobility and predisposes the individual to adapt it in a pathological way, therefore increasing the risk of articular injury.

In the study of Monteiro et al. [51], the authors compared plantar pressure parameters (peak pressure and absolute impulse) between obese and non-obese women, considering the existence of obesity from the cutoff value of the body mass índex (BMI) of 25.5 kg/m^2, as established by [52] in Portuguese postmenopausal womenThe obese women presented higher peak pressure values compared to the non-obese group in the metatarsal 4, midfoot, medial heel and lateral heel and higher absolute impulses in the metatarsal 1, metatarsal 4 and midfoot. They conclude that in obese postmenopausal women, the metatarsal 4 and the midfoot are the most overloaded areas, in comparison to the women with normal values of adiposity.

With the objective to analyse the association of plantar pressure parameters (maximum peak pressure and absolute impulses) with age and body composition (BMI; FFM, fat-free mass; SM, skeletal muscle mass; SMI, skeletal muscle mass index), Monteiro et al. [53] observed moderate associations in the midfoot for BMI and SMI with maximum peak pressure and absolute impulses. From the selected predictors, all of them revealed an ability to explain the maximum peak pressure and absolute impulses variation (except toe 1 and metatarsus 1). Consequently, they suggest that the work with this population must target the BMI reduction accompanied with special focus in the muscle condition maintenance or improvement, reducing the foot pain and increasing the predisposition to physical activities.

In relation to the influence of hormone therapy and the nature of menopause (natural or induced) in maximum peak pressure and absolute impulse values, the study of Monteiro et al. [54] revealed that the women with induced menopause have, comparatively to those that have a natural menopause, less dynamic arch index, less medial heel absolute impulse and less lateral heel absolute impulse. Those results suggested that the postmenopausal women with induced menopause apply more strength in the heel's stability, in comparison to those that had a natural menopause and have a larger midfoot area. The hormonal therapy used does not seem to influence the plantar pressure parameters studied.

FUTURES WORK DIRECTIONS

After the considerations that were conducted, certain suggestions arose naturally for future work with the aim to improve the assessments based on plantar pressure beyond the present state of the art. More precisely, concerning the definition of the interest areas, Pataky et al. [55] show that caution is prudent when defining areas boundaries and that areas peak pressure sensitivity should be considered when making statistical inferences regarding foot function. The authors suggest that improvements are needed in the identification of the areas of interest automatically defined based on the position of the markers placed on appropriate anatomical landmarks on the foot, making it possible to link the loading distribution under the foot and the position of the overlying anatomical structure. For instance developing new solutions starting from the work done by Giacomozzi et al. [43], that proposed an innovative method integrating pressure, force and kinematics measurements, where the position of each reflective marker placed on proper anatomical landmarks on the foot is projected vertically onto the footprint at a point corresponding to mid-stance, in order to link the loading distribution under the foot and the position of the overlying anatomical structure. With this approach every foot joint can be reliably identified over the footprint, and local loads can be accurately associated with the specific joint. On the other hand, the development of equipments that permit valid and reliable shear forces data with adequate spatial and temporal resolutions are expected to be done in the future.

All of those suggestions aim to improve the assessments based on plantar pressure in order to get a deeper biomechanical knowledge of the foot behaviour during several kinds of bipedal locomotion tasks. In this framework, the computational simulation, while it is difficult, costly or even invasive to obtain biomechanical measurements of the human body, the computational approach provides an efficient and objective alternative to predict tissue deformation, interfacial pressure, joint and bone movement, internal load distribution, etc [56]. Therefore, this kind of approach can strongly contribute to the improvement in the prediction of the plantar pressure during several kinds of walking tasks.

REFERENCES

[1] Burns, J., Crosbie, J., Hunt, A. & Ouvrier, R. (2005). The effect of pes caves on foot pain and plantar pressure. *Clinical Biomechanics, 20(9)*, 877-882.

[2] De Cock, A., De Clercq, D., Willems, T. & Witvrouw, E. (2005). Temporal characteristics of foot roll-over during barefoot jogging: reference data for young adults. *Gait Posture, 21(4)*, 432-439.

[3] MacWilliams, B. A., & Armstrong, P. F. (2000). Clinical applications of plantar pressure measurement in pediatric Orthopedics. 143-150.

[4] Pham, H., Armstrong, D. G., Harvey, C., Harkless, L. B., Giurini, J. M. & Veves, A. (2000). Screening techniques to identify people at high risk for diabetic foot ulceration: a prospective multicenter trial. *Diabetes Care, 23(5)*, 606-611.

[5] Van der Leeden, M., Steultjens, M., Dekker, J. H. M., Prins, A. P. A. & Dekker, J. (2006). Forefoot joint damage, pain and disability in rheumatoid arthritis patients with foot complaints: the role of plantar pressure and gait characteristics. *Rheumatology, 45(4)*, 465-469.

[6] Rodgers, M. M. (1988). Dynamic biomechanics of the normal foot and ankle during walking and running. *Physical Therapy, 68(12)*, 1822-1830.

[7] Nigg, B. M. (1994). Pressure distribution In B.M. Nigg and a.W. Herzog, *Biomechanics of the Musculo-Skeletal System, 1st edn* pp. 225-236). Chichester, Wiley.

[8] Hallemans, A., De Clercq, D., Van Dongen, S., & Aerts P. (2006). Changes in foot-function parameters during the first 5 months after the onset of independent walking: a longitudinal follow-up study. *Gait Posture, 23(2)*, 142-148.

[9] Eils, E., Behrens, S., Mers, O., Thorwesten, L., Volker, K. & Rosenbaum, D. (2004). Reduced plantar sensation causes a cautious walking pattern. *Gait Posture, 20(1)*, 54-60.

[10] Hills, A. P., Hennig, E. M., McDonald, M. & Bar-Or, O. (2001). Plantar pressure differences between obese and non-obese adults: A biomechanical analysis. *International Journal of Obesity, 25(11)*, 1674-1679.

[11] Abboud, R. J. (2002). Relevant foot biomechanics. *Current Orthopaedics*, *16(3)*, 165-179.

[12] Messier, S. P., Ettinger, W. H., Doyle, T. E., Morgan, T., James, M. K., OToole, M. L., & Burns, R. (1996). Obesity: Effects on gait in an osteoarthritic population. *Journal of Applied Biomechanics*, *12(2)*, 161-172.

[13] Messier, S. P., Thompson, D. C., & Ettinger, W. H. (1997). Effects of long-term aerobic or weight training regimens on gait in an older, osteoarthritic population. *Journal of Applied Biomechanics*, *13*, 205-225.

[14] Myers, A. M., Weigel, C. & Holliday, P. J. (1989). Sex- and age-linked determinants of physical activity in adulthood. *Canadian Journal Public Health*, *80*, 256-260.

[15] Humpel, N., Owen, N., Iverson, D., Leslie, E. & Bauman, A. (2004). Perceived environment attributes, residential location, and walking for particular purposes. *American Journal Preventive Medicine*, *26*, 119-125.

[16] Moreira, M. H. & Sardinha, L. B. (2003). Exercício Físico, Composição corporal e Factores de Risco Cardiovascular na Mulher Pós-Menopáusica Vila Real: Universidade de Trás-os-Montes e Alto Douro.

[17] Martyn-St James, M. & Carroll, S. (2009). A meta-analysis of impact exercise on postmenopausal bone loss: the case for mixed loading exercise programmes. *British Journal of Sports Medicine*, *43,* 898-908.

[18] Feskanich, D., Willett, W. & Colditz, G. (2002). Walking and leisure-time activity and risk of hip fracture in postmenopausal women. *Jama-Journal of the American Medical Association*, *288(18)*, 2300-2306.

[19] Morag, E. & Cavanagh, P. R. (1999). Structural and functional predictors of regional peak pressures under the foot during walking. *Journal of Biomechanics*, *32(4)*, 359-370.

[20] Chuckpaiwong, B., Nunley, J., Mall, N. & Queen, R. (2008). The effect of foot type on in-shoe plantar pressure during walking and running. *Gait & Posture*, *28(3),* 405-411.

[21] Gravante, G., Russo, G., Pomara, F. & Ridola, C. (2003). Comparison of ground reaction forces between obese and control young adults during quiet standing on a baropodometric platform. *Clinical Biomechanics*, *18(8)*, 780-782.

[22] Birtane, M. & Tuna, H. (2004). The evaluation of plantar pressure distribution in obese and non-obese adults. *Clinical Biomechanics*, *19(10)*, 1055-1059.

[23] Teh, E., Teng, L., Acharya U, R., Ha, T., Goh, E. & Min, L. (2006). Static and frequency domain analysis of plantar pressure distribution in obese and non-obese subjects. *Bodywork and movement therapies*, *10(2)*, 127-133.

[24] Scott, G., Menz, H. & Newcombe, L. (2007). Age-related differences in foot structure and function *Gait & Posture*, *26(1)*, 68 - 75.

[25] Willems, T., Witvrouw, E., Delbaere, K., De Cock, A. & De Clercq, D. (2005). Relationship between gait biomechanics and inversion sprains: a prospective study of risk factors. *Gait & Posture*, *21(4)*, 379-387.

[26] Finlay, O. & Beringer, T. (2007). Effects of floor coverings on measurement of gait and plantar pressure. *Physiotherapy, 93(2)*, 144-150.

[27] Wang, Y. & Watanabe, K. (2008). The relationship between obstacle height and center of pressure velocity during obstacle crossing. *Gait & Posture*, *27(1)*, 172-175.

[28] Maluf, K. S., Morley, R. E., Richter, E. J., Klaesner, J. W. & Mueller, M. J. (2004). Foot pressures during level walking are strongly associated with pressures during other

ambulatory activities in subjects with diabetic neuropathy. *Archives of Physical Medicine and Rehabilitation, 85(2)*, 253-260.

[29] McPoil, T. G., Cornwall, M. W., Dupuis, L. & Cornwell, M. (1999). Variability of plantar pressure data - A comparison of the two-step and midgait methods. *Journal of the American Podiatric Medical Association, 89(10)*, 495-501.

[30] Bus, S. & A. Lange (2005). A comparison of the 1-step, 2-step, and 3-step protocols for obtaining barefoot plantar pressure data in the diabetic neuropathic foot. *Clinical Biomechanics, 20(9)*, 892-899.

[31] Hughes, J., Pratt, L., Linge, K., Clark, P. & L. Klenerman (1991). Reliability of pressure measurements: the EM ED F system. *Clinical Biomechanics, 6(1)*, 14-18.

[32] Burnfield, J. M., Few, C. D., Mohamed, O. S. & Perry, J. (2004). The influence of walking speed and footwear on plantar pressures in older adults. *Clinical Biomechanics, 19(1)*, 78-84.

[33] Taylor, A., Menz, H. B. & A. Keenan (2004). The influence of walking speed on plantar pressure measurements using the two-step gait initiation protocol. *The Foot, (14)*, 49-55.

[34] Pataky, T. C., Caravaggi, P., Savage, R., Parker, D., Goulermas, J. Y., Sellers, W. I. & Crompton, R. H. (2008). New insights into the plantar pressure correlates of walking speed using pedobarographic statistical parametric mapping (pSPM). *Journal of Biomechanics, 41(9)*, 1987-1994.

[35] Rosenbaum, D. & Becker, H. (1997). Plantar pressure distribution measurements. Technical background and clinical applications *Foot and Ankle Surgery, 3(1)*, 1-14

[36] Lay, A. N., Hass, C. J. & Gregor, R. J. (2006). The effects of sloped surfaces on locomotion: A kinematic and kinetic analysis. *Journal of Biomechanics, 39(9)*, 1621-1628.

[37] Gabriel, R. C., Abrantes, J., Granata, K., Bulas-Cruz, J., Melo-Pinto, P. & Filipe, V. (2008). Dynamic joint stiffness of the ankle during walking: Gender-related differences. *Physical Therapy in Sport, 9(1)*, 16-24.

[38] McClellan, J. H., Schafer, R. W. & Yoder, M. A. (2003). *Signal Processing First International Edition* USA: Pearson Prentice Hall.

[39] Teyhen, D. S., Stoltenberg, B. E., Collinsworth, K. M., Giesel, C. L., Williams, D. G., Kardouni, C. H., Molloy, J. M., Goffar, S. L., Christie, D. S. & McPoil, T. (2009). Dynamic plantar pressure parameters associated with static arch height index during gait. *Clinical Biomechanics, 24(4)*, 391-396.

[40] Stebbins, J. A., Harrington, M. E., Giacomozzi, C., Thompson, N., Zavatsky, A. & Theologis, T. N. (2005). Assessment of sub-division of plantar pressure measurement in children. *Gait & Posture, 22(4)*, 372-376.

[41] Willems, T. M., De Clercq, D., Delbaere, K., Vanderstraeten, G., De Cock, A. & Witvrouw, E. (2006). A prospective study of gait related risk factors for exercise-related lower leg pain. *Gait & Posture, 23(1)*, 91-98.

[42] Orlin, M. N. & McPoil, T. G. (2000). Plantar pressure assessment. *Physical Therapy, 80(4)*, 399.

[43] Giacomozzi, C., Macellari, V., Leardini, A. & Benedetti, M. G. (2000). Integrated pressure-force-kinematics measuring system for the characterisation of plantar foot loading during locomotion. *Medical and Biological Engineering and Computing, 38(2)*, 156-163.

[44] Keijsers, N. L. W., Stolwijk, N. M., Nienhuis, B. & Duysens, J. (2009). A new method to normalize plantar pressure measurements for foot size and foot progression angle. *Journal of Biomechanics, 42(1)*, 87-90.

[45] Giacomozzi, C. & Martelli, F. (2006). Peak pressure curve: An effective parameter for early detection of foot functional impairments in diabetic patients. *Gait & Posture, 23(4)*, 464-470.

[46] Schrager, M. A., Metter, E. J., Simonsick, E., Ble, A., Bandinelli, S., Lauretani, F. & Ferrucci, L. (2007). Sarcopenic obesity and inflammation in the InCHIANTI study. *Journal of Applied Physiology, 102(3)*, 919-925.

[47] Caselli, A., Pham, H., Giurini, J. M., Armstrong, D. G. & Veves, A. (2002). The forefoot-to-rearfoot plantar pressure ratio is increased in severe diabetic neuropathy and can predict foot ulceration. *Diabetes Care, 25(6)*, 1066-1071.

[48] De Cock, A., Vanrenterghem, J., Willems, T., Witvrouw, E. & De Clercq, D. (2008). The trajectory of the centre of pressure during barefoot running as a potential measure for foot function. *Gait & Posture,27(4)*, 669-675.

[49] McCrory, J. L., Young, M. J., Boulton, A. J. M. & Cavanagh, P. R. (1997). Arch index as a predictor of arch height. *The Foot, 7*, 79-81.

[50] Razeghi, M. & Batt, M. E. (2002). Foot type classification: a critical review of current methods. *Gait Posture, 15(3)*, 282-291.

[51] Monteiro, M., Gabriel, R., Moreira, H., Maia, M. & Freitas, J. Comparisons of plantar pressures between obese and non obese postmenopausal women. in *13th annual congress of the European College of Sport Sciences*. 2008. Estoril: Faculdade de Motricidade Humana.

[52] Sardinha, L. & Teixeira, P. (2000). Obesity screening in older women with the body mass index: a receiver operating characteristic (ROC) analysis. *Science & Sports, 15*, 212-219.

[53] Monteiro, M., Gabriel, R. & Moreira, M. (2009). Biomechanic parameters of plantar pressure, age and body composition variables in postmenopausal women. *Maturitas, 63(Supplement 1)*, S130.

[54] Monteiro, M., Gabriel, R. & Moreira, M. (2009). Plantar pressure in postmenopausal women, hormonal replacement therapy and type of menopause. *Maturitas, 63(Supplement 1)*, S37.

[55] Pataky, T. C., Caravaggi, P., Savage, R. & Crompton, R. H. (2008). Regional peak plantar pressures are highly sensitive to region boundary definitions. *Journal of Biomechanics, 41(12)*, 2772-2775.

[56] Cheung, J. T. M. & Nigg, B. M. (2007). Clinical Applications of Computational Simulation of Foot and Ankle. *Sport-Orthopädie - Sport-Traumatologie - Sports Orthopaedics and Traumatology, 23(4)*, 264-271.

In: Overweightness and Walking
Editor: Caleb I. Black, pp. 75-86

Chapter 4

SPINAL AND SUPRASPINAL CONTROL OF HUMAN WALKING

Jonathan A. Norton

Pediatric Surgery, Department of Surgery, University of Alberta,
Edmonton, Alberta, Canada.

ABSTRACT

This review will focus on both the most recent evidence concerning the spinal and supraspinal control of human walking, in both health and disease, as well as the new and emerging techniques for performing these studies. In recent years our understanding of how humans control walking has undergone a revolution. Animal studies indicated that the spinal cord plays a critical role in the control of locomotion. Even in the absence of sensory input the spinal cord of cats and rats are capable of generating a 'locomotor rhythm'. Sensory input, such as that arising from a moving treadmill belt, can alter this rhythm such that animals will adapt the speed of the rhythm to match the treadmill, and can even decouple the two sides of the body so that one leg steps faster than the other. More recent studies from individuals with spinal cord injuries have indicated that although the spinal cord, and the circuitry within the spinal cord are critically important to human walking, the cortical drive to the spinal cord appears to be of greater importance in humans than other species.

In large part our change in understanding of the control of human walking has come apart because of studies utilising new, neurophysiological techniques, as well as studies on individuals with damage to their nervous system. These new approaches to studying the neural control of walking have included such methods as transcranial magnetic stimulation and temporal and spectral analysis of muscle activity (EMG) as well as the more established reflex approaches, many of which have been refined in recent years. These new and refined neurophysiological approaches will be described and the evidence they have provided will be presented and evaluated and emerging techniques described.

INTRODUCTION

Human walking is almost unique in that it is bipedal in nature, unlike virtually any other mammal walking. This makes for difficulties and challenges in studying mammalian walking and extrapolating to human walking. However, in recent years studies using both intact and reduced animal preparations and humans with and without neurological injuries we have been able to increase our understanding of how 'the simple act' of walking is controlled. It has become increasingly clear that in the human walking is controlled by neural centres located throughout the central nervous system, including the spinal cord and the motor cortex. This chapter will review the more recent evidence concerning this distributed control, as well the techniques used in the studies underlying this information. Taking an increasingly complex model approach we will start with the most reduced animal preparations, and move through to animal studies and human studies.

REDUCED ANIMAL PREPARATIONS

The basic action of walking involves an alternating pattern with the actions of one leg repeated by the opposite leg in the next phase of the step cycle (Nielsen JB, 2003). Essentially then, walking appears to be a rhythmical activity with alternating flexion and extension of the legs. This apparent simplicity has meant that greatly reduced neurophysiological preparations can be utilised to study the act of walking, since it is similar to many other forms of locomotion (Nielsen JB, 2003), although there are special features of human locomotion (Capaday C, 2002). The lamprey is a small water-born parasite, some of which are blood suckers. Ranging in length up to 1m they appear to bear little in common with humans. However, locomotion (propulsion) in lampreys occurs by flexing one side of its body, whilst extending the other, then extending the first, while the 2nd is flexed. This alternating pattern of flexion and extension is conceptually similar to that observed in human walking. Because of this, the ease of handling the lamprey in the laboratory and recording from its cells the lamprey has become a stable for neurophysiological investigations of locomotion (Grillner S, 1985).

The neonatal rat has become an increasingly important model for the study of locomotor control with the development of intracellular recording techniques capable of recording for prolonged periods of time. The neonatal rat spinal cord is so small that, with the brainstem attached, it can survive *ex vivo* for several hours in a bath of appropriate media, because the nutrients are able to diffuse throughout the cord. This makes it unique amongst mammalian preparations used for electrophysiological studies (Kjaerulff O & Kiehn O, 1996). The ability to manipulate pharmacological the spinal cord is enhanced by its small size and thus the model has become widely used to study network properties and the effects of pharmacological manipulations (Cowley KC & Schmidt BJ, 1995). Studies in rats have provided much of the evidence for the existence of central pattern generators (CPGs), basic building blocks of neural networks that produce a stepping pattern (Kiehn O, 2006).

CAT STUDIES

For over a century the cat has provided the model for physiological studies of the neural control of walking. Sherrington in the UK at the turn of the 20th century was instrumental in this development. His seminal series of papers on the control of locomotion (Sherrington CS, 1910), (Sherrington CS, 1913), (Sherrington CS, 1898) and his robust debate with Brown on the reflex vs pattern generator debate did much to formulate our understanding of how walking is controlled (Brown TG, 1911), (Brown TG, 1912). In addition to Brown, Denny-Brown (working at around the same time as Brown and Sherrington) also proposed that the rhythmical stepping pattern seen in cats after a spinal cord transaction may be the result of something intrinsic to the spinal cord, more akin to a network than just simple reflexes (Denny-Brown D, 1929). More recently it has been demonstrated that a cat with a chronic spinal cord injury can be re-trained to step on a moving treadmill belt (Barbeau H & Rossignol S, 1987). Analysis of the stepping pattern has shown how similar it is to the pattern exhibited by the same cat stepping on a treadmill prior to being spinalised. Furthermore the stepping pattern adapts to changes in treadmill speed and direction (Rossignol S & Bouyer L, 2004), and even differential changes in treadmill belt speed such that one leg is moving faster than the other, taking multiple steps for each one that the other leg takes. Intriguingly it is also observed that the hind limbs are never both in the swing phase of the gait cycle, which would cause the animal to fall. This is not true of the stance phase, and frequently both legs are in stance phase, which is a stable position (c.f. standing). This absence of double swing phase is seen in intact animals as well, but its persistence in the spinalised state suggests that inter-neurons, crossing within the spinal cord are largely responsible for this 'safety feature'. However, the taking of multiple steps with one leg whilst the other leg completes just one step (but without both legs being in swing phase at the same time) is not seen in neurologically intact animals, suggesting that this aspect of walking control is driven by the supraspinal centres.

Further evidence that walking or stepping may be controlled by neural circuits within the spinal cord came from studies in which the spinal cord was stimulated electrically through small electrodes placed at various locations within spinal cord (Barthelemy D et al., 2007), (Barthelemy D et al., 2006), (Guevremont L et al., 2006). Tonic activation or stimulation lead to a stepping pattern, even in the absence of a sensory input from a moving treadmill belt. Likewise pharmacological activation of the spinal cord with agents such as L-DOPA can result in a stepping pattern in the absence of sensory input (Pearson KG, 2000). In fact, this stepping pattern can be seen in electrophysiological recordings even in fictive locomotion preparations although sensory (proprioceptive) input can reset the stepping pattern (Conway BA et al., 1987). Both the pharmacological and electrical activation of spinal circuits responsible for stepping lead to stepping patterns that are similar, suggesting that the same neural networks are being activated by the two different mechanisms, although the mechanism of activating the network is not clear (Guevremont L et al., 2006), (Barthelemy D et al., 2007).

Fictive locomotion occurs in the absence of movement of the animal and hence natural sensory feedback. Such sensory feedback is a normal, critical part of walking and occurs from both intrinsic sources within the animal as well as a result of its' interaction with the external environment. For instance, feedback from muscle spindles is critical in regulating the duration of the stance phase of the gait cycle (Pearson KG, 2008), (Donelan JM & Pearson KG, 2004), (Hiebert GW *et al.*, 1996). In addition feedback from joints, specifically the hip joint plays a major role in the transitions between the phases of the step cycle (McVea DA *et al.*, 2005). In that study the hip angle was found to determine the transition from the swing phase to the stance phase. Similarly we found that spinalised animals that were previously trained to step on a moving treadmill and subsequently had their hip deafferented were no longer able to step (Guevremont L *et al.*, 2007).

Decerebration removes the cortex from the animal and allows the intact spinal cord and lower, supraspinal centres to be studied in the absence of anesthesia. Sherrington was, again, one of the first to exploit this procedure to study locomotor activity in the cat (Stuart DG, 2005). Although it allows us to study the animal in the absence of anesthesia, the removal of the cortical structures is hardly a physiological state. Despite the non-physiological nature of the preparation, it has produced considerable information concerning the control of locomotion, see (Whelan PJ, 1996). This is especially true concerning the transitions of the step cycle. However, perhaps surprisingly this preparation has also been used to study plasticity within the locomotor neural network. Decerebrate cats can adapt to their environment, including too different treadmill belt speeds, indicating that at least some of that control occurs below the level of the cortex (Whelan PJ, 1996).

Although it is widely accepted that a CPG is responsible for producing the locomotor pattern seen in the spinalised and/or decerebrate cat, the exact nature of the neural circuit has long remained unclear (Yakovenko S *et al.*, 2005). In a series of experiments in which they analysed both 'mistakes' in the stepping patterns of decerebrate cats and alterations in the pattern as a result of afferent stimulation, recorded over many years McCrea and colleagues built a reasonably complete model of a multi-level network that produces the neural pattern in their recordings (Rybak IA *et al.*, 2006b), (Rybak IA *et al.*, 2006a). This network has both a pattern-formation level and a rhythm generating level. In their model, the rhythm generator level of the network receives tonic drive from the mesencephalic locomotor region (MLR). This level then projects to a pattern formation level (Rybak IA *et al.*, 2006a), (McCrea DA & Rybak IA, 2008). It is this pattern formation level that projects to the motoneurons, as shown in figure 1 below (middle of the bottom row). The figure illustrates several iterations of the CPG theory from the original (top left) generated by Brown and Lundberg to increasingly complex models. Further details of the models can be found in (McCrea DA & Rybak IA, 2008).

There is considerable research into the ongoing control of locomotion, how the rhythm is maintained, the control between the two sides, the phase transitions etc... comparatively little has been paid to the initiation of locomotion. There is considerable evidence that the initiation of locomotion is controlled by a descending signal from supraspinal centres (Jordan LM *et al.*, 2008). Decerebrate preparations have also contributed to our understanding of this feature of the control of locomotion. Decerebrate locomotion has to be initiated by activation of the MLR. Depending on the level of the decerebration, and the extent of oedema within the residual brain this is either achieved with electrical stimulation or spontaneously. The MLR does not project directly to the spinal cord, but rather through a relay station, the medial medullary reticular formation, whose projections then travel within the ventrolateral funiculus of the spinal cord.

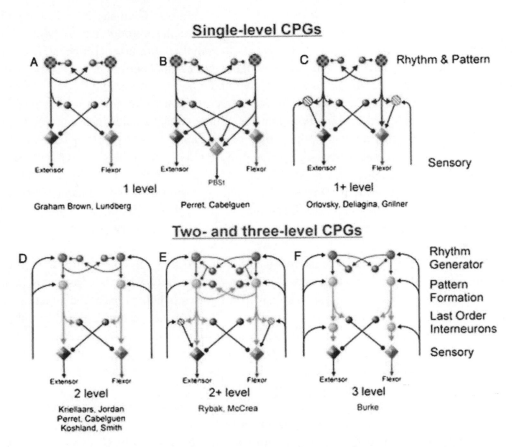

Figure 1. Schematic representations of half-center CPG models. Circles represent spinal interneuron populations and diamonds represent motoneuron populations. Excitatory and inhibitory connections are shown by lines ending with arrowheads and small filled circles, respectively. (A–C) Single-level half-center models in which rhythm generation is produced by two excitatory interneuron populations (green stippled populations) interconnected by reciprocal inhibition (purple). The same interneurons excite the corresponding motoneuron populations as well as inhibitory interneurons responsible for rhythmic inhibition of motoneurons during locomotion. (A) Classical half-center scheme. (B) More complex patterns of motoneuron activity can be produced by connections from both half-centers to some motoneuron populations (PBSt, posterior biceps semitendinosus). (C) Motoneurons receive excitation during locomotion from interneurons with sensory input (hatched circles) as well from the half-centres. (D–F) Two- and three-level CPG architectures with separate rhythm generator (dark green circles) and pattern formation (light green) circuitry. (E) As in panel C, a portion of motoneuron excitation during locomotion is mediated by interneurons with sensory input. There is reciprocal inhibition at both the rhythm generator and pattern formation levels. (F) A three-level CPG organization in which all locomotor excitation of motoneurons is mediated by interneurons with sensory input. From (McCrea DA & Rybak IA, 2008), with permission.

HUMAN STUDIES

Intuitively the best way to study human walking is to study humans walking. However, many of the studies described earlier are not possible in humans. However several animal studies have led directly to human studies or interventions. For instance the work by Barbeau and colleagues on treadmill training of spinal cord injured cats (Barbeau H & Rossignol S, 1987), showing a remarkable recovery of stepping led to the introduction of partial body weight supported treadmill training for humans with spinal cord injuries (Barbeau H & Blunt R, 1991), (Dietz V *et al.*, 1995). Individuals with complete spinal cord injuries (no anatomical connections from the brain to the lower limbs) are able to be re-trained to step on a moving treadmill belt (Dietz V & Harkema SJ, 2004). Early in the training period (although this is often months after a spinal cord injury in humans, unlike animal studies in which the training may start just hours after the injury), the pattern of muscle activity resembles a reflex pattern. With increased training this pattern changes and more closely resembles a CPG-type pattern (Dietz V, 2003), (Lunenburger L *et al.*, 2006), (Grillner S, 2002). This has been used as evidence for a central pattern generator for walking residing in the human spinal cord. Furthermore, epidural stimulation of the spinal cord has been demonstrated to produce a stepping pattern in those individuals with a complete spinal cord injury (Jilge B *et al.*, 2004), as it has in cats (Gerasimenko YP *et al.*, 2003).

What role then do supraspinal centres play? Although stepping has been re-trained on a treadmill in a human subject it is not clear that this is really what is considered human walking. Those subjects with complete spinal cord injuries (adults at least, the situation with children may be more complicated) are unable to walk off the treadmill. For that, subjects must have an incomplete spinal cord injury, i.e. have some connection between the brain and the spinal cord connected to the leg muscles (Yang JF & Gorassini MA, 2006). In a series of studies Monica Gorassini and colleagues showed that subjects required some corticospinal connection to the lower leg muscles (Thomas SL & Gorassini MA, 2005), that they should have some common cortical drive to their leg muscles (Norton JA & Gorassini MA, 2006) in order for them to generate functionally useful improvements in walking ability, which was mirrored by changes in EMG activity (Gorassini MA *et al.*, 2009). Clearly then, cortical control is important; at least in re-training walking ability after a spinal cord injury. However, individuals who have suffered a stroke (cerebral insult) are often left with a residual dropped foot that, if walking in humans was purely spinally controlled, should be corrected.

The initiation of the stepping pattern, seen only in individuals with an incomplete spinal cord injury, is most likely to arise from a supraspinal descending signal, as in other mammals (Jordan LM *et al.*, 2008). This would be part of the reason for the inability of individuals with complete spinal cord injuries to step overground, as opposed to on a moving treadmill belt, which would supply a sensory trigger to start stepping. Interestingly the corticospinal tract appears to be essential for the control of stepping in humans, especially for re-learning to step and walk. In cats, initiation of stepping (at least in the decerebrate preparation) is mediated via the ventrolateral funiculus and not the corticospinal tract.

Studies of human walking have demonstrated that, in a controlled environment, the pattern of walking is broadly similar between individuals. For many years the primary methods of studying human walking has been either to observe the kinematic and electrophysiological patterns or to study reflexes at various stages of the gait cycle. The study of reflexes during the gait cycle has shown that many of them are modulated during the gait cycle (Stein RB & Thompson AK, 2006). These modulations are over and above, and sometimes counter to, changes in the background level of muscle activity (which affects reflex amplitude in a static situation). For instance, the soleus H-reflex is larger during walking than stance, even when the background EMG level and the stimulus strength are equal in the two conditions (Capaday C & Stein RB, 1986). This was taken to assume the differential descending and segmental inputs to the alpha-motoneuron during standing and walking, and more so during the different phases of the step cycle.

More intriguingly, given that we tend to assume of human walking as being bipedal in nature, several studies have shown modulation in upper limb reflexes during movement of the legs (Baldissera F *et al.*, 2002). In this study subjects moved a foot, while the H-reflex in an upper limb was studied (flexor carpi radialis). The H-reflex was modulated in line with the movement of the leg. Cortical conditioning of the reflex by TMS facilitated this modulation. However when the reflex was triggered in the 'silent period' following TMS, no modulation of the reflex was seen. This appears to indicate not only some coupling between upper and lower limbs within the spinal cord, but also a linkage to the cortex that influences reflex responses. The impact of the cortex on reflex responses has been studied many times. Christenson and colleagues (Christensen LOD *et al.*, 1999) showed that even the cutaneous reflex pathway in tibialis anterior muscle (a flexor) is likely to have a transcortical element during walking. The stretch reflexes, which may contribute to stability in the gait cycle may also be partly cortical in origin according to a study from the same group (Christensen LOD *et al.*, 2001). Using cycling as a model of walking (recpriocal activity of flexors and extensors) as well as treadmill walking Zehr showed that the any human CPG responsible for generating the alternating pattern in the legs also modulated reflexes in the arms (Zehr P *et al.*, 2004). Arm reflexes showed both modulation and phase reversal in line with the leg movements.

More recently new analytical techniques have emerged that have allowed a greater understanding of the contribution of suparspinal centres to the control of human walking. Whilst reflex studies impose a perturbation on the gait cycle and study the response, analysis of the EMG obtained during gait imposes no such disturbance to the gait pattern (Nielsen JB, 2002). As Neilsen argues, this allows for the study of how locomotion is controlled rather than the neural response to perturbations. Examination of the frequency content of EMG and more specifically cross-correlating the frequency content from two signals (coherence) allows information to be gained concerning the common neural drive to the signals. Coherence in the β-band (15-35Hz) between a pair of muscles or two signals from the same muscle is assumed to indicate common cortical drive to the muscle(s) (Mima T & Hallet M, 1999). Such signals have been found to be reduced in the tibialis anterior muscle in individuals who have had a spinal cord injury (Hansen NL *et al.*, 2005). Interestingly, we found that during training, in those subjects with an incomplete spinal cord injury who showed an improvement with training, there was an increase in the β-band intermuscular coherence (Norton JA & Gorassini MA, 2006). Neurologically intact subjects, however had much lower levels of coherence. Using this techniques Halliday and colleagues were able to show that the coupling between motor units altered during the step cycle (Halliday DM *et al.*, 2003).

Although we are able to determine the origin of the β-band coherence as the cortex (Pohja M *et al.*, 2005), (Mima T & Hallet M, 1999), it is less clear where other frequency bands originate. In particular there is often seen coherence in the 10Hz region during these recordings. Does this represent just alpha-motoneuron firing, or is it from other sources? Some evidence suggests it may be vestibular in origin (Blouin JS *et al.*, 2006), but it has also been observed in subjects with a complete spinal cord injury who have been standing passively (Norton JA *et al.*, 2003).

These approaches have those far used the Fourier transform, which has considerable limitations when applied to walking data, such as the need for large amounts of stationary data. However, with newer algorithims, such as wavelets, starting to be used more and more information from these sorts of studies will be sure to come in the next few years (Brittain JS *et al.*, 2007).

Earlier, we showed that animals with a complete spinal cord lesion can be induced to step on a moving treadmill belt with a disconnect between the legs so that one leg took many steps to a single step taken by the other leg. Whilst neurologically intact human subjects do now show a similar phenomena, those with a complete spinal cord injury can be induced to step in a similar manner, and so can young infants (Yang JF *et al.*, 2005). This may be taken as evidence for both independent step generators in the spinal cords of humans, but also that the corticospinal tract, which is very immature in young infants mediates the inhibition that, in later life stops this form of stepping.

Aside from the spinal cord and the motor cortex, there are many other supraspinal centres which play a role in the control of walking. Patients with cerebellar disorders have difficulties in motor learning (Bastian AJ, 2008). This extends to problems in walking and learning of motor tasks (Morton SM & Bastian AJ, 2006), (Morton SM & Bastian AJ, 2004). Individuals with a cerebellar lesions have an increased postural sway which extends into a wide-based gait, often described as a 'drunken' gait. Although the cerebellum is involved in both balance and coordination of movements in general the balance issues are more significant in gait than the motor control and coordination issues (Morton SM & Bastian AJ, 2004). Interestingly though, many patients with cerebellar lesions show a breakdown in their complex movements into the smaller, individual component movements. Patients with cerebellar lesions also show an impaired ability to learn motor tasks, such as walking with prism goggles (reviewed in (Morton SM & Bastian AJ, 2004)).

The extent to which supraspinal structures are important in the control of human walking can be seen by the broad range of neural conditions which have gait disturbances as part of their recognised, and often archetypal, clinical manifestations. Parkinson's disease for instance (Rivlin-Etzion M *et al.*, 2006) has a characteristic gait pattern, the exact relationship of which with the underlying pathology in the thalamic region is unclear. Hydrocephalus, a cause of enlarged ventricles, with or without increased pressure in the brain, has a different gait abnormality (Johnston IH *et al.*, 2001).

CONCLUSION

So, where is human walking controlled? The control of human walking is complex in nature. Increasingly it is becoming apparent that whilst neural circuits within the spinal cord are responsible for low-level neural control of walking, such as the basic alternating pattern and reflex adjustments to perturbation. However, in humans more so than any other animal studied in detail to date, the supraspinal control centres exert a great deal of influence. The essential neural circuitry responsible for activating the muscles lies within the spinal cord. Sensory feedback from the legs activates reflexes within the cord. Supraspinal centres are involved in the higher level processing of movement intention, but also are involved in long-loop reflexes. Critically however, the supraspinal centres are required to initiate the stepping pattern. Cerebellar inputs play a role in the moment-to-moment control of balance, of potentially higher importance in bipedal humans than in quadripedal animals. The cerebellum is also involved in the learning of new motor patterns on a day-to-day and longer basis.

REFERENCE

Baldissera, F., Borroni, P., Cavallari, P., & Cerri, G. (2002). Excitability Changes in Human Corticospinal Projections to Forearm Muscles During Voluntary Movement of Ipsilateral Foot. *Journal of Physiology, 539*, 903-911.

Barbeau, H. & Blunt, R. (1991). A Novel Interactive Locomotor Approach Using Body Weight Support to Retrain Gait in Spastic Paretic Subjects. In *Plasticity of Motoneuronal Connections*, ed. Wernig A, 461-474.

Barbeau, H. & Rossignol, S. (1987). Recovery of Locomotion After Chronic Spinalization in the Adult Cat. *Brain Research, 412*, 84-95.

Barthelemy, D., Leblond, C. & Rossignol, S. (2007). Characteristics and Mechanisms of Locomotion Induced by Intraspinal Microstimulation and Dorsal Root Stimulation in Spinal Cats. *J Neurophysiol, 97*, 1986-2000.

Barthelemy, D., Leblond, H., Provencher, J., & Rossignol, S. (2006). Nonlocomotor and Locomotor Hindlimb Responses Evoked by Electrical Microstimulation of the Lumbar Cord in Spinalized Cats. *J Neurophysiol, 96*, 3273-3292.

Bastian, AJ. (2008). Understanding Sensorimotor Adaptation and Learning for Rehabilitation. *Current Opinion in Neurology 21*, 628-633.

Blouin, J. S., Inglis, J. T., & Siegmund, G. P. (2006). Startle Responses Elicited by Whiplash Perturbations. *Journal of Physiology, 573*, 857-867.

Brittain, J. S., Halliday, D. M., Conway, B. A., & Nielsen, J. B. (2007). Single-Trial Multiwavelet Coherence in Application to Neurophysiological Time Series. *IEEE Transaction on Biomedical Engineering, 54*, 854-862.

Brown, T. G. (1911). The Intrinsic Factors in the Act of Progression in the Mammal. *Proceedings of the Royal Society of London, 84*, 308-319.

Brown, T. G. (1912). The Factors in Rhythmic Activity of the Nervous System. *Proceedings of the Royal Society of London, 85*, 278-289.

Capaday, C. (2002). The Special Nature of Human Walking and its Neural Control. *Trends in Neuroscience, 25*, 370-376.

Capaday, C. & Stein, R. B. (1986). Amplitude Modulation of the Soleus H-Reflex in the Human During Walking and Standing. *Journal of Neuroscience, 6*, 1308-1313.

Christensen, L. O. D., Andersen, J. B., Sinkjaer, T., & Nielsen, J. B. (2001). Transcranial Magnetic Stimulation and Stretch Reflexes in the Tibialis Anterior Muscle during Human Walking. *Journal of Physiology, 531*, 545-557.

Christensen, L. O. D., Morita, H., Peterson, N., & Nielsen, J. B. (1999). Evidence Suggesting that a Transcortical Reflex Pathway Contributes to Cutaneous Reflexes in the Tibialis Anterior Muscle During Walking in Man. *Experimental Brain Research, 124*, 59-68.

Conway, B. A., Hultborn, H., & Kiehn, O. (1987). Proprioceptive Input Resets Central Locomotor Rhythm in the Spinal Cat. *Experimental Brain Research, 68*, 643-656.

Cowley, K. C. & Schmidt, B. J. (1995). Effects of Inhibitory Amino Acid Antagonists on Reciprocal Inhibitory Interactions During Rhythmic Motor Activity in the In Vitro Neonatal Rat Spinal Cord. *J Neurophysiol*, *74*, 1109-1117.

Denny-Brown, D. (1929). On the Nature of Postural Reflexes. *Proceedings of the Royal Society of London*, *104*, 252-301.

Dietz, V. (2003). Spinal Cord Pattern Generators for Locomotion. *Clinical Neurophysiology*, *114*, 1379-1389.

Dietz, V., Colombo, G., Jensen, L., & Baumgartner, L. (1995). Locomotor capacity of spinal cord in paraplegic patients. *Annals of Neurology*, *37*, 574-582.

Dietz, V. & Harkema, S. J. (2004). Locomotor Activity in Spinal Cord-Injured Persons. *J Appl Physiol*, *96*, 1954-1960.

Donelan, J. M. & Pearson, K. G. (2004). Contribution of Sensory Feedback to Ongoing Ankle Extensor Activity During the Stance Phase of Walking. *Canadian Journal of Physiology and Pharmacology*, *82*, 589-598.

Gerasimenko, Y. P., Avelev, V. D., Nikitin, O. A., & Lavrov, I. A. (2003). Initiation of Locomotor Activity in Spinal Cats by Epidural Stimulation of the Spinal Cord. *Neuroscience and Behavioural Physiology*, *33*, 247-254.

Gorassini, M. A., Norton, J. A., Nevett-Duchcherer, J. M., Roy, F. D., & Yang, J. F. (2009). Changes in Locomotor Muscle Activity after Treadmill Training in Subjects with Incomplete Spinal Cord Injury. *J Neurophysiol*, *101*, 969-979.

Grillner, S. (1985). Neurobiological Bases of Rhythmic Motor Acts in Vertebrates. *Science 228*, 143-149.

Grillner, S. (2002). The Spinal Locomotor CPG: A Target After Spinal Cord Injury. In *Spinal Cord Trauma: Regeneration, Neural Repair and Functional Recovery*, eds. McKerracher L, Doucet G, & Rossignol S.

Guevremont, L., Norton, J. A., & Mushahwar, V. K. (2007). A Physiologically-based Controller for Generating Overground Locomotion using Functional Electrical Stimulation. *J Neurophysiol*, *97*, 2499-2510.

Guevremont, L., Renzi, C., Norton, J. A., Kowalczewski, J., Saigal, R., & Mushahwar, V. K. (2006). Locomotor-Related Networks in the Lumbosacral Enlargement of the Adult Spinal Cat: Activation through Intraspinal Microstimulation. *IEEE Transactions on Neural Systems and Rehabilitation Engineering*, *14*, 266-272.

Halliday, D. M., Conway, B. A., Christensen, L. O. D., Hansen, N. L., Peterson, N., & Nielsen, J. B. (2003). Functional Coupling of Motor Units is Modulated During Walking in Human Subjects. *J Neurophysiol 89*, 960-968.

Hansen, N. L., Conway, B. A., Halliday, D. M., Hansen, S., Pyndt, H. S., Biering-Sorensen, F., & Nielsen, J. B. (2005). Reduction of Common Synaptic Drive to Ankle Dorsiflexor Motoneurones During Walking in Patients with Spinal Cord Lesion. *J Neurophysiol 94*, 934-942.

Hiebert, G. W., Whelan, P. J., Prochazka, A., & Pearson, K. G. (1996). Contribution of Hind Limb Flexor Muscle Afferents to the Timing of Phase Transitions in the Cat Step Cycle. *J Neurophysiol*, *75*, 1126-1137.

Jilge, B., Minassian, K., Rattay, F., Pinter, M. M., Gerstenbrand, F., Binder, H., & Dimitrijevic, M. R. (2004). Initiating Extension of the Lower Limb in Subjects with Complete Spinal Cord Injury by Epidural Lumbar Cord Stimulation. *Experimental Brain Research*, *154*, 308-326.

Johnston, I. H., Duff, J., Jacobson, E. E., & Fagan, E. (2001). Asymptomatic Intracranial Hypertension in Disorders of CSF Circulation in Childhood - Treated and Untreated. *Pediatric Neurosurgery, 34*, 63-72.

Jordan, L. M., Liu, J., Hedlund, P. B., Akay, T., & Pearson, K. G. (2008). Descending Command Systems for the Initiation of Locomotion in Mammals. *Brain Research Reviews, 57*, 183-191.

Kiehn, O. (2006). Locomotor Circuits in the Mammalian Spinal Cord. *Annual Review of Neuroscience, 29*, 279-306.

Kjaerulff, O. & Kiehn, O. (1996). Distribution of Networks Generating and Coordinating Locomotor Activity in the Neonatal Rat Spinal Cord *In Vitro* : A Lesion Study. *Journal of Neuroscience, 16*, 5777-5794.

Lunenburger, L., Bolliger, M., Czell, D., Muller, R., & Dietz, V. (2006). Modulation of Locomotor Activity in Complete Spinal Cord Injury. *Experimental Brain Research in press.*

McCrea, D. A. & Rybak, I. A. (2008). Organization of Mammalian Locomotor Rhythm and Pattern Generation. *Brain Research Reviews, 57*, 134-146.

McVea, D. A., Donelan, J. M., Tachibana, A., & Pearson, K. G. (2005). A Role for Hip Position in Initiating the Swing-to-Stance Transition in Walking Cats. *J Neurophysiol, 94*, 3497-3508.

Mima, T. & Hallet, M. (1999). Corticomuscular Coherence: A Review. *Journal of Clinical Neurophysiology, 16*, 501-520.

Morton, S. M. & Bastian, A. J. (2004). Cerebellar Control of Balance and Locomotion. *The Neuroscientist, 10*, 247-259.

Morton, S. M. & Bastian, A. J. (2006). Cerebellar Contributions to Locomotor Adaptations During Splitbelt Treadmill Walking. *Journal of Neuroscience, 26*, 9107-9116.

Nielsen, J. B. (2002). Motoneuronal Drive During Human Walking. *Brain Research Reviews 40*, 192-201.

Nielsen, J. B. (2003). How we Walk: Central Control of Muscle Activity during Human Walking. *The Neuroscientist, 9*, 195-204.

Norton, J. A. & Gorassini, M. A. (2006). Changes in Cortically Related Inter-muscular Coherence Accompanying Improvements in Locomotor Skills in Incomplete Spinal Cord Injury. *J Neurophysiol, 95*, 2580-2589.

Norton, J. A., Wood, D. E., Marsden, J. F., & Day, B. L. (2003). Spinally Generated Electromyographic Oscillations and Spasms in a Low-Thoracic Complete Paraplegic. *Movement Disorders, 18*, 101-106.

Pearson, K. G. (2000). Neural Adaptation in the Generation of Rhythmic Behaviour. *Annual Review of Physiology, 62*, 723-753.

Pearson, K. G. (2008). Role of Sensory Feedback in the Control of Stance Duration in Walking Cats. *Brain Research Reviews, 57*, 222-227.

Pohja, M., Salenius, S., & Hari, R. (2005). Reproducibility of Cortex-Muscle Coherence. *NeuroImage, 26*, 764-770.

Rivlin-Etzion, M., Marmor, O., Heimer, G., Raz, A., Nini, A., & Bergman, H. (2006). Basal Ganglia Oscillations and Pathophysiology of Movement Disorders. *Current Opinion in Neurobiology, 16*, 629-637.

Rossignol, S. & Bouyer, L. (2004). Adaptive Mechanisms of Spinal Locomotion in Cats. *Intergrative and Comparative Biology, 44*, 71-79.

Rybak, I. A., Shevtsova, N. A., Lafrenier-Roula, M., & McCrea, D. A. (2006a). Modelling Spinal Circuitry Involved in Locomotor Pattern Generation: Insights from Deletions During Fictive Locomotion. *Journal of Physiology, 577*, 617-639.

Rybak, I. A., Stecina, K., Shevtsova, N. A., & McCrea, D. A. (2006b). Modelling Spinal Circuitry Involved in Locomotor Pattern Generation: Insights from the Effects of Afferent Stimulation. *Journal of Physiology, 577*, 641-658.

Sherrington, C. S. (1898). On the Spinal Animal and the Nature of Spinal Reflex Activity. *Philosophical Transactions of the Royal Society of London (B) 190.*

Sherrington, C. S. (1910). Flexion-reflex of the Limb, Crossed Extension-reflex and Reflex Stepping and Standing. *Journal of Physiology, 40*, 28-121.

Sherrington, C. S. (1913). Nervous Rhythm Arising from Rivalry of Antagonistic Reflexes. Reflex Stepping as Outcome of Double Reciprocal Innervation. *Proceedings of the Royal Society of London, 86*, 233-261.

Stein, R. B. & Thompson, A. K. (2006). Muscle Reflexes in Motion: How, What, and Why? *Exercise and Sport Sciences Reviews, 34*, in press.

Stuart, D. G. (2005). Integration of Posture and Movement: Contributions of Sherrington, Hess, and Bernstein. *Human Movement Science, 24*, 621-643.

Thomas, S. L. & Gorassini, M. A. (2005). Increases in Corticospinal Tract Function by Treadmill Training after Incomplete Spinal Cord Injury. *J Neurophysiol, 94*, 2844-2855.

Whelan, P. J. (1996). Control of Locomotion in the Decerbrate Cat. *Progress in Neurobiology, 49*, 481-515.

Yakovenko, S., McCrea, D. A., Stecina, K., & Prochazka, A. (2005). Control of Locomotor Cycle Durations. *J Neurophysiol, 94*, 1057-1065.

Yang, J. F. & Gorassini, M. A. (2006). Spinal and Brain Control of Human Walking: Implications for Retraining of Walking. *The Neuroscientist, 12*, 379-389.

Yang, J. F., Lamont, E., & Pang, M. Y. C. (2005). Split-Belt Treadmill Stepping in Infants Suggests Autonomous Pattern Generators for the Left and Right Leg in Humans. *Journal of Neuroscience, 25*, 6869-6876.

Zehr, P., Carroll, T. J., Chua, R., Collins, D. F., Frigon, A., Haridas, C., Hundza, S. R., & Thompson, A. K. (2004). Possible Contributions of CPG Activity to the Control of Rhythmic Human Arm Movement. *Canadian Journal of Physiology and Pharmacology, 82*, 556-568.

In: Overweightness and Walking
Editor: Caleb I. Black, pp. 87-100

ISBN: 978-1-60741-298-4
© 2010 Nova Science Publishers, Inc.

Chapter 5

NORDIC WALKING IN KINESITHERAPY OF OSTEOPOROTIC PATIENT

*J. Wendlová**

University Derer´s Hospital and Policlinic, Osteological Centre, Bratislava, Slovakia

ABSTRACT

This article brings the biomechanical analysis of sport – Nordic walking – for patients with osteoporotic fractured vertebrae and shows that it is suitable for them.

Based on the biomechanical model of skeletal load we have developed a method of walking movement for patients, different from the method of walking movement for healthy people. And so came into being the "first sport"for patients with osteoporotic fractures. They can go for regular walks in easy terrains outdoors with friends and family, and so be liberated from social isolation. It requires only one-off financial costs of buying the poles and special footwear.

Keywords: osteoporosis – fractured vertebra – biomechanics – exercise - Nordic walking.

INTRODUCTION

Patients with Fractured Vertebra and Sport?

I have put the question mark deliberately, as it could seem absurd to some people without it. However, I know from my clinical experience that most of these patients strive to defy the heavy odds and want to overcome their handicap by physical activity. Many patients are aware that inactivity will aggravate their health, their muscles will slacken and their efficiency will diminish, and the back pain will get worse. The patients will have to rely on the help of other people or a care service, which they often cannot afford for financial

---

* Corresponding author: Email: jwendlova@mail.t-com.sk.

reasons. This is the reason why there is a growing interest in regular motion activities. I often hear in my surgery statements like *"Could you advise me some group exercise for people with the same handicap I have?"* The best exercise for patients with osteoporotic vertebra fractures is a regular group exercise lead by an experienced physiotherapist as well as exercise in a swimming pool (excluding swimming).

Unfortunately, there are not many towns and villages where the patients have the opportunity to participate in regular and long-term exercise organised by experienced physiotherapists. Other sport activities are not suitable for patients with osteoporotic vertebra fractures, either for the increased risk of injury or for increased strain on weakened skeleton.

When we pondered over the questions asked by my patients and considered what easy sport would be suitable for them, we have chosen – Nordic Walking. This assumption was confirmed by a biomechanical analysis. Based on the biomechanical model of skeletal load we have developed a method of walking movement for patients, different from the method of walking movement for healthy people. And so came into being the "first sport" suitable for patients with osteoporotic fractures. They can go for regular walks in easy terrains outdoors with friends and family, and so be liberated from social isolation. It requires only one-off financial costs of buying the poles and special footwear.

Nordic Walking – Walking with Supporting Poles

Nordic Walking is a dynamic fitness walking outdoors in different terrains, using a pair of special telescopic poles with exchangeable tips for different surfaces. When walking on less concrete surfaces, such as grass or dirt, the poles with classical spike tips are used, on hard surfaces, such as asphalt, the poles with rubber tips are used. The stride rhythm is given by swinging opposite arms and legs alternately forward and backward.

The correct pole length should represent about 70 – 72% of the body height and to calculate it there is a simple formula using one's own height multiplied by 0.66. The walker's elbow should be at approximately a 90° angle when holding the pole by the grip with the tip on the ground. We have chosen the Nordic Walking as a suitable sport for patients with osteoporosis, especially for patients with osteoporotic vertebra fractures. This conclusion was reached on the basis of biomechanical analysis of vertebra load. Firstly, we simulated the vertebra load as a patient with kyphosis walked with outstretched arms without supporting poles, to demonstrate the lever arms and components of the force of gravity of the upper part of the body acting upon the vertebra. Consequently, we unloaded the upper part of the body by poles held in arms extended forward during walking.

BIOMECHANICAL ANALYSIS

Calculation of Static Load of Vertebra during Mild Trunk Bending without the Support of the Poles [1–8, 14]

Model example no.1
   We are interested in static load, e.g., of the Th12 vertebra (12th thoracic vertebra) by the force of gravity of the upper part of the body above the mentioned vertebra, if both elbows of upper limbs are held at a 90° angle (i.e., without being supported by poles).

Mathematical definitions:

mass: $m = \dfrac{G}{g}$ (kg)

force of gravity: $G = m \times g$ $(kgms^{-2})$

acceleration due to gravity $g = 9.80665 ms^{-2}$

gravity force moment $M = G \times r$

r – arm, to which the force is applied

Solution
Static load will be calculated for the Th12 vertebra.
Patient's weight is m = 70 kg, his force of gravity is $G = m \times g \approx 700$ N
Bending forward, the spine is bent at a 15° angle.

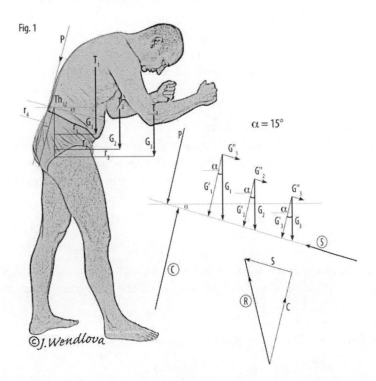

Figure 1. Static load of vertebra Th12 during mild trunk bending without the support of the poles

Table 1. The Mass Ratio of Different Body Parts to the Whole Body in Percentage
(Body mass = 100%) [13]

Body Part	The Ratio of the Body Part Mass to the Whole Body in % (according to Fischer)	The Ratio of the Body Part Mass to the Whole Body in % (according to Dempster)
Head	8.8	8.1
Torso	45.2	49.7
Thigh	11.0	9.9
Crus	4.5	4.6
Leg	2.1	1.4
Arm	2.8	2.8
Forearm	2.0	1.6
Hand	0.8.	0.6

When bending forward, there are four forces (G_1, G_2, G_3, P) acting upon the Th 12 vertebra:

1. G_1 - resultant gravity force of the upper part of the torso and head G_1 (over the Th12 vertebra), producing approx. 50% of the body mass (Table 1). $G_1 = 350N$, is applied in the gravity centre of the upper torso T_1.
2. G_2 , G_3 - resultant gravity forces of both upper limbs stretched forward with elbows held at a 90° angle, producing 5.6% x 2 = 11.2% of body mass. $G_2 = 39.20$ N acting upon the gravity centre of the left upper limb (UL) T_2.
3. $G_3 = 39.20$ N acting upon the gravity centre of the right UL T_3. P - is force produced by the contraction of erector spinae muscles (consisting of muscles: • m. iliocostalis thoracis, • m. spinalis thoracis, • m. longissimus thoracis). The magnitude of the P force is unknown; we know only its direction and the point of application (it is an imaginary point in erector spinae muscles above the Th12 vertebra body).

Calculation of the P Force Magnitude

All four forces, namely G_1, G_2 , G_3, P, are acting upon arms of different length (r_1, r_2, r_3, r_4) related to the imaginary point in Th12, producing four bending moments for this point.

Arms, on which the forces are applied, are real distances measured on the patient

$$r_1 = 0.25 \text{ m}, r_2 = 0.30 \text{ m}, r_3 = 0.40 \text{ m}, r_4 = 0.05 \text{ m}$$

Explanatory note to symbols used in equations
The clockwise acting force moment is called a positive moment, marked by the symbol (+), the counter clockwise acting force moment is called a negative moment and marked by the symbol (-).

Forces of gravity G_1, G_2 and G_3 produce positive bending moments.

$$M_1 = G_1 \times r_1$$

$$M_2 = G_2 \text{ x } r_2$$

$$M_3 = G_3 \text{ x } r_3$$

The contraction force P in m. erector spinae produces a negative bending moment

$$- M_4 = P \text{ x } r_4$$

Bending moment M_4 is the counterbalancing moment to bending moments M_1, M_2, M_3. The P force magnitude is calculated from the first condition of equilibrium:
The sum of the moments in the plane acting upon a given point is equal to zero.

$$\sum_{i=1}^{4} M_i = 0$$

$$M_1 + M_2 + M_3 + (- M_4) = 0$$

$$G_1 \text{ x } r_1 + G_2 \text{ x } r_2 + G_3 \text{ x } r_3 = P \text{ x } r_4$$

$$P = \frac{(G_1 \times r_1) + (G_2 \times r_2) + (G_3 \times r_3)}{r_4} = \frac{(350 \times 0.25) + (39.20 \times 0.30) + (39.20 \times 0.40)}{0.05} = 2298.80 N$$

$$P = 2298.80 \ N$$

Forces of gravity G_1, G_2 and G_3 are resolved in a polygon of forces into compressive forces G_1' G_2' G_3' and shearing forces G_1'', G_2'', G_3''. By both these forces the gravity forces G_1, G_2 and G_3 are acting upon Th12 vertebra at a 15° angle of bent back.

Calculation of Reactive Compressive Force C in Th12 Vertebra

Component compressive forces G_1', G_2', G_3' and the contraction force of muscles P, acting upon Th12 vertebra, condition the rise of the reactive compressive force C in the vertebra, which is in equilibrium with the forces G_1', G_2', G_3' and P (the equilibrium is upset in case of vertebra fracture).

The magnitude of the resultant reactive compressive force C in vertebra is unknown; we know only its direction and point of application. Its direction is opposite to the direction of G_1' G_2' G_3' and P forces, and its point of application is in Th 12 vertebra.

The C force is calculated from the second condition of equilibrium.

The sum of parallel forces in the plane is equal to zero.

$$\sum forces = 0$$

Magnitudes of component compressive forces G_1', G_2', G_3' are calculated from right-angled triangles by trigonometrical function for cosine:

$$\alpha = 15^0$$

$$\cos\alpha = \frac{G_1'}{G_1} \quad G_1' = \cos 15° \times G_1 = 0.966 \times 350 = 338.10 \text{ N}$$

$$\cos\alpha = \frac{G_2'}{G_2} \quad G_2' = \cos 15° \times G_2 = 0.966 \times 39.20 = 37.87 \text{ N}$$

$$\cos\alpha = \frac{G_3'}{G_3} \quad G_3' = \cos 15° \times G_3 = 0.966 \times 39.20 = 37.87 \text{ N}$$

$$(\cos 15° \times G_1) + (\cos 15° \times G_2) + (\cos 15° \times G_3) + P + (-C) = 0$$

$$C = (\cos 15° \times G_1) + (\cos 15° \times G_2) + (\cos 15° \times G_3) +$$
$$P = 338.10 + 37.87 + 37.87\text{N} + 2298.80 = 2712.64 \text{ N}$$

$$C = 2712.64 \, N$$

Calculation of reactive shearing force S in Th12 Vertebra

Component gravity forces G_1'', G_2'', G_3'' are shearing forces acting upon the vertebra, where the reactive shearing force S comes into being, in equilibrium with the forces G_1'', G_2'', G_3'' (the equilibrium is upset in case of vertebra fracture). The magnitude of the reactive shearing force S in the vertebra is unknown; we know only its direction and a point of application. It acts in the opposite direction than forces G_1'', G_2'', G_3'' and its point of application is in Th12 vertebra.

Magnitudes of component shearing forces G_1'', G_2'', G_3'' are calculated from right-angled triangles by trigonometrical function for sine:

$$\alpha = 15^0$$

$$\sin\alpha = \frac{G_1''}{G_1} \quad G_1'' = \sin 15° \times G_1 = 0.259 \times 350\text{N} = 90.65 \text{ N}$$

$$\sin\alpha = \frac{G_2''}{G_2} \quad G_2'' = \sin 15° \times G_2 = 0.259 \times 39.20 = 10.15 \text{ N}$$

$$\sin\alpha = \frac{G_3''}{G_3} \quad G'3'' = \sin 15° \times G3 = 0.259 \times 39.20 = 19.15 \text{ N}$$

The S force is calculated from the second condition of equilibrium.
The sum of parallel forces in the plane is equal to zero.

$$\sum forces = 0$$

$$G_1'' + G_2'' + G_3'' + (-S) = 0$$

$$S = G_1'' + G_2'' + G_3'' = 90.65 + 10.15 + 10.15 = 110.95 \text{ N}$$

$$S = 110.95 \, N$$

We calculated the magnitudes of reactions (reactive forces) C and S in the vertebra to compressive and shearing components of gravity forces G_1, G_2, G_3.

Calculation of Resultant Reactive Force R

As the forces C and S act perpendicularly upon each other, we can calculate the magnitude of their resultant R from the Pythagorean Theorem:

$$R = \sqrt{C^2 + S^2} = \sqrt{2712.64^2 + 110.95^2} = 864.94N$$

$$R = 864.94\ N$$

R is a resultant reactive force, produced in Th12 vertebra due to static load by the upper part of the body during bending the back at a 15° angle with upper limbs extended forward and elbows held at 90° angles. The direction of the action of the resultant force R is determined graphically by the composition of forces S and C.

The procedure for the calculation of static load for other dorsal vertebra is identical. The angle of action of component forces upon the vertebra changes as well as the magnitude of component forces depending upon the magnitude of resultant gravity force of the body part above the given vertebra. Less gravity force of the body acts upon proximally placed vertebra (upper vertebra) than upon distally placed vertebra (lower vertebra).

Forces Transferred into Poles during Nordic Walking [3, 4, 8–12, 14]

Model example no. 2

We start from the identical position of the trainee as in the example No. 1 – the spine is at a 15° angle during trunk bending (identical picture).

The force of gravity of the upper part of the torso and the head G_1 (the point of application is in the centre T_1) and forces of gravity of both upper limbs G_2, G_3 (acting upon the centres T_2, T_3) are transferred into poles during walking with the poles held in extended arms. We consider two independent solutions – the trainee supported with one vertical pole and the trainee supported with one deflected pole.

> *Solution A* Transfer of forces into the right-hand vertical pole.
> *Solution B* Transfer of forces into the left-hand pole, deflected from the vertical at an acute angle.

Solution A (Figure 2) Transfer of Forces into the Right-hand Vertical Pole

To find out how the forces are transferred into the pole, at first we have to determine the magnitude, direction and the point of application of the resultant gravity force R and then add a couple of forces in the pole to the force R. These two forces are formed by two equally large forces acting in the same beam and point of application; they are of an opposite direction, while it applies that:

$$R = R\,' = R\,''$$

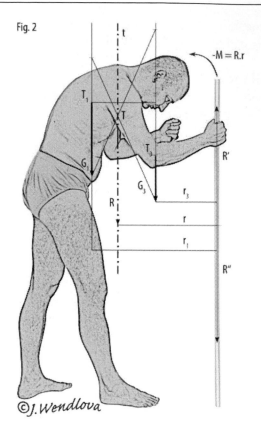

Figure 2. Solution A

The equilibrium status of forces is not changed, as the effects of both added forces are cancelled mutually. Vertical distances of centres T_1 and T_3 from the pole are arms r_1, r_3, upon which act the gravity forces G_1, G_3. We calculated them in the Model example No. 1. We find out the magnitude of the arm r, upon which acts the resultant of gravity forces R. The resultant of vertical gravity forces equals their sum.

$$G_1 = 350 \text{ N} \qquad G_3 = 29.20 \text{ N} \qquad r_1 = 0.52 \text{ m} \qquad r_3 = 0.30 \text{ m}$$

$$R = G_1 + G_3 = 350 + 29.20 = 379.20 \text{ N}$$

$$R = 379.20 \text{ N}$$

From the condition of equality of moments we calculate the arm, upon which acts the resultant R: The moment of the resultant set of forces in the plane to a given point equals the sum of moments of individual forces for this point

$$G_1 \times r_1 + G_3 \times r_3 = R \times r$$

$$r = \frac{G_1 \times r_1 + G_3 \times r_3}{R} = \frac{(350 \times 0.52) + (29.20 \times 0.30)}{379.20} = 0.503 m$$

$$r = 0.503 \text{ m}$$

We know now the resultant R, arm r, upon which acts the R and its direction (in the picture we determined its direction graphically), but we do not know its point of application – the centre T. The centre of the resultant R can be determined graphically or by calculation. This mathematical process is not the target of this analysis, because for physicians it is important to explain in a simple way the principle of the transfer of forces into poles, and the position of the centre T affects neither the magnitude of moments of gravity forces, nor the magnitude of the compressive force R'' transferred into the pole.

The resultant moment M is produced by the gravity force R, acting upon the arm r.

$$M = R \times r = 379.20 \times 0.503 = 190.74 \text{ Nm}$$

In the course of walking with a pole in an outstretched hand, the total resultant of gravity forces R of the upper part of the body is transferred as the compressive force R'' (379.20 N). To provide stability, a couple of forces R, R' (negative bending moment, - M = 190.74 Nm) are acting from the pole towards the upper part of the body against the forward inclination of the walker. Taking into consideration two vertical poles, while the distance of the centres of upper limbs from the poles is the same, a half of compressive force R'' of the resultant gravity force R is transferred into each pole.

Solution B (Figure 3) Transfer of forces into the left-hand pole, deflected from the vertical at an acute angle

The magnitude of the resultant force R of the upper part of the body is calculated in the same way as in Solution A, i.e., for an imaginary vertical left-hand pole.

$$G_1 = 350 \text{ N } G_2 = 29.20 \text{ N } r_1 = 0.43 \text{ m } r_2 = 0.30 \text{ m}$$

$$R = G_1 + G_2 = 350 + 29.20 = 379.20 \text{ N}$$

$$R = 379.20 \text{ N}$$

$$G_1 \times r_1 + G_2 \times r_2 = R \times r$$

$$r = \frac{G_1 \times r_1 + G_2 \times r_2}{R} = \frac{(350 \times 0.43) + (29.20 \times 0.30)}{379.20} = 0.42m$$

$$r = 0.42 \text{ m}$$

Equally as in the Solution A, we do not calculate the point of application of the force T, to make the analysis simpler. We know its magnitude, the arm, upon it acts and direction (determined graphically in the picture), which is sufficient for the explanation of application of forces.

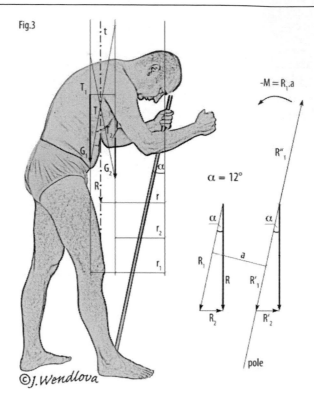

Figure 3. Solution B

The resultant force R is divided into two component forces R_1 a R_2.

The magnitude of component forces R_1 a R_2 is calculated from trigonometrical functions for sine and cosine of the angle:

$$\alpha = 12^0$$

$$\cos \alpha = \frac{R_1}{R_2} \quad R_1 = \cos 12° \times R = 0.978 \times 379.20 = 370.858 \text{ N}$$

$$\sin \alpha = \frac{R_2}{R} \quad R_2 = \sin 12° \times R = 0.208 \times 379.20 = 78.874 \text{ N}$$

$$R_1 = R_1{}' = R_1{}'' \quad a = r = 0.42 \text{ m}$$

$$- M = R_1 \times a = 370.858 \times 0.42 = 155.760 \text{ Nm}$$

The resultant force R, passing the axis of the gravity centre t, is transferred by its component R_1 at an 12° angle into the pole deflected from the vertical by 12°. We add to the component force R_1 of the resultant gravity force R two forces in the axis of the deflected pole, both of equal magnitude, acting in one beam but in the opposite direction. The equilibrium of forces does not change, because the effects of both added forces are mutually cancelled. The distance a is the distance of component force R_1 from the axis of the pole and simultaneously it creates the lever arm for two forces R_1 and $R_1{}''$. To provide stability, a couple of forces R_1 and $R_1{}''$ (negative bending moment, - M = 155.760 Nm) are acting from the pole towards the upper part of the body against the forward inclination of the walker. The remaining force R_1' (370.858 N) is the compressive component force R_1 of the resultant gravity force R transferred into the pole. The horizontal component force R_2 (78.874 N) of the resultant gravity force R prevents the sliding of the pole. If the two poles are deflected at the same angle and the axes of gravity force of upper limbs are at the same distance from the poles, then a half of the compressive component force R_1 of resultant gravity force R is transferred into each pole.

THE CONCLUSION OF BIOMECHANICAL SOLUTION OF FORCE TRANSFER INTO THE POLES

In the model example the Th12 vertebra of the trainee, bent in the spine at a 15° angle and stretching out the arms (without the poles) with elbows at a 90° angle, is loaded by a force of *864.94 N.*

If in the same position we put vertical poles in the trainee's hands, then *379.20 N* of the force of gravity of the upper part of the body is transferred into the poles; to provide stability two forces R and R' (negative bending moment) are acting from each pole towards the upper part of the body against the forward inclination of the walker. Using two vertical poles, the static load of the Th12 vertebra is reduced by 379.20 N and the vertebra is loaded by *485.74 N* force.

If we put into the trainee's hands two poles, deflected from the vertical at a 12° angle, then *370.858 N* of the force of gravity of the upper part of the body is transferred into the poles; to provide stability the two forces R_1 and R_1'' (negative bending moment) are acting from each pole against the forward inclination of the walker. Horizontal component forces of the resultant gravity force R, transferred into the poles, prevent their sliding. Using two poles, deflected from the vertical, the static load of the Th12 vertebra is reduced by 370.858 N and the vertebra is loaded by *494.08N* force.

EFFECTS OF NORDIC WALKING

Positive effects for osteoporotic patients with fractured vertebra:

strengthening the muscles of shoulders, arms, breast, abdomen, spine, and upper and
    lower limbs
stretching the muscles of the neck, shoulders and trunk
enlargement of the support area and improvement of stability while walking (Figure 5)
partial relief of vertebra from the gravity force of the head and trunk
reduction of tensile forces in spinal muscles by osteoporotic kyphosis
improvement of motion coordination → prevention of falls
improvement of muscle performance → improvement of mobility
sparing the knee and hip joints while walking
even longer walks do not worsen the back pain

Overall effects upon the organism:

up to a 20 to 50% increase in energy consumption compared with ordinary walking
    without poles
30% less load on the locomotory system compared with slow running combined with
    walking (jogging)
strengthening the cardiac muscle

Differences in the Walking Methods between Healthy Persons and Patients with Osteoporotic Vertebra Fractures

Healthy Person (Figure 4)

The motion rhythm is given by alternate diagonal walking. The right upper limb is forward, the left lower limb is extended backwards, the left upper limb is stretched backwards, the right lower limb is extended forward and in the next step the positions of the limbs alternate. There is a rotation of the axis of the left (right) shoulder joint against the axis of the left (right) hip joint.

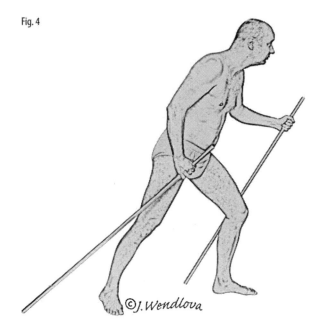

Fig. 4

©J. Wendlova

Figure 4. Regular motion activities stimulate new bone formation. The bone mineral density (BMD) and also the periosteal apposition of bone increase. The periosteal apposition brings the bone mineral further away from the central axis, the cross – sectional area (CSA) of bone and following the cross - sectional moment of inertia (CSMI) enlarge. Increasing in BMD and in CSMI improve the bone strength. Less than 1 mm increase in outer diameter can compensate for 10% loss in BMD [14].

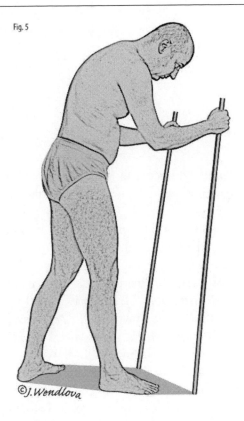

Fig. 5

©J. Wendlova

Figure 5.

Patient with Osteporotic Vertebra Fractures (Figure 5)

We suggest the same motion rhythm, given by alternate diagonal walking; however, the upper limbs are bent in the elbows and stay outstretched during walking to reduce partially the gravity force of the head and trunk upon the spine. The right upper limb is forward, left lower limb is extended backwards, the left upper limb is forward, but with the pole closer to the body as the right upper limb, the right lower limb is stretched forward. In the next step the positions of the limbs alternate. There is no counter-rotation of the axes of shoulder and hip joints and so the osteporotic spine is spared the stress of the torsion forces.

CONCLUSION

Based on the biomechanical analysis we recommend Nordic Walking as a suitable sport for patients with osteoporotic fractures, under the conditions of the change of the method of motion rhythm, as suggested in the article. Regular motion activities stimulate new bone formation. The bone mineral density (BMD) and also the periosteal apposition of bone increase. The periosteal apposition brings the bone mineral further away from the central axis, the cross – sectional area (CSA) of bone and following the cross - sectional moment of inertia (CSMI) enlarge. Increasing in BMD and in CSMI improve the bone strength. Less than 1 mm increase in outer diameter can compensate for 10% loss in BMD (15).

REFERENCES

[1] Wendlová, J. Biomechanika chrbtice a jej význam v pohybovej liečbe pri osteoporóze. (Biomechanics of spine and its signification in exercise therapy for osteoporotic patients) *Eurorehab,* 1999, vol.2, č. 3 – 4, 174 – 177.

[2] Wendlová, J. Odťaženie chrbtice o hmotnosť horných končatín v štádiu hojenia akútnej fraktúry stavca (Unloading the spine by the weight of upper extremities during healing of acute fracture of vertebra) *Rehabil fyz lék* 2004 vol.11, č. 2, 95 – 101.

[3] Obetková, V; Mamrillová, A; Košinárová, A. *Teoretická mechanika.Vydavateľstvo technickej a ekonomickej literatúry ALFA*, Bratislava, 1990, 30 – 94.

[4] Adamča, LF; Marton, P; Pavlík, M; Trávníček, F. *Teoretická mechanika. Vydavateľstvo technickej a ekonomickej literatúry ALFA*, Bratislava, 1992, 27 – 37.

[5] Homminga, J. Van-Rietbergen, B. Lochmuller EM. Weinans H. Eckstein F. Huiskes R: The osteoporotic vertebral structure is well adapted to the loads of daily life, but not to infrequent "error" loads. *Bone*, 2004, 34, 510-516.

[6] Bono, CM; Einhorn, TA. Overview of osteoporosis: Pathophysiology and determinants of bone strength. [Review] *Europ Spine J*, 2003, 12, 90-96.

[7] Lohfeld, S; Barron, V. Mc Hugh PE: Biomodels of bone: A review An of *Biomed Engineering*, 2005, 10, 145 – 150.

[8] Burr, DB. Biomechanics *Clin Reviews in Bone and Miner Metab*, 2006, 3, 112 – 117.

[9] Bouxein, ML. Biomechanics of osteoporotic fractures. *Clin Reviews in Bone and Miner Metab*, 2006, 3, 118 – 126.

[10] Ferguson, JS; Steffen, T. Biomechanics of the aging spine. *Europ Spinal J*, 2003, Suppl 2, 167 – 169.

[11] Özkaya, N; Nordin, M. *Fundamentals of biomechanics: Equilibrium, motion and deformation*, 2nd ed, Springer – Verlag, New York, 1999, 45 – 51.

[12] Fernandez, JW; Mithraratne, P; Thrupp, SF; Tawhai, MH; Hunter, PJ. Anatomically based geometric modeling of the musculo – sceletal system and other organs. *Biomech and Model in Mechanobiology*, 2004, 3, 444 – 450.

[13] Koniar, M; Leško, M. *Biomechanika Slovenské pedagogické nakladateľstvo*, Bratislava, 1992, 37.

[14] Wendlova J: Osteoporosis. Kinesitherapy. 1st ed, 2008 Bratislava, Sanoma Magazines Slovakia, 110-9.

[15] Faulkner, KG; Wacker, WK; Barden, HS; Simonelli, C; Burke, PK; Ragi, S; Del Rio, L. Femur strength index predicts hip fracture independent of bone density and hip axis length. *Osteoporos Int*, 2006, 4, 593 – 599.

In: Overweightness and Walking
Editor: Caleb I. Black, pp. 101-149

Chapter 6

BIPEDAL WALKING FROM NEUROLOGICAL AND BIOMECHANICAL PRINCIPLES

Sungho Jo and Andreas Hofmann
Computer Science and Artificial Intelligence Laboratory, Media Laboratory,
Massachusetts Institute of Technology

ABSTRACT

This chapter presents neurological and biomechanical principles of human bipedal walking and their potential application to humanoid walking robots by proposing two computational models. First, a computational model of cerebrocerebello-spinomuscular interaction during sagittal planar walking provides insight into each neural system's function based on neuro-anatomy and physiology. The neural systems substantially decouple gait cycle generation and postural stabilization, with a spinal pattern generator fulfilling the former function, and a cerebrocerebellar feedback system fulfilling the latter. A muscle synergy network facilitates control of redundant muscular actuators in descending pathways. Two control variables: horizontal position of the center of mass, and trunk pitch angle, are estimated from sensed information through the ascending neural pathways. Therefore, the space of the controller is simpler than the space of the actuators and plant. In this way, a simple control strategy is constructed.

The second computational model features a hierarchical task execution architecture that is suitable for control of a 3-D biped, for a variety of challenging walking tasks, including walking on difficult terrain with foot placement constraints. This approach supports exploration of performance limits based on biomechanical structure for such challenging tasks. The model uses an enhanced multivariable feedback linearizing controller, inspired by the muscle synergy approach used in the first computational model, to transform the biped into an abstracted plant that is easier to control. As with the first computational model, key control variables are the biped's center of mass, posture, and stepping foot position. The plant abstraction linearizes and decouples these variables, but the linearization has constraints based on actuation limits, and on limits of the biped's base of support. A reachability analysis is performed, in terms of the abstracted plant, in order to generate families of trajectories that satisfy task goals while observing constraints. Use of such trajectory sets supports high performance execution of difficult tasks such as kicking a soccer ball, or dynamic walking on a path of irregularly placed stones, while rejecting disturbances that may occur.

1. INTRODUCTION

Bipedal walking on level terrain is characterized by a regular pattern of rhythmic stepping movements, where each step involves coordination of multiple muscles. The control problem is one of moving the center of mass of the biped forward while maintaining balance and posture. Maintaining balance involves controlling the center of mass momentum with respect to the base of support provided by the biped's feet.

Our first model, the *hypothetical neural walking controller,* addresses the problems of generation of rhythmic movement patterns, coordination of multiple muscles, and balance control, using a computational model of cerebrocerebello-spinomuscular interaction during sagittal planar walking. Because this model is based on a plausible neural anatomy, it provides insight into the function of each anatomical structure for human walking. Additionally, it makes sense to investigate use of such neural-based approaches for artificial bipeds since such approaches leverage a design that has been perfected by nature over millions of years of evolution.

Experimental studies support the existence of rhythmic pattern generation in humans [Dimitrijevic et al., 1998; Grasso et al, 2004; Calancie et al., 1994; Dietz and Harkema 2004]. Even though no explicit neural circuitry for such rhythmic pattern generation has been confirmed, the high probability of its existence has encouraged use of such pattern generation models to describe human biped walking [Taga, 1995; Ogihara and Yamazaki, 2001].

With respect to multiple muscular activation during walking, it is useful to begin with neuro-mechanical principles. Observations of muscular activations during gaits at different speeds [Ivanenko et al., 2004] indicate that the electromyogram (EMG) pattern remains unchanged principally. Several investigations [Ivanenko et al., 2004; Ivanenko et al., 2005; Olree and Vaughan, 1995] have used factor analysis to extract four or five principal waveforms from the muscular activations and tried to interpret the waveforms in terms of functions. Experimental studies demonstrate that tonic stimulation of the spinal cord in frogs induces synergistic patterns of muscular activations [Tresch et al., 1999; Cheung et al., 2005; d'Avella et al., 2003; d'Avella and Bizzi, 2005]. Such a mechanism simplifies redundant muscle control by providing a lower dimensional control for each leg. The lower dimensional control can analytically construct a wealth of frog leg EMG activities and behaviors in a feed-forward manner.

Rhythmic pattern generation, and muscle activation using synergies are feed-forward mechanisms. They generate a regular pattern of muscle activation without considering the actual state of the muscles and limbs being moved. Because disturbances occur, the actual muscle and limb state will differ from that intended by the feed-forward mechanism. To correct for this difference, feedback mechanisms must be utilized. It has been shown, experimentally, that the cerebrum and cerebellum augment the muscle activations provided by simpler feed-forward mechanisms [Kandel et al., 2000]. These augmentations are critical for reacting to disturbances and maintaining balance. Furthermore, it has been experimentally shown that selective lesions of descending control from the motor cortex compromise fine control of swing leg trajectories in cats [Drew, 1993]. The motor cortex has also been shown to contribute to the structure and timing of the step cycle during locomotion in the intact cat [Bretzner and Drew, 2005]. Malfunction of the cerebellum due to either stroke or tumor in humans causes devastating effects in postural balance and locomotion [Porter and Lemon, 1993]. Thus, normal bipedal function in humans appears to depend significantly upon activity in transcerebral pathways [Nielsen, 2003; Peterson et al., 1998; Nathan, 1994]. Moreover, most cerebral activities during locomotion seem to be generated by sensory long-loop feedback mechanisms [Christensen et al., 2000; Nielsen, 2003]. For these reasons, a cerebrocerebellar long-loop feedback system must be considered in order to completely understand the neural mechanisms of human biped walking.

While it is important to understand walking fundamentals by studying normal human walking on level terrain, it is also important to understand and exploit the unique advantages provided by legged systems. The most obvious advantage of legged systems over wheeled vehicles is the ability to traverse un-even terrain. A normal human can traverse steps, climb rocks, cross brooks by stepping on stones, and in general, perform a wide variety of locomotion tasks that require irregular stepping patterns to traverse difficult terrain. The ability to perform such tasks is the primary reason for using legs, rather than wheels, for locomotion. Furthermore, humans perform such tasks in everyday life, and therefore, the ability to perform these tasks is a requirement for robotic devices intended for use in unstructured human environments.

For this reason, our second model focuses on execution of challenging locomotion tasks. This 3-dimensional, 18 degree of freedom model is used to investigate performance limits for such challenging tasks, taking into account the state and timing requirements of the tasks, and the actuation limits of the biped. As with the first model, the control architecture is functionally hierarchical, but it is not based on neural anatomy. Nevertheless, there are interesting parallels between the second model and the first at the functional level. The second model uses a *dynamic virtual model controller* to generate multiple actuation commands based on state goals. Thus, it performs a function similar to the synergistic muscle activation component in the first model. Above this controller in the functional hierarchy, the second model uses a task executive to monitor execution state and adjust control parameters. This function is analogous to that provided by the cerebrocerebellar long-loop feedback mechanism in the first model.

By comparing, and ultimately, merging key features of these two models, we expect to gain insight into the key principles of human walking, and how such principles can be used in the design of advanced artificial bipedal walking machines.

In the next section, we provide a review of common approaches used previously to control bipedal walkers, and we also review key requirements for bipedal balance control. In Section 3, we describe the first model, and in Section 4, we describe the second. Section 5 compares important features of each model, and discusses how these features could be merged in order to leverage the best features of both.

2. BACKGROUND

We begin this section with a brief review of previous control algorithms for walking bipeds. We then review the biomechanics of balance control, emphasizing the key requirements that all bipedal walking controllers must satisfy. This is important for understanding the function of the two models described subsequently.

2.1. Control of Walking Bipeds

Over the past decade, a number of humanoid robots capable of walking have been developed. These include the Honda P3 and Asimo robots [Hirai, 1997, 1998], the Sony SDR [Yamaguchi, 1999], and Tokyo University's H6 [Kagami, 2001]. These systems generate detailed joint trajectories offline using dynamic optimization algorithms that observe dynamic limitations. These trajectories are then tracked using simple high-impedance PD control laws. However, this approach is not very robust to disturbances, since it depends on close tracking of the joint reference trajectories. If a disturbance occurs, tracking error can easily become too large due to actuation limits related to imperfect ground contact, and the system can lose its balance [Pratt and Tedrake, 2005].

The main problem with this approach is that use of high-impedance position control to track predetermined, detailed, joint reference trajectories results in a lack of compliance and robustness to force disturbances. The tracking controller will try to follow the predetermined trajectory no matter what, even if the situation requires a completely different response, such as modifying stepping foot placement, or using non-contact limb movement. Humans, on the other hand, are compliant to force disturbances in that they yield, when necessary, and are robust in that they can take complex compensating actions.

Achieving human-like performance using the high-impedance tracking method would require it to either generate, or somehow find, a new reference trajectory, quickly, when a significant disturbance occurs. Since generation of such reference trajectories, is computationally expensive, and since a very large number of such trajectories is needed to cover a wide range of disturbances, achieving human-like compliance and robustness is an unsolved problem for this method. Thus, although the method achieves stable walking on level terrain, it is brittle in to force disturbances, and performance on rough, uneven terrain, is poor.

2.2. Biomechanics of Balance Control

Balance control is essential for performing walking tasks robustly. Balance control requires the ability to adjust the biped's linear and angular momentum. Due to conservation of momentum laws, such adjustment can only be achieved through force interaction with the environment. For a biped, this force interaction is comprised of gravity and the *ground reaction force*, the net force exerted by the ground against the biped. In this section, we present an analysis of physical constraints and requirements for balancing. This leads to a simple set of balance control requirements that specify coordination of control actions that adjust the ground reaction force, and therefore, the momentum of the biped.

To derive this set of requirements, we make use of a number of physical points that summarize the system's balance state. These points are the *center of mass* (CM), the *zero-moment point* (ZMP) [Vukobratovic and Juricic, 1969], and the *centroidal-moment point*

(CMP) [Popovic et al., 2005]. As we will discuss in more detail, the ZMP is a point on the ground that represents the combined force interaction of all ground contact points. The CMP is the point on the ground from which the ground reaction force would have to emanate if it were to produce no torque about the CM.

We define the biped's support base as the smallest convex polygon that includes all points where the foot or feet are in contact with the ground. The ground reaction force vector, $\mathbf{f}_{gr}$, is then defined as the integral, over the base of support, of the incremental ground reaction forces emanating from each point of contact with the ground. This is expressed as

$$\mathbf{f}_{gr} = \iint_{B.O.S} \mathbf{f}_{gr}(x, y)\, dxdy$$

where $\mathbf{f}_{gr}(x, y)$ is the incremental force at point x,y on the ground, and B.O.S refers to the base of support region.

The CM is the weighted mean of the positions of all points in the system, where the weight applied to each point is the point's mass. Thus, for a discrete distribution of masses m_i located at positions $\mathbf{r}_i$, the position of the center of mass is given by

$$CM = \frac{\sum_i m_i \mathbf{r}_i}{\sum_i m_i}.$$

A bipedal mechanism consists of a set of articulated links, each of which is a rigid body with mass m_i, and center of mass $\mathbf{r}_i$. The CM represents the effective mass of the system, concentrated at a single point. This is valuable because it allows us to simplify the balance control problem by reducing the problem to keeping the CM in the right place at the right time.

The ZMP [Vukobratovic and Juricic, 1969] also is a point that represents a combination of distributed points. It is defined as the point on the ground, where the total moment generated due to gravity and inertia is 0 [Takanishi et al., 1985]. This point has been shown to be the same as the *center of pressure* [Goswami, 1999], which is the point on the ground where the ground reaction force acts. Because the base of support is defined by the convex polygon of points in contact with the ground, and because the ZMP represents the average force contribution of these points, the ZMP is always inside the biped's base of support [Goswami, 1999].

The CMP [Popovic et al., 2005] is the point on the ground, not necessarily within the support base, from which the observed net ground reaction force vector would have to act in order to generate no torque about the CM. The relationship between the CM and CMP then indicates the specific effect that the net ground reaction force has on CM translation. Because the observed net ground reaction force always operates at the ZMP which is within the support base, whenever the net ground reaction force generates no torque about the CM, then the ZMP and CMP coincide, as shown in figure 2.2a. If the net ground reaction force generates torque, however, as shown in figure 2.2b, then the CMP and ZMP differ in location, as shown in figure 2.2c. In particular, the CMP may be outside the support base. In this case the displacement of the CMP from the ZMP reflects the increased ability of the net ground reaction force to affect translation of the CM.

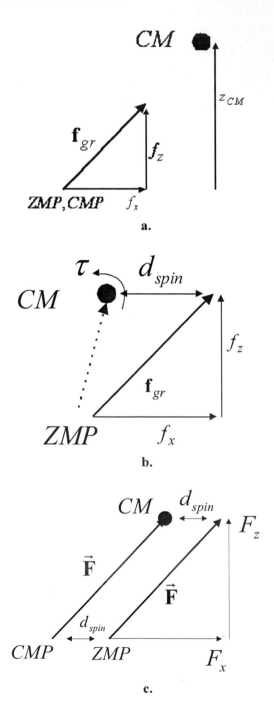

Figure 2.2.a. If the ground reaction force vector points from the ZMP directly toward the CM, no moment is generated about the CM, and the ZMP and CMP coincide. b. When $\mathbf{f}_{gr}$ does not point towards the CM, a torque is generated about the CM. c. The CMP is the point where the ZMP would have to be in order for the ground reaction force vector to pass through the CM.

This capability of producing torque about the CM comes at an expense, however. While translational controllability of the CM is improved, angular stability about the CM is sacrificed. Thus, for example, the torso may deviate from its upright posture. In many situations, such a sacrifice is worthwhile if the angular instability is bounded and temporary. For example, a tightrope walker will tolerate temporary angular instability if this means that he will not fall off the tightrope.

Expressing requirements for balance in terms of CM, ZMP, CMP, and the support base is extremely useful for planning and control, due to the simplicity of this representation. Balance control is then reduced to a problem of adjusting the base of support, adjusting the ZMP within the base of support, and, if necessary, performing motions that generate angular momentum, so that the CMP can be moved, temporarily, outside the base of support, in order to exert additional compensating force on the CM.

3. HYPOTHETICAL NEURAL CONTROL OF BIPEDAL WALKING

The impression of most investigators is that during human locomotion, higher systems drive and modulate spinal level systems that are responsible for much of the basic patterning of muscle activity. The precise hierarchical partitioning of function has not yet been determined. However, several observations are relevant.

Muscular activation and leg function during locomotion [Ivanenko et al., 2004] indicate that the *electromyogram* (EMG*)* pattern is consistent across movement speeds, with only duration and intensity changing.

Experimental observations support a spinal locus for important rhythmic locomotor EMG pattern generation in humans [Dimitrijevic et al., 1998; Grasso et al., 2004; Calancie et al., 1994; Dietz and Harkema, 2004] often in response to tonic electrical stimulation [Dimitrijevic et al., 1998].

Experimental stimulation of either the cerebellum or midbrain produces rhythmic locomotor movement in both intact and decerebrate cat with vigor and frequency that increase with stimulus intensity [Mori et al., 1999; Mori et al., 1998]. These locomotor regions both strongly recruit vestibulospinal, reticulospinal and other direct spinal efferent pathways [Shik and Orlovsky, 1976]. Either cerebellar or midbrain locomotor regions can presumably drive and potentially modulate a spinal locomotor control system [Grillner, 1975; Mori et al., 1999; Mori et al., 1998; Shik and Orlovsky, 1976; Kandel et al., 2000].

Tonic stimulation of a frog spinal cord demonstrates synergistic patterns of muscle activities [Tresch et al., 1999; Cheung et al., 2005; d'Avella et al., 2003; d'Avella and Bizzi, 2005]. Such a mechanism collapses multiple muscle control to a lower degrees of freedom control for each leg.

These findings suggest that a rhythmic central pattern generator, modulated by the supraspinal system, may interact with muscle control synergies to provide a simple and effective walking control.

3.1. Methods

3.1.1. Musculoskeletal model

Walking dynamics is implemented by repetitive interaction between body and ground in the gravitational field. In this study, we used rigid body dynamics to construct a human body model to implement sagittal planar walking motions. Three joints: ankle, knee, and hip, for each leg are connected with body segments: trunk with head, upper leg, and lower leg. The interaction between the feet and the ground is modeled by a nonlinear impedance as generally used for computational modeling [van der Kooij et al., 2003]. Each leg is surrounded by a total of nine muscles, that is to say, six mono- and three bi-articular muscles: dorsiflexor, plantarflexor, knee extensor, knee flexor, hip extensor, hip flexor, biarticular knee-hip extensor, biarticular knee-hip flexor, and biarticular ankle-knee flexor as indicated in figure 3.1.

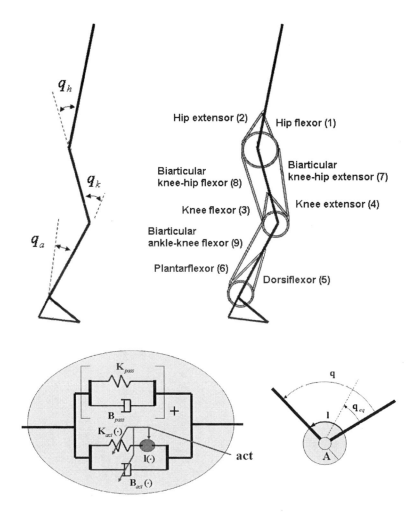

Figure 3.1. Body configuration: each leg has ankle (q_a), knee (q_k) and hip (q_h) joints and are surrounded by nine muscles. For simplicity, only one leg is illustrated. Each muscle is modeled as the circuit in the oval. Geometric relationship between joint angle and muscle length is also illustrated (For simplicity, they are expressed in scalars).

Each muscle consists of passive and active force generators. Each component is described by a nonlinear impedance, but the active one is activation-dependent as follows:

$$\mathbf{F}_{pass} = \left[\mathbf{K}_{pass}(\mathbf{l}_{eq} - \mathbf{l}) - \mathbf{B}_{pass}\dot{\mathbf{l}}\right]_{+}$$
$$\mathbf{F}_{act} = \mathbf{K}_{act}(\mathbf{act})\left[\mathbf{l}_{eq} - \mathbf{l}\right]_{+} - \mathbf{B}_{act}(\mathbf{act})\dot{\mathbf{l}} \tag{3.1}$$

where $\mathbf{l}$ is the muscle length vector; $\dot{\mathbf{l}}$ the muscle length change rate vector; $\mathbf{l}_{eq}$ intrinsic muscle length at equilibrium position; $\mathbf{K}_{pass}$, $\mathbf{B}_{pass}$ are respectively the passive muscle stiffness and viscosity matrices; $\mathbf{K}_{act}(\mathbf{act})$, $\mathbf{B}_{act}(\mathbf{act})$ are respectively the active muscle stiffness and viscosity matrices depending on activation signal $\mathbf{act}$ [Jo, 2006]; $\mathbf{l}(\mathbf{act}) = \mathbf{l}_{eq} + \mathbf{act}$ is computationally assumed.

The joint angles and muscle lengths hold the following relation through the moment arm matrix $\mathbf{A}$ as in figure 3.1 [Jo and Massaquoi, 2004].

$$\mathbf{l} = \mathbf{l}_{eq} + \mathbf{A}(\mathbf{q} - \mathbf{q}_{eq}) \tag{3.2}$$

where $\mathbf{q}$ is joint angle vector; $\mathbf{q}_{eq}$ is joint angle vector at equilibrium. Here, the moment arms are assumed to be constants over motions for computational simplicity [Ogihara and Yamazaki, 2001; Jo, 2006].

The generation of muscular activation by neural signal is approximately described by low-pass dynamics in the form of:

$$EC(s) = \frac{\rho^2}{(s+\rho)^2} \qquad \rho = 30 \text{ rad/sec [Fuglevand and Winter, 1993]},$$

and

$$\mathbf{act} = EC(s)\left(\mathbf{u}_{\alpha}\right) \tag{3.3}$$

where $\mathbf{u}_{\alpha}$ is the command from α motorneuron and s is the Laplace varaible.

3.1.2. Spinal pattern generator

For further simplicity and generality, a hypothetical pulse generator is considered to have binary output. At the level of the spinal pulse generator, the locomotor function is viewed in terms of five hypothetical *control epochs*: "loading" (LOA), "regulation" (REG), "thrust" (THR), "retraction" (RET) and "forward" (FOW) (figure 3.3). The last is almost, but not precisely coextensive with the actual swing phase. These epochs are empirically selected. If the command output of each epoch is designated $u_{PG,i}(t)$, then its periodic activation can be modeled as rectangular pulse:

Sungho Jo and Andreas Hofmann

$$u_{PG,i}(t) = \eta_{PG} \cdot 1\left[\cos(2\pi f_{PG}t - \phi_i) - h_i\right]_+ \quad i = 1,2,3,4. \qquad (3.4)$$

where $1[x]_+ = 1$ where $x > 0$ and 0 otherwise.

f_{PG} determines the pattern frequency, η_{PG} is an activation intensity factor, ϕ_i is the phase shift, and h_i activity discharge threshold. Specification of ϕ_i and h_i determines the sequence and potential overlap between the pulse activations. Figure 3.2 illustrates the four pulses corresponding to the control epochs.

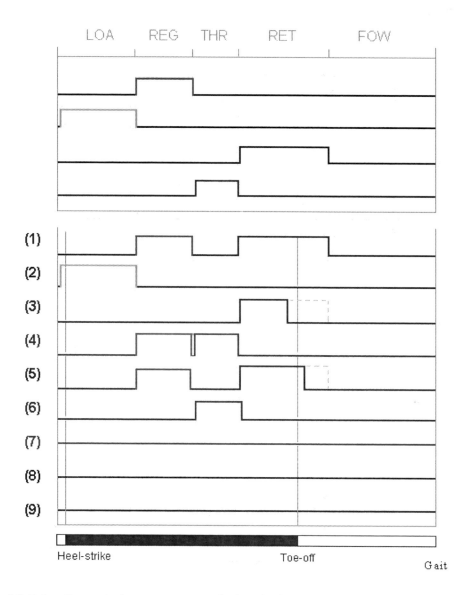

Figure 3.2. Pulses from spinal pattern generator (top) and spinal signals to muscles (bottom). Numbers indicate corresponding muscles in figure 3.1

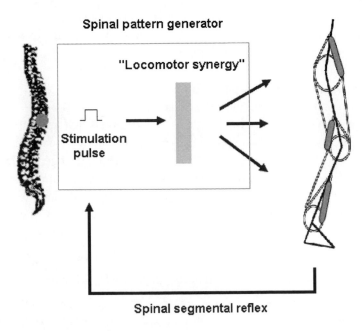

Figure 3.3. Locomotor synergy in the spinal pattern generator

It is proposed that pulse generator commands are distributed to the muscles through a spinal network represented by the matrix $\mathbf{W}_{pg}$ according to five functional epochs during the gait cycle. No command is activated during the fifth epoch so that the swing phase is almost passive.

$$\mathbf{u}_{sp} = \mathbf{W}_{pg}\mathbf{u}_{pg} \qquad (3.5)$$

where $\mathbf{u}_{pg}$ is the pulse command vector, and $\mathbf{u}_{sp}$ is the vector of spinal patterns to muscles.

The combination of the spinal pulse generator and the synergy distribution network can be considered a neural pattern generator (NPG). A major feature of the NPG is that only a few simple pulses are required to generate sequential activations over the whole muscles as in figure 3.3. The columns in the spinal network $\mathbf{W}_{pg}$ are comparable with synergies [Tresch et al., 1999; Cheung et al 2005; d'Avella et al., 2003] even though the concept is not exactly identical. We call each column in $\mathbf{W}_{pg}$ a locomotor synergy. For computational simplicity, synergies only related to the mono-articular muscle activities were formed for present research.

3.1.3. Supraspinal and Spinal Feedback Systems

Pure feedforward systems such as synergies are not effective due to lack of robustness. Feedback systems effectively compensate for unexpected disturbances or noise. We assume that two feedback systems in the human body are significant. One is called the supraspinal (long-loop) feedback system, circulating between muscle to the cerebrocerebellar system, and the other is called the spinal (segmental reflex) feedback system, indicating a pathway between muscle and spinal cord. Without feedback components, signals from the pattern generator have to be very accurate and sophisticated to implement stable walking; even small disturbances would easily destabilize walking.

3.1.3.1. Spinal (Segmental) Reflex Feedback

In viewpoint of the system, the spinal pattern generator provides pure feedforward commands to generate the stereotyped patterns. It is known that several spinal reflexes in reality effect the neural patterns to improve walking morphology by using peripherally sensed information [Baxendale and Ferrell, 1981; Brooke et al., 1997; Grillner, 1975; Duysens et al., 2000]. Peripheral segmental reflex modifies certain synergy components. In this way, a few number of simple feedforward patterns are synergetically sufficient to construct overall muscle activations. For the present model, a possible neural circuit, presynaptic inhibition, is embedded [Baxendale and Ferrell, 1981; Brooke et al., 1997; Rossignol et al., 2006; Duysens et al., 2000]. A descending signal conveys a tonic excitation $q_{th,j}$, $j = a,k,h$ (ankle, knee, hip) that inhibits the proprioceptive afferent q_j at joint j until superseded. Each $q_{th,j}$ is a constant threshold value. Thereafter, the interneuron is activated and the motor neuron activity is suppressed. It is speculated herein that such a mechanism could truncate activities in early FOW to prevent excessive leg retraction. This mechanism is empirically useful to improve the timing between knee and ankle motions to prevent ground contact during swing phase. The spinal reflex action is therefore modeled as:

$$\mathbf{u}_{reflex} = -\mathbf{W}_S \cdot 1\big[\mathbf{q}(\mathbf{t} - \mathbf{T}_{pr}) - \mathbf{q}_{th}\big]_+ \qquad (3.6)$$

where $\mathbf{q}_{th} = \begin{bmatrix} q_{th,a} & q_{th,k} & q_{th,h} \end{bmatrix}^T$, and $\mathbf{W}_S$ is a matrix that scales and distributes joint-related signals from the uniarticular muscles to the other muscles via the vector $\mathbf{u}_{reflex}$. $\mathbf{T}_{pr}$ represents neural transmission delays from spinal cord to muscle. The inhibitive effect of the reflex action is indicated by dotted lines in figure 3.2.

3.1.3.2. Supraspinal feedback

We implemented computational walking tests of our model for the case where the supraspinal system is missing. With only the pattern generator and spinal segmental reflex feedback, the computational model took several forward steps initially but soon fell down. Physiologically, an intact motor cortex is believed to be a prerequisite for bipedal walking, although conclusive data is still lacking [Nielsen, 2003]. It is observed that corticospinal cells are always modulated during walking, which means the supraspinal system participates in walking control somehow. Lesion studies support the necessity of the supraspinal feedback for integrated walking [Porter and Lemon, 1993; Nielsen, 2003; Peterson et al., 1998].

The cerebrocerebellar feedback system (supraspinal control) used in this study is illustrated in figure 3.4a. The model is adapted from a balance control model in Jo and Massaquoi, 2004. In figure 3.4a, the cortical integration represents the inherent input-output characteristic of the main neurons of the motor cortex as proposed in [Karameh and Massaquoi, 2005]. Gains A and B affect the relative balance of cortical and cerebellar circuitries. The activity related to the recurrent feedback circuit between the cerebellar output and input is implemented by integration [Massaquoi and Topka, 2002] and the local close-loop provides phase lead compensation to the cerebellar input signal. The signal on the projection pathway may be interpreted to comparably be "efference-copy" discharge [Allen and Tsukahara, 1974].

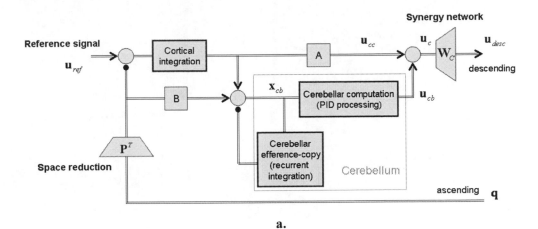

Figure 3.4. a. A model of the cerebrocerebellar feedback system (a filled circle indicates inhibition), b. the neural circuit of the cerebellar computation.

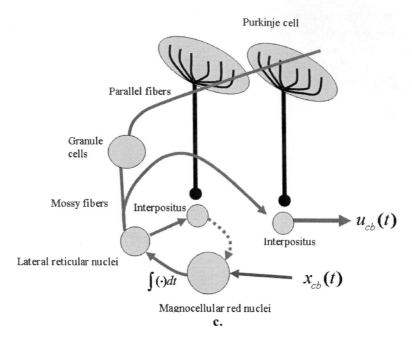

Figure 3.4. c. integration by precerebellar nuclei

Ito (1997) proposed that cerebellar processing is performed by functional corticonuclear microcomplexes. Under the framework, the cerebellum can be regarded to compute proportional scaling, integration, and differentiation [Massaquoi and Topka, 2002]. Figure 3.4b and c illustrate cerebellar neural circuitry. It does not include the climbing fiber-related neural circuitry known to process adaptation because the adaptation is beyond this chapter interest. The deep cerebellar nuclei conveys the output signal $u_{cb}(t)$. The output signals from the cerebellar computation are sent to other areas through different deep cerebellar nuclei depending on the regions of the cerebellum. Medial, intermediate and lateral regions, respectively, project via fastigial, interpositus, and dentate deep nuclei. It is known that the fastigial conveys information on upright stance and gait, and interpositus on reaching movements or alternating agonist and antagonist muscles, and dentate on coordinating movements [Thach, 1998]. The cerebellar input signal $x_{cb}(t)$ is transmitted through mossy fibers. The input excites the deep cerebellar nuclei directly and the Purkinje cell through parallel fibers. Then, the Purkinje cell inhibits the deep cerebellar nuclei. Therefore, there are two neural pathways between the input and output signals (figure 3.4b). The neural activities through the pathways are modeled as follows:

$$\lambda_1 x_{cb}(t) - \lambda_2 x_{cb}(t-\Delta) = \lambda_1 (x_{cb}(t) - x_{cb}(t-\Delta)) + (\lambda_1 - \lambda_2) x_{cb}(t-\Delta) \quad (3.7)$$

where Δ is neural transmission delay and constants λ_1, λ_2 represents intensity of activity.

The first term above on the right hand side is interpreted as a differential operation in the continuous domain, and the second as a scaling operation. As a result, the input and output signals of the cerebellar computational circuitry are in the relation of

$$u_{cb}(t) = g_d \dot{x}_{cb}(t) + g_p x_{cb}(t) \tag{3.8}$$

where g_d represents the cerebellar derivative gain, and g_p the cerebellar proportional gain.

In addition, it is suggested that signal processing from magnocellular red nuclei to lateral reticular nuclei is interpreted as integration [Jo and Massaquoi, 2004; Jo, 2006]. Then, the cerebellar input signal through mossy fibers now becomes $\int x_{cb}(t)dt$ where input $x_{cb}(t)$ is fed to the signal processing from magnocellular red nuclei to lateral reticular nuclei, and then transmitted to deep cerebellar nuclei (especially, interpositus in medial cerebellum) and also conveyed to granule cells through mossy fibers as in figure 3.4c [Allen and Tsukahara, 1974]. When Eq. (3.8) is applied to this new input, the output signal is in the form of

$$u_{cb}(t) = g_p x_{cb}(t) + g_i \int x_{cb}(t)dt \tag{3.9}$$

Therefore, the overall cerebellar computation, summation of Eq. (3.8) and (3.9), is represented as Proportional-Integral-Derivative (PID) signal processing.

$$u_{cb}(t) = g_p x_{cb}(t) + g_i \int x_{cb}(t)dt + g_d \dot{x}_{cb}(t) \tag{3.10}$$

A different set of PID gains will be selected to represent different regional signal processings for different behaviors. As mentioned previously, cerebellar computation is regionally distinguished. For example, arm motions are usually at higher frequencies than leg motions. Therefore, the derivative component will be more effective for arm motion control. For this walking model problem, it turns out empirically that proportional control mainly operates. Considering the lead compensation of the local closed-loop, the signal related to proportional control is velocity-like in fact.

The cerebellar PID gains are also adaptively tunable. Plasticities such as Long Term Depression (LTD) or Long Term Potentiation (LTP) etc [Ito, 2001] in the cerebellar cortex are computationally comparable with the gain tuning. This chapter does not go deeply into the adaptation but the manipulation of walking behavior. However, the second model may provide insights into automatic gain tuning.

It may be reasonable to assume that the supraspinal system manages the sensorimotor activities in specified coordinates rather than fully concerns the whole redundant sensory information though it is not completely verified yet. In this way, the control problem gets simplified because control variable dimensionality is reduced. Each columnar assembly in sensorimotor area 3a is expected to contain a specific feature presentation of sensory information [Huffman and Krubitzer, 2001]. Presumably it is the spot for such control space reduction. Further research is required for confirmation, however. Two control variables, the body's CM (x_{com}) and trunk pitch angle (q_{com}), are empirically chosen for the cerebrocerebellar control channels. Recent experimental study indicates the two variables are critical to regulate human postural balance [Freitas et al., 2006]. Presumably the supraspinal feedback system is still in charge of balance control during normal walking as it is during postural balance. It may be possible to regard walking as extension of postural balance in similar mechanical principle. In both walking and postural balance, the upper body desirably remains close to the vertical line so that the posture helps control the body's CM within stable supporting area [Gilchrist and Winter, 1997]. Walking requires a sequential postural balance control in dynamical manner. Precisely speaking, x_{com} indicates the forward position of the body's CM relative to the stance foot. It is assumed that the two control variables are approximately estimated from sensed information and represented in the form of:

$$\hat{x}_{com} = \mathbf{p}_1^T \mathbf{q}(\mathbf{t} - \mathbf{T}_{spr})$$
$$\hat{q}_{com} = \mathbf{p}_2^T \mathbf{q}(\mathbf{t} - \mathbf{T}_{spr})$$

(3.11)

where $\mathbf{T}_{spr}$ represents neural transmission delays from muscle to supraspinal system.

A weighted linear combination of sensory information as above is the inner product of a population vector $\mathbf{p}$ and a vector of sensory information [Georgopoulos, 1988]. Their tonic reference signals $x_{com,ref}$ and $q_{com,ref}$ are specified in cortical cortex. For a steady walking, constant offset $x_{com,ref}$ and verticality of head-trunk segment, $q_{com,ref} = 0$, are desired.

The cerebrocerebellar signal processing is applied separately to each control variable, therefore, two long-loop feedback pathways are coexistent. Still, it is possible to walk or even run with the trunk bent forward or backward, and during running the trunk is maintained erect even while there is no ground contract. Therefore, it is plausible that regulations of trunk pitch and relative CM position are managed by separate neural circuits. The interpositus nucleus projects to the cortex and could be involved in the cerebrocerebellar coordination. The interpositus also is known to be involved in arm and leg control. Therefore, it may be related to the CM relevant control loop. The fastigial nucleus receives direct connections from spinal cord connects the vestibular nucleus and then back down to spinal cord, therefore, perhaps it is involved with the trunk pitch control loop.

When $\mathbf{u}_c$ represents the neural output from the cerebrocerebellar system, $\mathbf{u}_{cc}$ the output from parietal or motor cortices that bypass the cerebellum, and $\mathbf{u}_{cb}$ the output from the cerebellar signal processing,

$$\mathbf{u}_c = \mathbf{u}_{cc} + \mathbf{u}_{cb}$$

and

$$\mathbf{u}_{desc} = \mathbf{W}_c \mathbf{u}_c(\mathbf{t} - \mathbf{T}_{sp})$$

(3.12)

where $\mathbf{W}_c$ is a matrix to represent the distribution network presumably in cerebral cortical area 4, and $\mathbf{u}_{desc}$ the descending signal from the supraspinal system to muscles.

The distribution network functions as if it is the inverse of the space reduction $\mathbf{p}^T = [\mathbf{p}_1 \quad \mathbf{p}_2]^T$ so that it spreads out neural signals to the whole muscles. We call it the supraspinal synergy network. $\mathbf{T}_{sp}$ represents neural transmission delays from supraspinal to spinal systems.

The alpha motor neuronal signal $\mathbf{u}_{\alpha}$ is obtained by summing the overall neural signals from supraspinal and spinal systems (Eq. (3.5), (3.6) and (3.12)):

$$\mathbf{u}_{\alpha} = \mathbf{u}_{desc} + \mathbf{u}_{sp} + \mathbf{u}_{reflex} \qquad (3.13)$$

The alpha motor command is applied to Eq. (3.3) to produce muscular activations.

3.2. Result

Neural systems explained in the previous section are integrated as in figure 3.6 to build the whole biped walking model. The model is designed under the following assumptions for tractability of the initial study and simple requirements.

1. Movements will be mainly driven by monoarticular muscle activations.
2. Spinal rhythmic patterns are represented by a sequence of on-off pulses.
3. Inter-leg coordination is achieved by 180 degree phase difference between the pattern generators in each leg.

With a set of initial conditions, model parameters are determined to achieve stable walking simulations. At the first step, neural control only with feedforward spinal pattern generation is simulated. The parameters in the pattern generator are tuned for the model to take a couple of steps before falling. Then, the spinal segmental feedback is added to achieve smooth swing motions. Finally, the supraspinal feedback is added to maintain stable walking motions. No optimization for tuning parameters is intended because the goal of the study is the explanation of the principles behind the system and its performance, rather than achieving optimal performance.

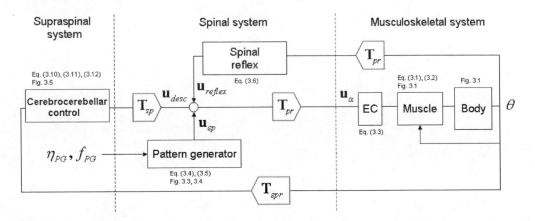

Figure 3.5. Integrated neural system for walking simulation.

The overall system for walking simulation is illustrated in figure 3.5. Principally, the neural system consists of two feedback controls and one feedforward command generator to control behavior of the body. Figure 3.6 demonstrates simulated walking tests using the proposed model. Elimination of either spinal or supraspinal neural feedback results in a fall. Unstable walking with no spinal reflex feedback is caused because the left leg swings too excessively. In comparison, walking with no supraspinal feedback failed postural balance to support the body. As for normal walking pattern, the steady state motion at speed of 1.21m/s is simulated after initial transient responses even though the model includes phase lag components such as neural delays and EC coupling. Moreover, the model does not require any detailed dynamic information like an internal model but a few rudimentary feedforward pulses.

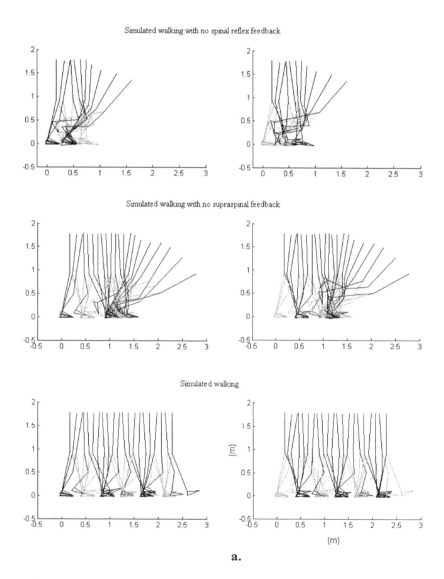

a.

Figure 3.6. a. stick plot of biped walking. (top): simulation with no spinal reflex feedback, (middle): simulation with no supraspinal feedback, and (bottom): simulation of nominal walking. Left columns highlights left leg motions, and right columns right leg motions

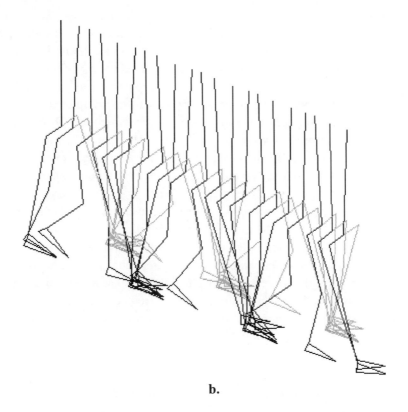

b.

Figure 3.6. b. three-dimensional illustration.

The major feature of the model is the functional decoupling over the hierarchical neural control circuits even though the functions are not perfectly separate. The NPG executes gaits, and supraspinal system controls dynamic postural balance. Segmental reflex in the level of spinal cord helps regulate interlimb movement. The supraspinal system concerns the processing of two sensed variables, i.e., the location of CM and trunk pitch angle. The control channel relevant to the location of CM plays a main role as the postural control of the lower limb, and trunk pitch angle as that of the upper limb. The decoupling scheme makes it possible to avoid the overall complicated recomputation of motor program when the body responses to environment or elicit a new behavior. A simple adjustment of the relevant local neural system may enable simply the achievement of behavioral adaptation.

4. EXECUTION OF CHALLENGING BIPEDAL LOCOMOTION TASKS

A particularly challenging example of an autonomous robot in an unstructured environment is a bipedal walking machine. An example task for such a system is to walk to a moving soccer ball and kick it. Stepping movement must be synchronized with ball movement so that the kick happens when the ball is close enough. More generally, such tasks require that the biped be in the right location at an acceptable time. This implies spatial and temporal constraints for such tasks. There are also important dynamic balance constraints that limit the kinds of movements the biped may make without falling down.

If the system encounters a disturbance while performing a task, it will have to compensate in some way in order to successfully carry out the task. In the soccer example, the disturbance may cause a delay, allowing another player to kick the ball, or it may interfere with movement synchronization. For example, a trip causes disruption of synchronization between the stepping foot, and the overall forward movement of the system's CM. This synchronization must be restored in order for the task to be completed. A second example task is walking on a constrained foot path, such as stones across a brook, or on a balance beam. As with the soccer ball example, this task has spatial, temporal, and dynamic constraints, but in this case, the spatial constraints are more stringent; the biped must reach its goal using foot placements that are precisely constrained. A biped walking over blocks also constrains foot placement in a similar manner. When foot placement is constrained, the stepping pattern cannot be changed arbitrarily to compensate for a disturbance. For example, if a lateral push disturbance occurs, rather than stepping the leg out to the side, other compensating techniques, such as angular movement of the body and swing leg must be used.

In these examples, and others like them, the key challenge is to move a complex, dynamic system to the right place, at the right time, despite actuation limits, and despite disturbances. The system should be able to recover from disturbances such as slips, trips, pushes, and ground contact instability due to soft terrain, even when foot placement is constrained.

4.1. Locomotion Task Execution Problem Statement

A control system for tasks such as those discussed in the previous examples must be capable of guiding a robotic biped through a series of walking task goals, in the presence of disturbances. The system must accept as input a high-level specification of where it should be, and by what time, and then automatically figure out the details of how to move to accomplish these goals. If a disturbance occurs during execution of the task, the system should attempt to compensate in order to avoid a fall, and should still try to complete the task on time. If this is not possible, the system should detect this as soon as possible after the disturbance, and issue a warning to a higher-level control authority.

4.1.1. Specification of Task Goals

There are two kinds of task constraints: state and temporal. We specify state constraints as bounds on key position and velocity variables that summarize the state of the biped, such as the CM, and foot placement positions. For example, to specify state constraints for the soccer example, we specify a set of constraints on foot placement locations, corresponding to a series of steps leading up to the soccer ball, as shown in figure 4.1. To ensure that the body is in an appropriate position, we additionally specify a constraint on the CM so that it is close to the soccer ball.

We specify temporal constraints as bounds on durations of tasks. For example, we specify a lower and upper bound on the duration allowed for the biped to reach the ball. This synchronizes movement of the biped with movement of the ball.

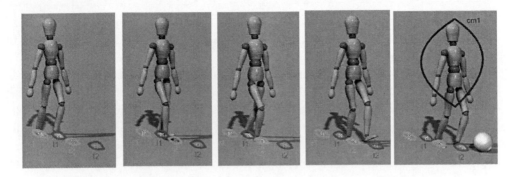

Figure 4.1. State constraints for foot placement and CM for kicking a soccer ball

Note that state and temporal constraints specified for a task are distinct from state and temporal limitations inherent in the biped itself. The latter are due to actuation and dynamic limitations of the biped; they arise from the fact that the biped is a complex, articulated mechanism, where movement is achieved by applying torques to the joints, which accelerate the segments in the mechanism. Acceleration is limited by segment inertias, limitations of the joint actuators, and by the fact that the support base on the ground is limited. The state and temporal constraints specified for a task interact with, and often conflict with, the state and temporal limitations of the biped; a key challenge of the control system is to resolve this fundamental tension between task requirements and robot capabilities.

4.1.2. Task Execution

The task execution problem can be stated in the following way. Given a set of task constraints, and given a particular biped with actuation limits, generate a sequence of control actions that are within the biped's actuation limits, and that result in state trajectories that satisfy the task constraints. Thus, the generated state trajectories must pass through the goal regions at acceptable times. If it is not possible to generate such a control sequence, the system should issue a warning indicating that the task is not feasible. For example, if the soccer ball is moving too quickly or is too far away, it may not be possible to kick it.

4.2. Challenges

There are two key challenges to solving the task execution. First, a biped is a high-dimensional, highly-nonlinear, tightly coupled system, so computing control actions that achieve a desired state is a challenging problem. Second, a biped is under-actuated and has significant inertia, so future state evolution is coupled to current state through dynamics that limit acceleration, and the executive must consider how current state and actions may limit achievement of future desired state.

Bipeds have multiple articulated joints, and therefore, have a large number of degrees of freedom. For example, the biped model used here has 12 actuated joints, and 18 degrees of freedom, resulting in a system with 36 state variables, and 12 control input variables. Furthermore, movement dynamics are highly nonlinear and tightly coupled, so computing control actions that achieve a desired state is a challenging problem.

The second challenge, under-actuation, is due to the fact that a biped has significant inertia, and limited ability to generate force against the ground. This results in limits on the biped's ability to accelerate its center of mass.

The principal actuation limit is the horizontal force that can be applied to the biped's CM. This is due to its high center of mass and limited base of support. Because the contact surface of the feet with the ground is limited, particularly in single support, the feet may slip or roll if inappropriate actuation forces are used. To avoid this, horizontal force exerted by the feet against the ground must be limited, but this also limits acceleration of the center of mass, and thus, the ability to control its position when there are disturbances. Thus, unlike manipulators, walking machines are under-actuated because they do not have a firm base of support, and therefore, are very sensitive to balance disturbances.

A further complicating factor is due to the inherent nature of walking tasks. Bipeds operate in a sequence of discrete modes defined by contact of the feet with the ground. At transitions between these modes, the base of support changes discontinuously. Thus, at toe-off, the base of support is instantly reduced because the biped transitions from double to single support. At heel-strike, the base of support is instantly enlarged because the biped transitions from single to double support. These discontinuous changes in support base imply discontinuous changes in actuation limits. The control system must take these discontinuous changes in actuation limits into account when generating control actions and projecting evolution of state trajectories over the future time horizon.

The support base limitations imply that walking is an inherently unstable process, where the system is constantly in a state where it is about to fall. The mode transitions due to stepping, which change the base of support, simply defer the fall; for fast walking, these modes do not have a stable equilibrium point. This is a direct consequence of the actuation constraints, and the fact that the biped has significant momentum during fast walking. This means that the biped cannot stop instantly, in the middle of a gait cycle. Rather, the system must first slow down to a slower walk, and then come to a rest in a standing position, a mode that does have a stable equilibrium point. Thus, for such walking plans, the executive must guide the system through a sequence of inherently unstable states to get to a goal state that is stable.

4.3. Approach and Innovations

To address the difficulty of determining the effect of control actions on biped state, we use a model-based approach, where a model of the biped is used to predict this effect. Thus, we use a *model-based executive* [Williams and Nayak, 1997; Leaute, 2005] to interpret task goals, monitor biped state, and compute joint torque inputs for the biped, as shown in figure 4.2.

We address the challenges described in the previous section with three key innovations. To address the first challenge (nonlinearity, high dimensionality, and tight coupling), we linearize and decouple the biped system into a set of independent, linear, single-input single-output second-order systems, resulting in an abstraction of the biped that is easier to control. We accomplish this through a novel controller called a *dynamic virtual model controller* [Hofmann, et. al., 2004]. The linearization and decoupling provided by this controller allows points of interest on the biped, such as the center of mass and the stepping foot, to be controlled directly, as if the biped were a puppet, as shown in figure 4.3.

To address the second challenge (actuation limits and sensitivity to balance disturbances), we perform a reachability analysis that defines sets of feasible trajectories for the state variables and control parameters in the abstracted biped. These trajectory sets, called flow tubes, represent bundles of state trajectories that take into account dynamic limitations due to under-actuation, and also satisfy plan requirements. Additionally, our system uses a novel strategy that employs angular momentum to increase the horizontal force that can be applied to the system's center of mass, and thus, to enhance its balance controllability. This strategy is particularly useful for tasks where foot placement is constrained.

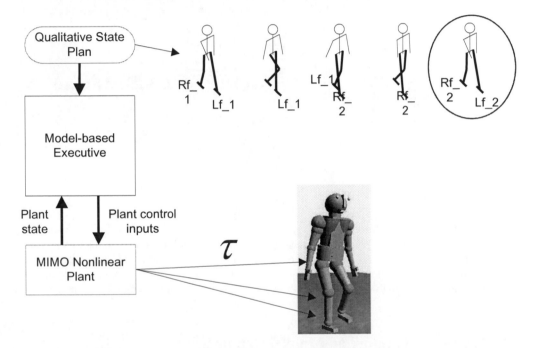

Figure 4.2. A model-based executive computes a sequence of joint torques for the biped that results in the achievement of the successive qualitative state goals

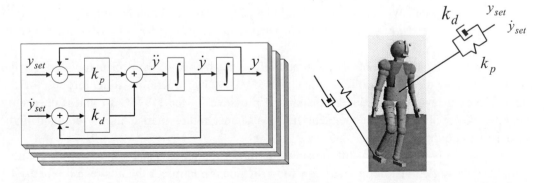

Figure 4.3. A dynamic virtual model controller provides a linear abstraction so that the reaction points move as if they were independent, linear second-order systems, controlled by the virtual elements.

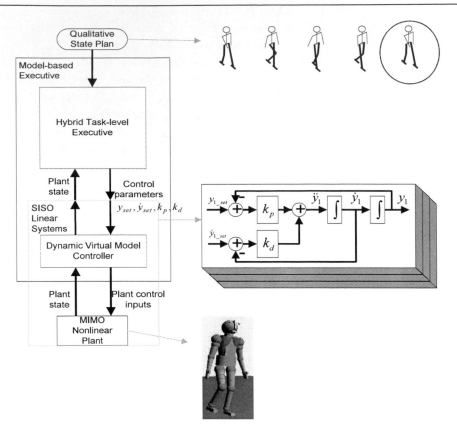

Figure 4.4. The model-based executive consists of a hybrid task-level executive and a dynamic virtual model controller. The hybrid executive controls the biped by adjusting control parameters of the linear virtual element abstraction provided by the controller. The hybrid executive sets control parameters to guide state variables through successive goal regions, while satisfying timing and balance constraints.

4.4. Control Architecture and Implementation

To achieve correct plan execution, the model-based executive must generate a control trajectory that satisfies all future goal region and temporal constraints specified in the qualitative state plan. We accomplish this by using a two-part architecture, consisting of a *hybrid task-level executive*, and a *dynamic virtual model controller* (DVMC), as shown in Figure 4.4.

The hybrid executive controls the biped indirectly, by setting control parameters for the dynamic virtual model controller, rather than directly, by generating joint torques for the biped. Thus, it leverages the linear abstraction provided by the DVMC so that it need only consider the evolution of independent linear systems, rather than a tightly-coupled high-dimensional nonlinear system.

In order to project the feasible future evolution of the biped's state, the hybrid executive computes *flow tubes* that define valid operating regions in terms of the abstracted biped. The flow tubes represent bundles of state trajectories that satisfy plan requirements, and also take into account dynamics and actuation limitations. The flow tubes observe the discontinuous changes in actuation constraints due to ground contact events. Once the flow tubes have been computed, the hybrid executive executes the plan by adjusting control parameters in the abstracted biped in order to keep trajectories within the tubes.

Because computation of flow tubes is time consuming, and because the hybrid executive must run in real time, we perform this step off-line, as a compilation. Thus, the hybrid executive consists of two components: a *plan compiler*, and a *dispatcher*. The plan compiler outputs a *qualitative control plan*, which contains the flow tubes for all state variables in the abstracted biped.

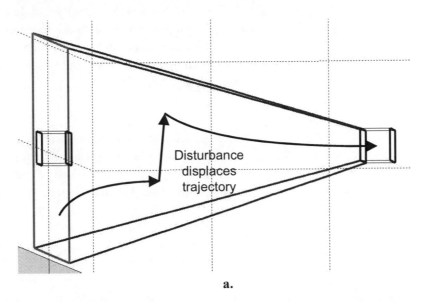

a.

Figure 4.5.a. If a disturbance is not too large, the trajectory remains inside the tube. This means that the dispatcher will be able to adjust control parameters so that the trajectory reaches the goal at an acceptable time.

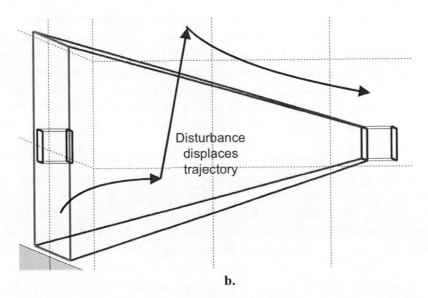

b.

Figure 4.5. b. If a disturbance is too large, it pushes the trajectory outside its tube, and the plan fails

The dispatcher monitors the state of the abstracted biped, adjusting control parameters based on the specifications in the qualitative control plan to keep trajectories in their flow tubes. The dispatcher monitors plan execution by monitoring the abstracted biped's state relative to the plan. In this way, it checks whether each trajectory is in its tube. If a disturbance occurs, the dispatcher attempts to adjust the SISO control parameter settings in order to compensate, so that the trajectory remains inside the tube, as shown in figure 4.5a. If the disturbance has pushed the trajectory outside its tube, as shown in figure 4.5b, then the dispatcher aborts, indicating to a higher-level planner that plan execution has failed.

We next describe the qualitative state plan, the input that specifies the locomotion task to be performed. We then discuss the dynamic virtual model controller, which provides the abstracted biped. Plan compilation of the qualitative state plan and dispatching of the resulting qualitative control plan are then discussed.

4.4.1. Qualitative state plan

For most practical applications, a precise specification of state and temporal goals is not necessary. Rather, a loose specification, in terms of state space regions and temporal ranges, is preferable in that it admits a wider set of possible solutions. This may be exploited, for example, to improve optimality or to adapt to disturbances. An example state space goal is for the biped's center of mass position to be within a particular region. An example temporal goal is that this state space goal be achieved after 5 seconds, but before 6.

Reaching a goal location may require the biped to take a sequence of steps. Such steps represent transitions through a sequence of fundamentally different states, defined by which feet are in contact with the ground. Thus, a stepping sequence consists of alternating between double support phases, where both feet are on the ground, and single support phases, where one foot (the stance foot) is in contact with the ground, and the other foot (the swing foot) is taking the step. These phases represent qualitatively different system states, with correspondingly different behaviors.

We define a qualitative state as an abstract constraint on desired position, velocity, and temporal behavior of the biped. A qualitative state indicates which feet are on the ground, and includes constraints on foot position. It may also include state constraints on quantities like the biped's center of mass, and temporal constraints specifying time ranges by which the state space goals must be achieved. Thus, a qualitative state is a partial specification of desired behavior for a portion of a walking gait cycle. A sequence of qualitative states represents intermediate goals that lead to the final overall task goal. Such a sequence forms a qualitative state plan.

For example, a plan for a biped walking cycle is a sequence of qualitative states representing single and double support gait phases. Such a plan is shown in figure 4.6. In this plan, the first qualitative state represents double support with the left foot in front, the second, left single support, the third, double support with the right foot in front, and the fourth, right single support. The fifth qualitative state repeats the first, but is one gait cycle forward.

A qualitative state plan has a set of *activities* representing constraints on desired state evolution of workspace state variables. Activities are indicated by horizontal arrows in figure 4.6, and are arranged in rows corresponding to their associated state variables. In figure 4.6, the activities *left foot ground 1* and *left foot step 1* are for the left foot, *right foot ground 1*, *right foot step 1*, and *right foot ground 2* are for the right foot, and CM1 – 4 are for the center of mass.

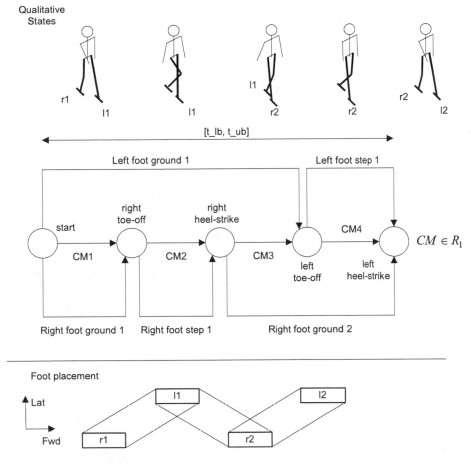

Figure 4.6. Example qualitative state plan for walking gait cycle. Circles represent events, and horizontal arrows between events represent activities. Activities may have associated state space constraints, such as the goal region constraint $CM \in R_1$, which specifies a goal for CM position and velocity. Foot placement constraints are indicated at the bottom; for example, rectangle r1 represents constraints on the first right foot.

Every activity starts and ends with an *event*, represented by a circle in figure 4.6. Events in this plan relate to behavior of the stepping foot. Thus, a *toe-off* event represents the stepping foot lifting off the ground, and a *heel-strike* event represents the stepping foot landing on the ground. Events define the boundaries of qualitative states. Thus, the right toe-off event defines the end of the first qualitative state (double support), and the beginning of the second qualitative state (left single support).

The qualitative state plan in figure 4.6 has a temporal constraint between the start and finish events. This constraint specifies a lower and upper bound, $[lb, ub]$, on the time between these events. Such temporal constraints are useful for specifying bounds on tasks consisting of sequences of qualitative states. The temporal constraint in figure 4.6 is a constraint on the time to complete the gait cycle, and thus, can be used to specify walking speed.

In addition to temporal constraints, qualitative state plans include state constraints. These are associated with activities, and are specified as rectangles in position/velocity state space. Such rectangles can be used to specify required initial and goal regions. In figure 4.6, the goal region constraint $CM \in R_1$ represents the requirement that the CM trajectory must be in region R_1 for the CM movement activity to finish successfully.

In addition to initial and goal regions, an activity may also have operating region constraints that specify valid regions in state-space where the trajectory must be over the entire duration of the activity. These are of the form $g(y_i, \dot{y}_i) \leq 0$, and they may be linear or nonlinear. Such constraints are used to express actuation limits. For example, CM movement in the plan of figure 4.6 is represented by four separate activities: CM1 – CM4. Only CM4 has a goal region. However, each of these activities have different operating regions. This is due to the discontinuous changes in the base of support resulting from the foot contact events; the base of support in double support is very different from the one in single support. Thus, for CM1, the base of support is the polygon defined by r1 and l1 in figure 4.6. For CM2, it is the polygon defined by l1 only.

The base of support has a strong effect on the maximum force that can be exerted on the CM. This is why these operation constraints must be defined; they represent actuation limits for the CM activities. This is why CM movement in the plan of figure 4.6 is represented by four activities instead of only one.

4.4.2. Dynamic virtual model controller

The *dynamic virtual model controller* (DVMC), the component of the model-based executive that interacts directly with the biped. The DVMC simplifies the job of the hybrid executive component of the model-based executive by providing the linear abstraction.

The DVMC provides the task executive with a simple way to control the biped's forward and lateral CM position. This allows the executive to maintain the system's balance, and to move the biped forward during walking, by specifying desired CM movement. Additionally, the DVMC provides the hybrid executive with a simple way to control movement of the stepping foot, and to maintain the upright posture of the torso.

The abstraction provided by the DVMC allows the hybrid executive to control the biped like a puppet, using virtual linear spring-damper elements. These virtual elements are attached at key reaction points, like the center of mass, and the stepping foot, as shown in figure 4.3. The virtual elements don't actually exist. However, the biped will move as if they did. In particular, the hybrid executive can assume that the motion of a reaction point will be that of a linear system with spring and damping parameters corresponding to the virtual elements. This greatly simplifies the planning and control functions of the hybrid executive because it does not have to be concerned with the nonlinear dynamics of the actual biped, or with computing joint actuator torques. The hybrid executive lets the dynamic virtual model controller worry about these details.

Our use of virtual elements is similar, in concept, to the one used in a virtual model controller [Pratt et al., 1997]. An important difference is that our dynamic virtual model controller takes dynamics into account, while a virtual model controller does not. A virtual model controller uses a Jacobian transformation to translate the desired forces at the reaction points, specified by the virtual elements, into joint torques that produce these forces. This works well for static or slow-moving mechanisms, but can break down as movements become faster because the controller does not take into account the dynamics of the system. Therefore, movement of the reaction point is not necessarily in line with the desired virtual force. In contrast, our dynamic virtual model controller uses a dynamic model to account for the biped's dynamics. This results in a linear system, where reaction points move as if they were simple linear second order systems, controlled by the virtual elements, as shown in figure 4.3.

The DVMC performs four key functions. First, it uses a model-based input-output linearization algorithm [Slotine and Li, 1991] to linearize and decouple the plant. Second, the controller performs a geometric transform from joint space to workspace coordinates in order to make state variables relevant to balance control, such as center of mass position, directly controllable, as the state variables of a simple linear system. Third, the controller prioritizes goals in order to accommodate actuation constraints. Such actuation constraints may cause the overall system to become over-constrained. To address this problem, our controller automatically sacrifices lower-priority goals when the system becomes over-constrained in this way. For example, the system may temporarily sacrifice goals of maintaining upright posture in order to achieve balance goals. Fourth, the DVMC addresses the problem of model inaccuracy by incorporating a sliding control algorithm [Slotine and Li, 1991].

The linearization and goal prioritization approach of our controller is similar, in concept, to the recently developed whole-body control algorithm [Khatib et al., 2004]. However, the whole-body controller relies heavily on an accurate model; it does not account for model inaccuracy. Our controller accounts for this inaccuracy using the sliding control approach. Recently, the whole-body control approach has been used to regulate a biped's linear and angular momentum [Kajita et al., 2001; Yokoi et al., 2001; Sugihara et al., 2002; Nishiwaki et al., 2002]. A key point of difference is that our model is able to purposely sacrifice angular momentum control goals in order to achieve linear control goals when both cannot be met.

4.4.2.1. Linearization and State Transformation

A geometric transform, $\mathbf{h}$, is used to convert from the joint state to the workspace state representation, according to

$$\left[\mathbf{y}^T, \dot{\mathbf{y}}^T\right]^T = \mathbf{h}\left[\mathbf{x}^T, \dot{\mathbf{x}}^T\right]^T \tag{4.1}$$

where $\left[\mathbf{x}^T, \dot{\mathbf{x}}^T\right]$ is the joint state vector, and $\left[\mathbf{y}^T, \dot{\mathbf{y}}^T\right]$ is the workspace state vector. Elements of $\mathbf{x}$ include joint angle positions, such as left knee joint angle, and elements of $\mathbf{y}$ include forward and lateral CM position. The controller uses a feedback linearizing transformation to convert desired workspace variable accelerations, $\ddot{\mathbf{y}}$, into corresponding joint torques, $\boldsymbol{\tau}$, as shown in figure 4.7. Application of these torques results in a new joint state, $\left[\mathbf{x}^T, \dot{\mathbf{x}}^T\right]$. The multivariable controller then uses the transformation, $\mathbf{h}$, to convert from joint to workspace state.

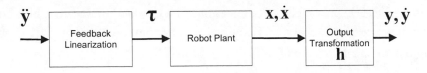

Figure 4.7. Feedback linearization and output transformation

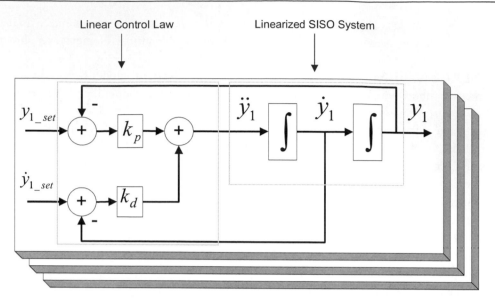

Figure 4.8. Linear virtual element abstraction consisting of a set of SISO systems with associated linear control laws

If we draw a black box around the series of transforms in figure 4.7, the *multiple-input multiple-output* (MIMO) nonlinear plant appears to be a set of decoupled SISO linear 2nd-order systems, as shown in figure 4.8. Each element, y_i of position vector $\mathbf{y}$, can be viewed as the output of one of the SISO systems, with the corresponding acceleration element, $\ddot{y}_i$, being the input. Each SISO system can be controlled by a simple linear control law, such as the proportional-differential (PD) law shown in figure 4.8. The set of SISO systems, with associated linear control laws, forms the linear virtual element abstraction. The solution trajectory for each SISO system is defined by a linear second-order differential equation, so the trajectory value at any time can be computed analytically.

Linearization of the plant dynamics is accomplished using the standard dynamics equation for an articulated body [Craig, 1989]:

$$\mathbf{H}(\mathbf{q})\ddot{\mathbf{q}} + \mathbf{C}(\mathbf{q},\dot{\mathbf{q}}) + \mathbf{g}(\mathbf{q}) = \boldsymbol{\tau} \qquad (4.2)$$

Thus, for a particular joint state $\begin{bmatrix} \mathbf{q}^T, \dot{\mathbf{q}}^T \end{bmatrix}$, this gives joint torques as a linear function of joint accelerations:

$$\mathbf{H}_1\ddot{\mathbf{q}} + \mathbf{G}_1 = \boldsymbol{\tau} \qquad (4.3)$$

Plant outputs are expressed as a nonlinear function of plant joint state, using Eq. (4.1). A linear relation between workspace accelerations, $\ddot{\mathbf{y}}$, and joint accelerations, $\ddot{\mathbf{q}}$, is obtained by computing the second derivative of $\mathbf{y}$.

$$\ddot{\mathbf{y}} = \frac{\partial^2 \mathbf{h}(\mathbf{q},\dot{\mathbf{q}})}{\partial(\mathbf{q},\dot{\mathbf{q}})^2} \tag{4.4}$$

resulting in an equation of the form

$$\ddot{\mathbf{y}} = \mathbf{\Psi}\ddot{\mathbf{q}} + \mathbf{\Psi}_{const} \tag{4.5}$$

It is assumed that this linear system can be solved for $\ddot{\mathbf{q}}$ given $\ddot{\mathbf{y}}$, at least for the region of state space in which the controller is operating.

Now, suppose we add a linear controller that computes a control input of the form

$$\ddot{\mathbf{y}}_{des} = \mathbf{f}_{controller}\left(\mathbf{y}_{des}, \mathbf{y}, \dot{\mathbf{y}}_{des}, \dot{\mathbf{y}}\right) \tag{4.6}$$

Eq. 4.5 is then used to convert to desired joint accelerations:

$$\ddot{\mathbf{q}}_{des} = \mathbf{\Psi}^{-1}\left(\ddot{\mathbf{y}}_{des} - \mathbf{\Psi}_{const}\right) \tag{4.7}$$

These are then substituted into Eq. (4.2), with $\ddot{\mathbf{q}} = \ddot{\mathbf{q}}_{des}$, in order to get the desired control torques

The result is a a two-stage linearization, where setpoints are specified in terms of the desired output variables, as shown in the figure 4.9. In this two-stage linearization, output variable accelerations are converted to joint accelerations by the first linearization, and then joint accelerations are converted to torques by the second, inverse dynamics, linearization.

Further details of the derivation of the feedback linearization and output transformation can be found in [Hofmann, 2005] and [Hofmann et al., 2004].

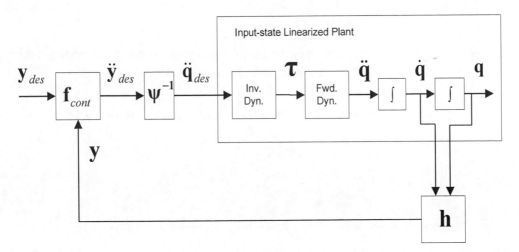

Figure 4.9. Two-stage Linearization

4.4.2.2. Goal Prioritization

We chose the following outputs to be elements of the $\mathbf{y}$ vector.

forward CM position
lateral CM position
stance knee joint angle
torso roll angle
torso pitch angle
torso yaw angle
forward swing foot position
lateral swing foot position
swing knee joint angle
swing foot roll
swing foot pitch
swing hip joint yaw angle

The forward and lateral CM positions are important variables to control for balancing, so it makes sense to include these in the output vector. Similarly, swing foot placement determines the shape of the support polygon, and is therefore also crucial for balance control. Thus, it makes sense to include swing foot forward and lateral position in the output vector. It is desirable to maintain an upright torso position, so torso orientation should also be included. Note that vertical CM and swing foot position are not included in the output vector, in order to avoid singularities that may occur with these quantities. Instead, stance and swing knee joint angles are controlled, and vertical CM and swing foot positions emerge from these.

With this choice of outputs, the system given by Eq. (4.5) is square, because there are 12 inputs (the torques to the 12 joints), and there are 12 outputs. As long as $\mathbf{\Psi}$ is invertible, the system will appear to be completely linearized and decoupled to the outer controller $\mathbf{f}_{cont}$. Thus, the outer controller can specify elements of $\ddot{\mathbf{y}}_{des}$ as if they were independent, and a corresponding $\ddot{\mathbf{q}}_{des}$ can always be computed.

Next, consider what happens when bounds on plant inputs due to saturation limits are added. If $\mathbf{f}_{cont}$ does not take these bounds into consideration, it could generate values for $\ddot{\mathbf{y}}_{des}$ that cause the bounds to be violated.

To avoid this type of infeasibility, slack variables, $\ddot{\mathbf{y}}_{slack}$, are introduced for each element of $\ddot{\mathbf{y}}_{des}$, so that the new controller output, $\ddot{\mathbf{y}}_{cont\_out}$, is

$$\ddot{\mathbf{y}}_{des} = \ddot{\mathbf{y}}_{cont\_out} + \ddot{\mathbf{y}}_{slack} \qquad (4.8)$$

Use of these slack variables provides flexibility in that $\ddot{\mathbf{y}}_{des}$ conforms to the $\mathbf{f}_{cont}$ linear control law, without regard to the actuation bounds, while $\ddot{\mathbf{y}}_{cont\_out}$, the true output of the controller, does obey actuation bounds. The goal of the overall control system is then to minimize $\ddot{\mathbf{y}}_{slack}$, taking into account the relative importance of each element.

This minimization is accomplished by formulating the control problem as a quadratic program (QP), and then using a QP optimizer to solve it. The relative importance of the slack variables is expressed in the cost function for the QP. Slack variables associated with important outputs are given higher cost than slack variables for less important outputs. This causes the optimizer to prioritize goals by minimizing the slack variables for the most important outputs first, and therefore, setting $\ddot{y}_{cont\_out}$ to be as close as possible to $\ddot{y}_{des}$, in Eq. (4.8), for these outputs. For example, slack variables associated with the CM position output are given higher cost than those associated with torso orientation.

Details of the formulation are provided in [Hofmann, 2005; Hofmann et al., 2004].

The linearization described previously can be problematic for real plants because it assumes a perfect plant model. The sliding control algorithm, [Slotine and Li], addresses this problem with additional corrective control terms used to compensate for model inaccuracy. Details of our incorporation of this algorithm are provided in [Hofmann, 2005; Hofmann et al., 2004].

4.4.3. Qualitative control plan and flow tubes

A QCP augments the input QSP by adding flow tubes which represent feasible trajectory sets [Bradley and Zhao, 1993; Frazzoli, 2001]. Flow tubes are associated with QSP activities; they represent feasible trajectories that result in successful execution of the associated activities. Thus, a flow tube depends on the activity's constraints, and the dynamics of the activity's SISO system.

An example flow tube is shown in figure 4.10a. A flow tube can be characterized as a set of cross-sectional regions in position-velocity phase space, one for each time in the interval $[t_0, t_g]$. Thus, such a cross section, r_{cs}, is a function of the flow tube, and of time: $r_{cs} = CS(Y,t): t_0 \leq t \leq t_g$. Figure 4.10b depicts cross sections for times t_0, t_1, and t_g.

Next, consider the set, R_{cs}, of all cross sections in an interval $[t_0, t_1]$, where $t_0 \leq t_1 \leq t_g$. We use this set to investigate conditions under which the associated activity can be executed successfully for any start time in the interval $[t_0, t_1]$. If an allowed initial region, r_1, is a subset of every cross section in R_{cs}, then the duration of the activity is controllable over the interval $[l, u]$, where $l = t_g - t_1$, and $u = t_g - t_0$. Conversely, each cross section of Y of which r_1 is a subset corresponds to a controllable duration of the activity.

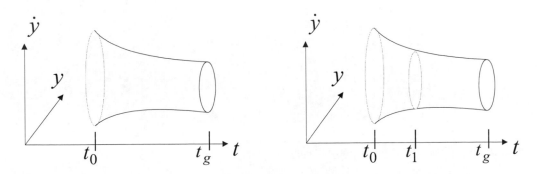

Figure 4.10.a. Example flow tube over interval $[t_0, t_g]$; b. cross sections at t_0, t_1, and t_g.

In this way, if the initial state of the system is in r_1, the controllable duration of the activity is known. This controllable duration is the temporal constraint due to the plant dynamics. It is added to the temporal constraints specified explicitly in the QSP.

4.4.4. Plan compilation

Flow tubes have a complex geometry. Therefore, any tractable flow tube representation will be an approximation of the feasible set. In order to ensure that any trajectory chosen by the dispatcher leads to plan execution success, we require our flow tube representation to include only feasible trajectories; the representation may include a subset of all feasible trajectories, but not a superset [Kurzhanski and Varaiya, 1999].

Our flow tube approximation uses polyhedral cross sections at discrete time intervals [Vestal, 2001]. The time interval chosen matches the control increment of the dispatcher. Therefore, the dispatcher will always be able to access flow tube cross sections for exactly the correct time. Figure 4.11 shows a flow tube cross-sectional region in position-velocity phase space, and its polyhedral approximation. Note that the approximation is a subset of the true region; the approximation does not include points in state-space that do not belong to feasible trajectories.

In order to generate the polyhedral cross-sections, the plan compiler performs a *reachability analysis* that, for every vertex position, computes extreme corresponding velocities such that the resulting polygon contains only feasible trajectory points for the time associated with the cross section. We accomplish this reachability analysis by formulating constraints on cross section vertices as a linear program (LP).

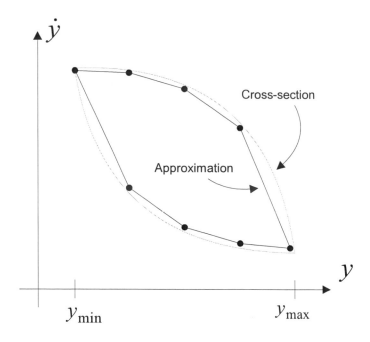

Figure 4.11. Flow tube cross section and approximation

The LP formulation is based on the analytical solution of a 2nd-order linear differential equation, with analytic solution:

$$y = e^{\alpha t}\left(K_1 \cos \beta t + iK_2 \sin \beta t\right) + u/c$$

$$\dot{y} = e^{\alpha t}\left(\beta\left(-K_1 \sin \beta t + iK_2 \cos \beta t\right) + \alpha\left(K_1 \cos \beta t + iK_2 \sin \beta t\right)\right)$$

(4.9)

where

$$K_1 = y(0) - u/c, \ K_2 = (i/\beta)\left(\alpha K_1 - \dot{y}(0)\right)$$
$$K_1 = y(0) - u/c, \ K_2 = (i/\beta)\left(\alpha K_1 - \dot{y}(0)\right)$$
$$\alpha = -k_d/2, \beta = \left(-i\sqrt{k_d^2 - 4k_p}\right)/2, u = k_p y_{set} + k_d \dot{y}_{set}$$

This is the solution for an SISO system in figure 4.3. If we set the time, t, in Eq. (4.9) to a particular duration, d_i, corresponding to a particular cross section of interest, and if we fix gains k_p and k_d, then Eq. (4.9) can be expressed as

$$y = f_1\left(y(0), \dot{y}(0), y_{set}, \dot{y}_{set}\right)$$
$$\dot{y} = f_2\left(y(0), \dot{y}(0), y_{set}, \dot{y}_{set}\right)$$

(4.10)

where f_1 and f_2 are linear for a particular setting of t, k_p, and k_d. Eq. (4.10) forms a set of equality constraints in the LP formulation. We also include a set of inequality constraints of the form

$$y_{set\_min} \leq y_{set} \leq y_{set\_max}$$
$$\dot{y}_{set\_min} \leq \dot{y}_{set} \leq \dot{y}_{set\_max}$$

(4.11)

to represent the actuation limits, specified for the activity in the QSP. Further, we use a set of equality constraints to express

$$\langle y, \dot{y} \rangle \in R_{goal}$$

(4.12)

to ensure that state at the end of duration d_i is in the goal region, specified for the activity in the QSP. The formulation of (4.12) as a set of linear inequalities is straightforward because R_{goal} is required to be convex.

To compute a cross section for a particular R_{goal} and d_i, the plan compiler uses the formulation described by Eqs. (4.10 - 4.12), and sets the LP cost function to minimize $y(0)$. Solving this formulation yields the minimum initial position, y_{min}, shown in figure 4.11.

Repeating this process with the cost function set to maximize $y(0)$ yields the maximum initial position, y_{max}. The compiler then establishes vertex positions at regular increments between y_{min} and y_{max}. For each such vertex position, the compiler solves the LP formulation with the cost function set to first minimize, and then maximize, $\dot{y}(0)$, in order to find the minimum and maximum velocities for that position. This results in a set of vertices in position-velocity state space, which form the polyhedral approximation, as shown in figure 4.11.

The compiler computes cross section approximations for every d_i in the temporal range $[l, u]$, where this range is given for each activity by the minimum dispatchable graph. This set of cross sections approximates a flow tube, such as the one shown in figure 4.10.

4.4.5. Dispatcher

In order to execute a QCP, the dispatcher must successfully execute each activity in the QCP. The dispatcher accomplishes this by setting control parameters for each activity such that the associated trajectory reaches the activity's goal region at an acceptable time.

In order to execute an activity, the dispatcher performs three key functions: initialization, monitoring, and transition. Initialization is performed at the start of an activity's execution, monitoring is performed continuously during the activity's execution, and transition is performed at the finish of the activity's execution.

For initialization, assuming that all trajectories begin in the flow tube of their activity, the dispatcher chooses a goal duration for the control activity that is consistent with the activity's temporal constraints, and sets control parameters such that the state trajectory is predicted to be in the activity's goal region after the goal duration. The initialization function formulates a small *quadratic program* (QP) and solves it in order to determine these control parameters. This formulation is given in figure 4.12. Key to this formulation's simplicity is the fact that the analytic solution of Eq. (4.10) (functions f_1 and f_2) is used to predict the future state of the SISO system associated with the activity, and the fact that the formulation is guaranteed to produce a feasible solution, because the trajectory is within its flow tube. Further, presence of the trajectory in the flow tube guarantees that there exists a set of feasible control settings for all remaining activities in the plan, if there are no further trajectory disturbances.

After initializing an activity, the dispatcher begins monitoring execution of that activity. To monitor execution, the dispatcher continually checks whether the state trajectory remains in its flow tube. If this is not the case, then plan execution has failed, and the dispatcher aborts to a higher-level control authority. Such a control authority might issue a new plan in response to such an abort. For example, the biped trying to kick the soccer ball may give up on this goal if it is no longer feasible.

If the state trajectory is in its flow tube, the dispatcher checks whether it is on track to be in the goal region at the end of the goal duration. This check is accomplished by evaluating Eq. (4.10) for the current state, and checking whether the predicted state is within the goal region. If this is not the case, the dispatcher corrects this situation by adjusting control parameters using the QP formulation of figure 4.12. Note that because the state trajectory is in its flow tube at this point, such a correction will always be possible.

FormulateControlQP($R_{goal}, y_{curr}, \dot{y}_{curr}, t_s, t_f$)

Parameters to optimize: $y_{pred}, \dot{y}_{pred}, y_{set}, \dot{y}_{set}$
Equality constraints: Eq. (3)
Inequality constraints: Eqs. (4, 5)
  (Eq. (5) requires that trajectory prediction be within goal region)
Cost function
$$y_{goal} = \left(y_{min}\left(R_{goal}\right) + y_{max}\left(R_{goal}\right)\right)/2$$
$$\dot{y}_{goal} = \left(\dot{y}_{min}\left(R_{goal}\right) + \dot{y}_{max}\left(R_{goal}\right)\right)/2$$

Figure 4.12. Dispatcher QP formulation.

As part of the monitoring function, the dispatcher also continually checks whether an activity's completion conditions are satisfied. Thus, it checks whether the state trajectory is in the activity's goal region, and whether the state trajectories of other activities whose completion must be synchronized are in their activity's goal regions. If all completion conditions for a control activity are satisfied, the dispatcher switches to the transition function.

If the activity being executed has a successor, the transition function invokes the initialization function for this successor. When all activities in the QCP have been executed successfully, execution terminates.

4.5. Results

4.5.1. Biped simulation
The controller was tested using a high-fidelity biped simulation, serving as the plant to be controlled. This simulated biped, shown in figure 4.6, is three-dimensional with 18 degrees of freedom (6 representing the position and orientation of the trunk, and 12 corresponding to the leg joints, which can exert torques). Each leg was modeled with a ball-and socket hip joint (3 degrees of freedom), a pin knee joint (one degree of freedom), and a saddle-type ankle joint (two degrees of freedom). The upper body (head, arms and torso), upper leg and lower leg were modeled with cylindrical shapes, and the feet were modeled with rectangular blocks.

The total mass was divided among the segments according to morphological data from the literature [Clauser et al., 1969; Brown, 1987]. The dimensions of each model segment were obtained by considering morphological data that describe average human proportions [Tilley and Dreyfuss, 1993; Winters, 1990]. Ground contact force was modeled using a nonlinear spring-damper system at four points per stance leg, located at each corner of the rectangular foot. Further details of this simulated biped are given in [Hofmann, 2005].

4.5.2. Balance tests
The ability to balance on one leg is an important prerequisite for walking, expecially when foot placement is constrained. Therefore, a series of experiments was performed to evaluate the DVMC's ability to stabilize the biped in single-support mode, that is, standing on

one leg. Thus, these tests exercise the DVMC component of the execution system, independently of the task executive.

Balance recovery was tested by initializing the simulated biped in a motionless position, but with the horizontal position of the center of mass (CM) outside the support polygon, defined by the stance foot. For such an initial condition, stance ankle torque alone is insufficient for restoring balance. The maximum stance ankle torque that can be exerted without having the foot roll places the ZMP point at the edge of the support polygon, but not beyond it. Since the CM is beyond this point, this is insufficient for generating an appropriate corrective horizontal component of the ground reaction force, as explained previously. The biped is sufficiently out of balance that it becomes necessary to perform dynamic movement of non-contact segments in order to generate spin torque about the CM. This augments the horizontal ground reaction force provided by the stance ankle torque, by moving the CMP outside the edge of the support polygon. This action can help the system restore balance, by bringing the horizontal position of the CM back to the center of the support polygon, but it also causes a disturbance in the angular stability (upright posture) of the biped. The controller, therefore, must judiciously sacrifice angular stability temporarily, in order to bring the CM back under control, after which, it corrects for the angular disturbance.

The initial condition used here for testing results in an instability that is similar to the one that occurs when the system is pushed near its CM. Thus, it is a good indicator of how the system will perform when disturbed in this way.

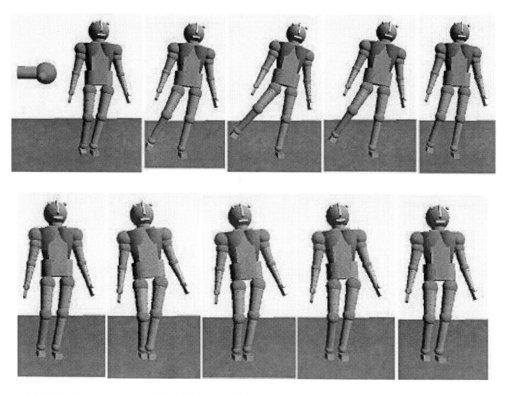

Figure 4.13. Motion sequence of biped for lateral disturbance while standing on left leg

Figure 4.13 shows the system's response to a lateral disturbance, that is, where the lateral position of the CM starts beyond the left-most limit of the system's support polygon, while standing on level ground. The counter-clockwise rotation of the upper body and right (non-stance) leg results in spin angular momentum about the CM. By conservation of angular momentum, this results in an orbital angular momentum of the CM about the support point, which augments the angular momentum produced by stance ankle torque. This pushes the CM toward the system's right.

Figure 4.14 shows the ZMP (in blue), and the CMP (in red) during this maneuver. The left-most limit of the support base is at 0.05 meters. The ZMP stays within this limit, so that the foot does not roll, but the CMP starts outside of it. The angular movement of the upper body and non-stance leg provides enough equivalent horizontal ground reaction force to bring the horizontal position of the CM back to the center of the support base. Note that after about 0.8 seconds, the ZMP is no longer pegged at the limit. This is an indication that the CM is under control, and that the controller can turn its attention to correcting the angular disturbance.

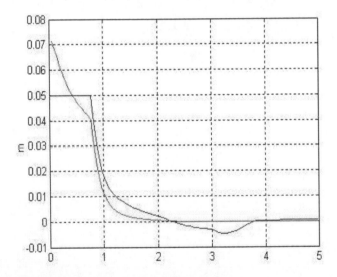

Figure 4.14. Lateral (leftward) direction ZMP in blue, CMP in red.

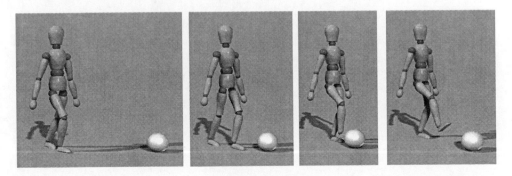

Figure 4.15. Walking to a moving soccer ball and kicking it.

4.5.3. Kicking a moving soccer ball

Consider the previously described example task of walking to a moving soccer ball and kicking it. Such a task exercises the execution system's ability to synchronize movement of the biped with an externally applied temporal constraint; the biped must be in the right place at the right time to kick the ball.

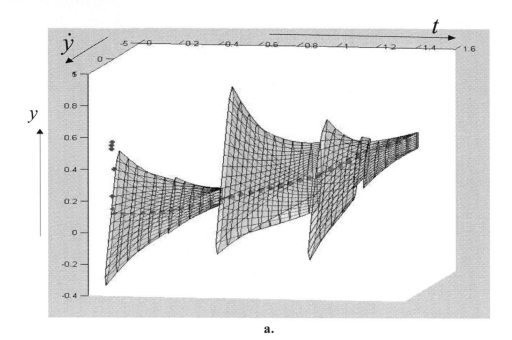

a.

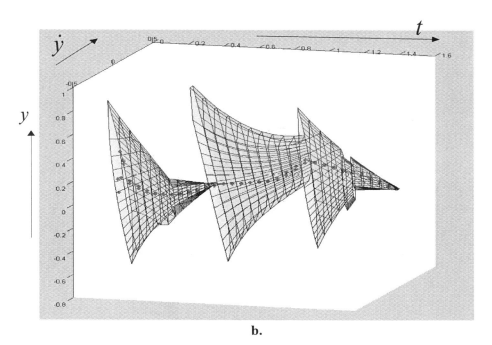

b.

Figure 4.16. Flow tubes and state trajectories for forward CM (a.) and lateral CM (b.)

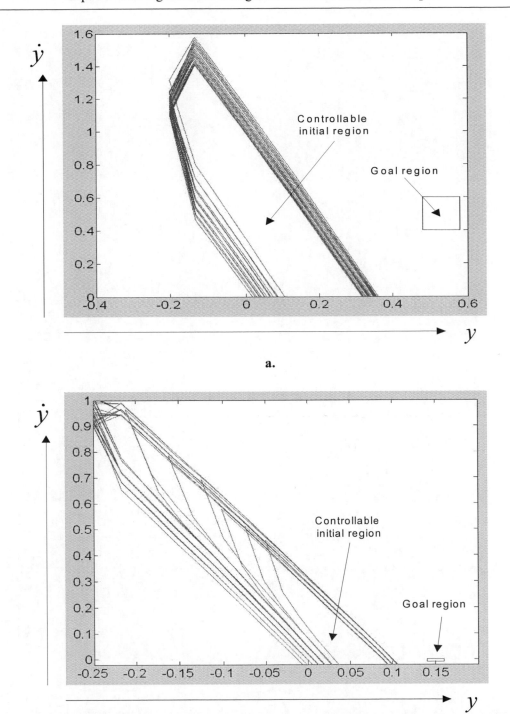

Figure 4.17. Initial flow tube cross sections for soccer ball kicking task.

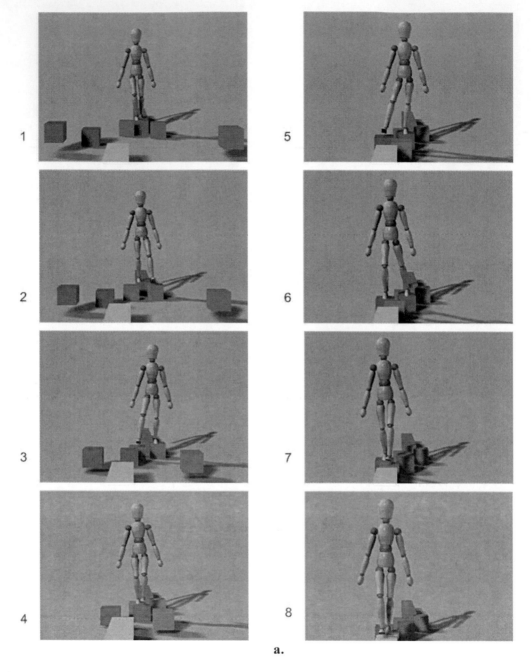

a.

Figure 4.18.a. Walking by stepping on slowly moving blocks: 1) biped starts on long, narrow path; 2) steps with left foot onto the brown block; 3) steps with right foot onto the other brown block; 4) steps with left foot onto the green block; 5, 6) steps with right foot onto the other green block; 7) steps with left foot onto blue block; 8) finished.

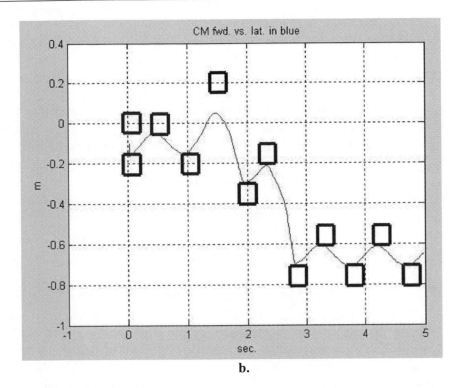

b.

Figure 4.18.a. Walking by stepping on slowly moving blocks: 1) biped starts on long, narrow path; 2) steps with left foot onto the brown block; 3) steps with right foot onto the other brown block; 4) steps with left foot onto the green block; 5, 6) steps with right foot onto the other green block; 7) steps with left foot onto blue block; 8) finished. b. Foot placement and CM trajectory for irregular foot placement test.

Figure 4.15 shows the result of a test execution of this type of task. The QSP is similar to that for walking, except that there is a kick at the end. Figure 4.16 shows the corresponding flow tubes for forward and lateral CM movement, and the state trajectories within these tubes. Figure 4.17 shows initial cross sections for all flow tube sets for the task shown in figure 4.15. If the initial state of the biped is in the controllable initial region, then the task can be achieved in any duration ranging from 0.8 to 1.2 seconds. Such controllability can be used to adjust biped speed depending on the speed of the moving soccer ball, so that the biped arrives at the ball at the right time. If the initial state of the biped is in a subset of the cross sections, then this temporal controllability is more restricted; it is restricted to a tighter range than [0.8, 1.2], and synchronization with the moving soccer ball may be more difficult.

4.5.4. Walking on restricted terrain

Figure 4.18a shows the result of a test where the task requires walking on terrain where foot placement is restricted. The irregular stepping pattern is necessary due to the irregular foot placements required by the blocks that the biped is walking on. These blocks move slowly, so the timing of foot placement, as well as the positioning is important. Timing requirements force the biped to move at a relatively fast speed, of about 0.8 m/s. At this speed, the biped can't just balance statically on each block; the fast speed requires dynamic balancing and coordination of the center of mass trajectory. Figure 4.18b shows the CM trajectory and foot placements for this test. The dynamic nature of this task is indicated by the fact that the CM trajectory barely touches the foot placement polygons, and in one case, is 0.1 m away. This indicates that the system is not statically stable in this pose, and is relying on the subsequent foot placement sequence to maintain balance.

In a subsequent series of tests, we subjected the simulated biped to lateral force disturbances as it was executing this task. Due to the limited base of support in the lateral direction, such a test exercises the system at its weakest point. These tests showed recovery from disturbances as high as 40 N, even if they occurred at in-opportune times. For example, a push from the right to the left when the biped is in left single support is a worst-case test because the right (stepping) foot cannot be placed further to the left to catch the biped. The right foot must be placed on the next available block, which is to the right. Thus, the biped must compensate by moving the ZMP and CMP appropriately, using the techniques demonstrated in Section 5.2.

5. CONCLUSION

This chapter introduced two computation control strategies of biped walking that potentially provide either neuron- or bio- mechanical principles. The first model is to propose a human walking mechanism based on the functional and anatomical plausibilities of neurobiological systems, and the second to propose a hierarchical execution algorithm for biped walking under disturbance by achieving sequential goal tasks.

Each model provides useful insights into biped walking control. The first model proposes a functionally decoupled system of gait execution and balance control. A feedforward pattern generator constructs gait execution while feedback neural systems control balance. The spinal feedback system provides activation synergies that facilitate control by reducing control dimensionality. This allows the gait pattern generator to provide only a few neural command signals, which are then expanded, according to the synergies, into muscle activation signals. The viscoelasticity of the muscles smoothes the effects of command inputs and enables stable and compliant contact with the ground without explicit computation of joint torques or foot forces.

The second model uses an advanced multivariable controller to transform a tightly coupled nonlinear system into a loosely coupled system of local controllers that is much easier to control. This decoupling allows for definition of plan success in terms of synchronized presence of key control variables in goal regions at key points in the gait cycle. Compilation of the qualitative state plan into a qualitative control plan results in a precise specification of operating regions and synchronization requirements that result in successful execution of the plan.

The two models have several common points which we consider to be principal elements for controlling high-performance biped walkers.

First, a gait is represented in terms of distinct control epochs: segmentation of neural command signals into five distinct epochs over a gait cycle in the first model (figure 3.2) is comparable with the five qualitative states in the qualitative state plan in the second model (figure 4.3). This suggests that a human gait is achieved through a sequence of distinct control actions that guide the biped through a corresponding sequence of control epochs. For the first model, this control sequence is generated by the neural pattern generator, for the second model, it is generated by the dispatcher sequencing through the qualitative states. Augmenting the control epochs for a standard gait cycle with new ones enables modified gait behaviors, including ones for kicking moving soccer balls, and for traversing difficult terrain using irregular stepping patterns. The control epochs are defined by events, such as ground contact events, and represent qualitative regions in which important parameters and model structures remain constant. In particular, piecewise linearization according to the control epochs is a powerful concept, utilized by both models.

A second common point between the two models is their hierarchical organization. For the first model, muscle activation is controlled by the spinal feedback system, which provides a layer of control abstraction. This abstraction is used by the neural pattern generator, allowing for generation of fewer control signals. At the highest level, the cerebro-cerebellar (supra-spinal) feedback system ensures that the key balance variables, CM position and body orientation, are close to their desired values. For the second model, the DVMC provides a control abstraction similar to the one provided by the spinal feedback system in the first model. The DVMC provides synergies by automatically converting control signals for key balance variables like CM position and body orientation into joint control signals. The task executive in the second model performs the control epoch sequencing and long loop feedback functions performed by the neural pattern generator and supra-spinal feedback system in the first model. Thus, a key feature of both models is the simplification provided by the lower-level synergistic control layers. In both cases, these synergistic control layers are not dominantly demanding because they are not concerned with gait pattern generation; they simply map higher level gait generation signals into muscle activation or joint control signals. Nevertheless, they provide an important simplification for the higher control levels. Thus, the decoupling provided by the lower levels splits the task of walking control into manageable parts.

A third common point between the two models is that they both focus on control of two important variables: horizontal CM position, and body orientation. Horizontal CM position is important for achieving translational balance control, whereas body orientation is important for maintaining angular stability. In both models, the higher control layers monitor these variables, and issue control actions that directly affect these variables. These control actions are translated into muscle activation or joint control signals by the lower control layers. An important point of difference between the two models is that the second model adds explicit control of the stepping foot, whereas in the first model, stepping foot behavior emerges indirectly. Such an indirect approach is appropriate for level ground walking, but the direct approach used by the second model is necessary for challenging tasks like kicking a moving soccer ball, or working on terrain with constrained foot placements.

A fourth common point between the two models is extensive use of linearization. The first model uses a simple linearization about a small number of possible operating points. The linearization is simple, and as a result, has some error over the entire range of operation. Nevertheless, this simple linearization is adequate for stable walking on level terrain, even in the presence of disturbances, as discussed previously. The DVMC in the second model uses an input-output linearization approach, which is more precise, but which is subject to model error, and can be computationally intensive. From a neuro-physiological standpoint, it is unlikely that humans perform such precise computations [Georgopouls, 1988]. These considerations suggest that it may be worth investigating a more approximate, biologically compatible table-lookup linearization approach for the DVMC. This would replace the computationally intensive input-output linearization, making the DVMC computation faster, but possibly less accurate. The results from the first model suggest that such a loss of accuracy is not crucial for adequate performance.

6. REFERENCES

Allen, G. I. & Tsukahara, N. (1974). Cerebrocerebellar communication systems, *Physiological Review, 54,* 957-1006.

Baxendale, R. H., Ferrell, W. R. (1981). The effect of knee joint afferent discharge on transmission in flexion reflex pathways in decerebrate cats, *Journal of Physiology (London), 315,* 231-242.

Bretzner, F. & Drew, T. (2005). Contribution of the motor cortex to the structure and the timing of hindlimb locomotion in the cat: A microstimulation study, *Journal of Neurophysiology, 94,* 657-672.

Brooke, J. D., Chen, J., Collins, D. F., Mcilroy, W. E., Misiaszek, J. E. & Staines, W. R. (1997). Sensori-sensory afferent conditioning with leg movement: gain control in spinal reflex and ascending paths, *Progress in Neurobiology, 51,* 393-421.

Brown, G. A. (1987). Determination of body segment parameters using computerized tomography and magnetic resonance imaging MIT Master of Science in Mechanical Engineering Thesis.

Calancie, B., Needham-Shropshire, P., Jacobs, P., Willer, K., Zych, G. & Green, B. A. (1994). Involuntary stepping after chronic spinal cord injury: Evidence for a central rhythm generator for locomotion in man, *Brain, 117,* 1143-1159.

Cheung, V., d'Avellar, A., Tresch, M. & Bizzi, E. (2005). Central and sensory contributions to the activation and organization of muscle synergies during natural motor behaviors, *Journal of Neuroscience, 25(27),* 6419-6434.

Clauser, C. E., Mcconville, J. T. & Young, J. W. (1969). Weight, Volume, and Center of Mass Segments of the Human Body. Technical Report AMRL Tech. Report 69-70, Wright-Patterson Air Force Base, OH.

d'Avella, A. Bizzi, E. (2005). Shared and specific muscle synergies in natural motor behaviors, *Proceedings of the National Academy of Sciences of the United States of America, 102(8),* 3076-3081.

d'Avella, A., Saltiel, P. & Bizzi, E. (2003). Combinations of muscle synergies in the construction of a natural motor behavior, *Nature Neuroscience, 6(3),* 300-308.

Dietz, V. & Harkema, S. J. (2004) Locomotor activity in spinal cord-injured persons, *Journal of Applied Physiology, 96,* 1954-1960.

Dimitrijevic, M. R., Gerasimenko, Y. & Pinter, M. M. (1998). Evidence for a spinal central pattern generator in humans, *Annals of the New York Academy of Sciences, 860,* 360-376.

Drew, T. (1993). Motor cortical activity during voluntary gait modifications in the cat. I. Cells related to the forelimbs, *Journal of Neurophysiology, 70,* 179-199.

Duysens, J., Clarac, F. & Cruse, H. (2000). Loading-regulating mechanisms in gait and posture: comparative aspects, *Physiological Review 80(1),* 83-133.

Freitas, S., Durate, M. & Latash, M. L. (2006). Two kinematic synergies in voluntary whole-body movements during standing, *Journal of Neurophysiology 95*, 636-645.

Fuglevand, A. J. & Winter, D. A. (1993) Models of recruitment and rate coding organization in motor-unit pools, *Journal of Neurophysiology 70(6)*, 2470-2488.

Georgopouls, A. P. (1988) Neural integration of movement: role of motor cortex in reaching, *FASEB J, 2*, 2849-2857.

Gilchrist, L. A. & Winter, D. A. (1997) A multisegment computer simulation of normal human gait, *IEEE Transaction on Rehabilitation Engineering 5(4)*, 290-299.

Goswami, A. (1999) Postural stability of biped robots and the foot rotation indicator (FRI) point. *International Journal of Robotics Research, July/August*.

Grasso, R., Ivanenko, Y. P., Zago, M., Molinari, M., Scivoletto, G., Castellano, V., Macellari, V. & Lacquaniti, F. (2004). Distributed plasticity of locomotor pattern generators in spinal cord injured patients, *Brain, 127(5)*, 1019-1034.

Hirai, K. (1997) Current and future perspective of Honda humanoid robot *Proceedings of the 1997 IEEE/RSJ International Conference on Intelligent Robot and Systems* Grenoble, France:IEEE, New York, NY, USA. 500-508.

Hirai, K., Hirose, M., Haikawa, Y. & Takenaka, T. (1998). The development of Honda humanoid robot. *IEEE International Conference on Robotics and Automation (ICRA)*

Hofmann, A. (2005) Robust execution of bipedal walking tasks from biomechanical principles. Ph.D. Thesis, Massachusetts Institute of Technology, Cambridge, Massachusetts, USA.

Hofmann, A., Massaquoi, S., Popovic, M. & Herr, H. (2004) A sliding controller for bipedal balancing using integrated movement of contact and non-contact limbs. *Proc. International Conference on Intelligent Robots and Systems* (IROS). Sendai, Japan.

Huffman, K. J. & Krubitzer, L. (2001). Area 3a: Topographic organization and cortical connections in marmoset monkeys, *Cerebral Cortex, 11(9)*, 849-867.

Ito, M. (1997). Cerebellar microcomplexes, in The cerebellum and cognition. J. D. Schmahmann, Academic Press, 41, 475-487.

Ivanenko, Y. P., Cappellini, G., Dominici, N., Poppele, R. E. & Lacquaniti, F. (2005). Coordination of locomotion with voluntary movements in humans, *Journal of Neuroscience, 25(31)*, 7238-7253.

Ivanenko, Y. P., Poppele, R. E. & Lacquaniti, F. (2004). Five basic muscle activation patterns account for muscle activity during human locomotion, *Journal of Physiology, 56*, 267-282.

Jo, S. (2006). *Hierarchical neural control of human postural balance and bipedal walking in sagittal plane*, Ph.D. Thesis, Massachusetts Institute of Technology, Cambridge, Massachusetts, USA.

Jo, S. & Massaquoi, S. (2004). A model of cerebellum stabilized and scheduled hybrid long-loop control of upright balance, *Biological Cybernetics, 91*, 188-202.

Kagami, S., Kanehiro, F., Tamiya, Y., Inaba, M. & Inoue, H. (2001). AutoBalancer: An online dynamic balance compensation scheme for humanoid robots, in *"Robotics: The Algorithmic Perspective"*, Donald, B. R., Lynch, K. M., and Rus, D., editors, A. K. Peters Ltd. 329 – 340

Kandel, E. R., Schwartz, J. H. & Jessell, T. M. *Principles of neural science*, fourth edition, McGraw-Hill, 2000.

Karameh, F. N. & Massaquoi, S. G. (2005). A model of nonlinear motor cortical integration and its relation to movement speed profile control, *Proceeding of 2005 IEEE Engineering in Medicine and Biology*, 27th Annual conference, Shanghai, China.

Khatib, O., Sentis, L., Park, J. & Warren, J. (2004) Whole body dynamic behavior and control of human-like robots, *International Journal of Humanoid Robotics, 1(1),* 1-15.

Kurzhanski, A. & Varaiya, P. (1992) Ellipsoidal techniques for reachability analysis: Internal approximation, *Systems and Control Letters.*

Leaute, T. (2005) Coordinating agile systems through the model-based execution of temporal plans. Master's Thesis, MIT

Massaquoi, S. G. (1999) Modelling the funcito of the cerebellum in scheduled linear servo control of simple horizontal planar arm movements, PhD thesis, *Electrical Engineering and Computer Science*, MIT, Cambridge, MA.

Massaquoi, S. G. & Topka, H. (2002). Models of cerebellar function. *The cerebellum and its disorders*, M. Pandolfo and M. Manto, Cambridge, U.K., Cambridge University Press, 69-94.

Nathan, P. W. (1994). Effects on movement of surgical incisions into the human spinal cord, *Brain, 117(Pt2)*, 337-346.

Nielsen, J. B. (2003) How we walk: central control of muscle activity during human walking, *Neuroscientist, 9(3)*, 195-204.

Ogihara, N. & Yamazaki, N. (2001). Generation of human bipedal locomotion by bio-mimetic neuron-musculo-skeletal model, *Biological Cybernetics, 84,* 1-11.

Olree, K. S. & Vaughan, C. L. (1995). Fundamental patterns of bilateral muscle activity in human locomotion, *Biological Cybernetics, 73*, 409-414.

Peterson, N. T., Christensen, L. O. & Nielsen, J. (1998). The effect of transcranial magnetic stimulation on the soleus H reflex during human walking, *Journal of Physiology (London) 513(Pt 2)*, 599-610.

Popovic, M., Goswami, A. & Herr, H. (2005) Ground reference points in legged locomotion: definitions, biological trajectories, and control implications. *International Journal of Robotics Research, 24(12)*, 1013-1032.

Porter, R. & Lemon, R. *Corticospinal function and voluntary movement*, New York, Oxford University Press, 1993.

Pratt, J., Dilworth, P. & Pratt, G. (1997). Virtual model control of a bipedal walking robot, *Proc. International Conference on Robotics and Automation (ICRA)*

Rossignol, S., Dubuc, R. & Gossard, J. P. (2006). Dynamic sensorimotor interactions in locomotion, *Physiological Review, 86*, 89-154.

Slotine, J. & Li, W. (1991). *Applied Nonlinear Control*. Ch. 6, Prentice Hall, NJ, USA

Taga, G. (1995). A model of the neuron-musculo-skeletal system for human locomotion I. Emergence of basic gait, *Biological Cybernetics 73,* 97-111.

Takanishi, A., Ishida, M., Yamazaki, Y. & Kato, I. (1985) The realization of dynamic walking by the biped robot WL-10RD. In *International Conference on Advanced Robotics, Tokyo,* 459-466.

Thach, W. T. (1998) What is the role of the cerebellum in motor learning and cognition? *Trends in Cognitive Science, 2,* 331-337.

Tilley, A. R. & Dreyfuss, H. (1993). The measure of man and woman. Whitney Library of Design, an imprint of Watson-Guptill Publications, New York.

Tresch, M. C., Saltiel, P. & Bizzi, E. (1999). The construction of movement by the spinal cord, *Nature Neuroscience, 2*, 162-167.

van der Kooij, H., Jacobs, R., Koopman, B. & van der Helm, F. (2003). An alternative approach to synthesizing bipedal walking. *Biological Cybernetics, 88(1),* 46-59.

Vestal, S. (2001). A new linear hybrid automata reachability procedure. *Hybrid Systems: Computation and Control (HSCC).*

Vukobratovic, M. & Juricic, D. (1969). Contribution to the synthesis of biped gait. *IEEE Transactions on Bio-Medical Engineering, BME-16(1),* 1 – 6.

Williams, B. & Nayak, P. (1997). A reactive planner for a model-based executive. *Proceedings of the International Joint Conference on Artificial Intelligence (IJCAI)*

Winters, D. A. (1990). *Biomechanics and Motor Control of Human Movement.* John Wiley and Sons, Inc., New York.

Yamaguchi, J., Soga, E., Inoue, S. & Takanishi, A. (1999). Development of a bipedal humanoid robot -control method of whole body cooperative dynamic biped walking, *ICRA '99, IEEE,* 368 – 374.

In: Overweightness and Walking
Editor: Caleb I. Black, pp. 151-176

ISBN: 978-1-60741-298-4
© 2010 Nova Science Publishers, Inc.

Chapter 7

GENETIC DETERMINANTS OF OVERWEIGHT RELATED WITH CARDIOVASCULAR DISEASE

Zhaoxia Wang and Tomohiro Nakayama[*]

Nihon University School of Medicine, Tokyo, Japan

ABSTRACT

Overweight is defined as an excess accumulation of body fat. Overweight is a chronic multifactorial complex disease resulting from a long-term positive energy balance, in which both genetic and environmental factors are involved. It increases the risks of cardiovascular disease (CVD), type 2 diabetes, dyslipidemia, arthritis, and certain cancers and ultimately reduces the average life expectancy.

The purpose of the present review focuses on the current status of our knowledge concerning the genetic determinants of overweight related with CVD, including heart disease, vascular disease, atherosclerosis, stroke and hypertension. The review describes the anthropometric measurements of overweight, the sex steroid hormones involved in the distribution of adipose tissues and the occurrence of CVD, the pathogenesis of overweight, the relationship between overweight and CVD, and the environmental and genetic factors involved in regulating overweight development.

Simple anthropometric measurements of overweight that can be used to measure not only the total amount of fat but also the distribution of fat in the body include BMI, waist circumference, and fat mass, among others. Currently, adipose tissue is recognized not only as a storage deposit of excess energy but also as a major endocrine and secretory organ. Sex steroid hormones including the estrogen, progesterone and androgen receptors are involved in the metabolism, accumulation and distribution of adipose tissues. With a decrease in sex steroid hormones, there is a tendency to increase overweight, which is a major risk for CVD. Based on the current knowledge of the pathogenesis of overweight, genetic factor involvement in the development of overweight is estimated to be at the 30-70% level. There are several plausible mechanisms for a causative role for overweight in

[*] Corresponding author: Tomohiro Nakayama, M.D. Ph.D. Division of Laboratory Medicine, Department of Pathology and Microbiology, Nihon University School of Medicine, Nihon University School of Medicine. 30-1 Ooyaguchi- kamimachi, Itabashi-ku, Tokyo 173-8610, Japan. Tel: +81 3-3972-8111 (Ext. 8205); Fax: +81 3-5375-8076. E-mail: tnakayam@med.nihon-u.ac.jp

producing CVD. These include changes in blood pressure, lipids, glucose metabolism, and systemic inflammation. In addition, evidence is emerging that factors produced by adipose tissue in overweight can directly impact the atherogenic environment of the vessel wall through the regulation of gene expression and function in the endothelial cells, arterial smooth muscle, and macrophage cells. There is also substantial support in the literature that adipose tissue distribution plays an important role in atherosclerotic risk. The heredity of overweight is usually due to an interaction of more than 30 multiple candidate genes that are found at different locations on the gene map, and therefore, is considered to be polygenic in nature. At the present time, research is still attempting to determine the gene variants that cause most cases of overweight.

1. INTRODUCTION

Overweight is defined as an excess accumulation of body fat [1]. Over the last two decades, overweight prevalence has increased significantly and has become a global epidemic [2]. In the US, the prevalence of overweight was recently reported to occur in as much as 61% of the population [3]. Overweight is a chronic multifactorial complex disease resulting from a long-term positive energy balance, in which both genetic and environmental factors are involved [4]. It increases the risks of cardiovascular disease (CVD), type 2 diabetes, dyslipidemia, arthritis, and certain cancers and ultimately reduces the average life expectancy [5]. Recently, the rapid development of molecular biology has led to remarkable progress in studies on candidate genes of overweight. This review focuses on the genetic determinants of overweight related with CVD. It will discuss the anthropometric measurements of overweight, the sex steroid hormones involved in the distribution of adipose tissues and the occurrence of CVD, the pathogenesis of overweight, the relationship between overweight and CVD, and the environmental and genetic factors in the regulation and development of overweight.

2. MEASUREMENTS OF OVERWEIGHT

The original definition of overweight for males (android type) and females (gynoid type) dates from the first clinical observations made by J. Vague in 1947. The greatest health risk is associated with fat distribution in the central or upper body (android) parts. Recent research has shown there is an insulin resistance and that hyperinsulinism is the metabolic basis for accelerated atherosclerosis in overweight android types of subjects. Findings have indicated that it is not only the total amount of fat that an individual carries that is important, but also where the fat is distributed within the body. It is difficult to measure fat in the body accurately, and at the present time there is no easily available method for routine clinical use.

Table 1. The numbers of the candidate genes and studies related with the phenotype of overweight

Phenotype/Measurement	Number of genes	Number of studies
BMI	82	230
Obesity	45	76
Body weight	35	66
Body fat	34	48
Waist circumference	28	39
Waist-to-hip ratio	25	32
Fat mass	23	38
Leptin	14	23
Fat-free mass	11	13
Abdominal visceral fat	10	12
Skin folds	10	12
Abdominal subcutaneous fat	7	9
Hip circumference	7	7
Lean mass	7	7
Overweight	6	8
Sagittal abdominal diameter	6	6
Respairatory quotient	5	7
Abdominal total fat	5	6
Basal metabolic rate	5	5
Lipolysis	4	4
Adipocyte size	3	4
Trunk-to-extremity ratio	1	2
Waist-to-height ratio	1	1

Note: Data were calculated based on the last edition of the Human Obesity Gene Map (2005).

There are many methods that can be used to evaluate body fat [6]. Table 1 lists the measurements that have been used to examine overweight. While anthropometric measurements of weight-for-height have been traditionally used to evaluate overweight, more recently, body mass index (BMI) has become the standard parameter. BMI is defined as weight in kilograms divided by height in meters squared. The normal range is 19-24.9 kg/m^2, with overweight defined as 25-29.9 kg/m^2, and obesity as $\geq$30 kg/m^2. In this review, we use a wider concept to define 'overweight', which includes the traditional measurements for being overweight and obese. However, BMI is not always a reliable measurement of body composition in individuals, particularly in older and younger people. Unfortunately, BMI does not give any insight into the regional body fat distribution. There are simple anthropometric measurements that can be used, for example, waist circumference. This parameter can be used to determine a valid index of visceral fat accumulation in addition to being able to serve as an indicator of health risks associated with visceral obesity. A waist circumference of greater than 1020 mm in men or 880 mm in women is a risk factor for CVD. A particularly important anthropometric parameter that has been increasingly applied in recent years is the use of sagittal abdominal diameter (SAD). By using a simple caliper that was originally constructed by Kahn, this anthropometric indicator can measure just the visceral fat tissue. As for other techniques, one of the first that should be considered is the measuring of body density, as this provides information on the relationship between the body mass and the volume. With tetrapolar bioelectric impedance analysis, data is obtained by measuring the resistance of the body exposed to the impact of an alternating current of 50 kHz at a strength of 800 microA. Double photon absorptiometry and X-ray absorptiometry are also precise methods that can be used to determine the body composition, although they require expensive equipment. Additionally, X-ray absorptiometry also exposes the organism to various types of radiation. Radioisotopic techniques use deuterium or tritium as markers to measure the total body liquid and total body potassium. Infrared spectrometry is a simple although not a particularly reliable method that is based on the application of two sources of monochromatic light. Ultrasonographic measuring of fat tissue is currently a very favored technique by which one can measure both the subcutaneous and visceral fat tissue. Measurements are carried out by using a transducer of 7.5 mHz for the subcutaneous and 3.5 mHz for the visceral fat tissue. The most accurate way to measure central overweight is through the use of magnetic resonance imaging or computer-assisted tomography scanning. Unfortunately, this approach is too expensive for routine use.

3. THE ROLE OF SEX STEROID HORMONES IN THE REGULATION OF OVERWEIGHT AND CVD

CVD, which includes heart disease, vascular disease, atherosclerosis, stroke and hypertension, is the most critical global health threat, contributing to more than one-third of the global morbidity. The American Heart Association reports that CVD is the leading cause of death in the United States and causes more than half of all mortality in the world's developed countries [7]. In most cases, these clinical conditions result from atherosclerosis, which is a progressive disease of the arterial wall that is characterized by focal thickening and luminal obstruction [8]. The most important independent risk factors for CVD include overweight, dyslipidemia along with hypertension, sedentary lifestyle, diabetes and chronic inflammation. Furthermore, often times there is a further increased risk when a combination of these independent risk factors are present at the same time.

Health problems associated with being overweight generally are related more to the central (abdominal, omental, visceral) distribution of fat rather than to the amount of fat. The distribution of fat is different between males and females [9]. Men have a more central accumulation of fat, whereas women have a more gluteal/femoral accumulation. Men also have a higher incidence of CVD than women, although menopause in women increases the incidence of CVD and the central distribution of adipose tissue [10]. This epidemiological and clinical evidence strongly suggests a major role for sex steroid hormones in the regulation of adipose tissue distribution. Sex steroid hormones are involved in the metabolism, accumulation and distribution of adipose tissues. As it is now known that the estrogen, progesterone and androgen receptors exist in the adipose tissues [11–15], they may be directly involved with the adipose tissue. Sex steroid hormones employ both genomic and nongenomic mechanisms when carrying out their functions in the adipose tissues [16]. For the genomic mechanism, the sex steroid hormone binds to its receptor with the steroid–

receptor complex then regulating the transcription of the given genes. Leptin and lipoprotein lipase are two key proteins in the adipose tissues that are under the transcriptional control of the sex steroid hormones. A further discussion on the functions and other related studies that have been done on these two proteins is presented in parts 5.3.1 and 5.3.6 of this review. In the nongenomic mechanism, after the sex steroid hormone binds to its receptor in the plasma membrane, second messengers are formed [17].

Normal distribution of body fat exists when sex steroid hormones are present. When a decrease in sex steroid hormones occurs, such as that seen during ageing or gonadectomy, there is a tendency for overweight states to increase, in addition to increases in major risks for CVD, type 2 diabetes and certain cancers. Since sex steroid hormones regulate the amount and distribution of adipose tissues, administration of the hormones or adipose tissue-specific selective receptor modulators could possibly be used to ameliorate overweight conditions. In fact, hormone replacement therapy in postmenopausal women and testosterone replacement therapy in older men appears to reduce the degree of central overweight. However, since these therapies can have numerous side effects, their use is somewhat limited. Therefore, selective receptor modulators of the sex steroid hormones that have fewer side effects and that are more specific for adipose tissues need to be developed.

4. ENVIRONMENTAL AND BEHAVIORAL FACTORS OF OVERWEIGHT RELATED WITH CVD

Overweight is a multifactorial complex disease resulting from environmental, behavioral and genetic factors. Over the last two decades, both our environment along with our behaviors have undergone crucial changes. Both technical conditions and social environments, such as reliance on cars for transportation, computerization within the workplace and at home, building design, lack of sidewalks, advertisements, and pressure to consume, among other things, have created the current global obesogenic environment. Our current lifestyles now favor the adoption of many obesogenic behaviors such as high-fat diets, high intake of simple sugars, sedentarism due to low levels of habitual physical activity, and more time spent watching TV and sitting in front of computers [18]. All these environments and behaviors can significantly influence CVD.

Furthermore, epidemiological studies have recently shown that various drugs, chemicals, and pollutants can also affect the prevalence of CVD [19,20], insulin resistance, metabolic syndrome and diabetes [21–24]. Exposure to tobacco smoke, which contains the carcinogenic environmental agents arsenic and dioxin, along with exposure to ionizing radiation have been proven to be atherogens [25,26]. In addition, air pollution exposure is increasingly being recognized as a risk factor for the development of specific cardiac events [27], including life-threatening arrhythmia [28,29] and myocardial infarction [30]. However, the mechanisms of the vascular injury and proatherogenic effects from environmental toxins have yet to be fully clarified. Many of the mechanisms of adverse cardiovascular effects are believed to be associated with inflammation and oxidative stress [31].

5. POLYGENETIC FACTORS OF OVERWEIGHT RELATED WITH CVD

Interactions between genes and environmental factors can result in overweight and CVD. The polygenic nature of overweight and related cardiovascular risk makes it unlikely that just a single gene could be responsible for the development of these diseases. It is more plausible that there are multiple genes, each with their own small effect, that when combined with other factors lead to modifications that ultimately cause disease development.

5.1. The Pathogenesis of Overweight

In overweight subjects, excess adipose tissue and serum lipoprotein have a close relationship. Although an excess of energy is sufficiently buffered and stored in the adipose tissue initially, evidence of overload is already present at this point. An increased production of apoB-containing lipoprotein particles that transport triglycerides to adipose tissue can lead to an increase in LDL (low-density lipoprotein) particles if the adipose tissue is able to maintain a fast conversion of the VLDL (very low-density lipoprotein) compartment to higher densities via extraction of triglycerides. Due to this conversion, the newly secreted apoB can be rapidly shifted to the LDL fraction [32]. When adipose tissue capacity is surpassed by the buffering demands, the conversion of VLDL and similar particles slows down, and patients exhibit a well-known increase in triglyceride rich particles. Eventually, new surrogate storage depots, such as the liver and to a lesser extent the skeletal muscle, are used for the excess fat. Fatty liver disease further leads to steatohepatitis, which is the generic response of an overloaded system.

Today, adipose tissue is now recognized as not only a storage depot for excess energy but also as a major endocrine and secretory organ [33]. This organ can release a wide range of protein factors and signals, termed adipokines, in addition to fatty acids and other lipid moieties [34]. These factors are derived from adipocyte or non-adipocyte fractions, and include proteins, metabolites and hormones [35]. Adipose tissue areas also seem to differ with regard to their main functions. While all of the areas appear to share common properties and capacities, apparently the visceral fat is more active in terms of accepting and releasing free fatty acids [36,37]. Visceral fat is in a privileged situation for receiving fat input and releasing free fatty acids in a metabolically secured circulation. The liver processes the blood from this area [38] and thus, the rest of the body is prevented from an excessive exposure to these free fatty acids. Since massive energy storage takes place in the subcutaneous adipose tissue, the buffering capacity of the visceral adipose tissue is preserved. However, when storage capacity of the former becomes exhausted, the visceral area is then forced to take over and its buffering capacity is blunted. Individual and gender differences determine the subcutaneous fat capacity and therefore, the point at which the energy starts to be stored in visceral fat can vary [39]. Although men have an inferior subcutaneous fat storage capacity due to evolutionary requirements of reproduction biology [40], men start to accumulate fat in the visceral depot far earlier than women [41]. If a sequential repletion of adipose depots occurs, this would explain the coincidence of increased visceral adiposity that is seen in the syndrome in addition to the apparent protection that is derived from the increased subcutaneous (and mainly lower-body) deposits [42,43]. In fact, in overweight subjects, the whole body fat mass contributes to an increased glucose uptake that somehow is able to compensate for the insulin resistance effect [44]. Therefore, while visceral obesity can be linked to the syndrome phenomenologically, it is only partially causative.

5.2. The Relationship between Overweight and CVD

Overweight is an independent risk factor for CVD. The link between overweight and the development of atherosclerosis that results in CVD has been well established. The mechanism of this relationship is indicated in Figure 1. The link between overweight and macrovascular disease has been demonstrated by using imaging approaches. This discovery has led to the expansion of opportunities for investigating potential mechanisms by which excess adipose tissue adversely impacts the vessel wall and for evaluating how adipose tissue distribution or reduction (weight loss) impact atherosclerosis. In overweight subjects, there are a number of consequences that have been shown to accelerate atherosclerosis, including hypertension, diabetes, and dyslipidemia [45,46].

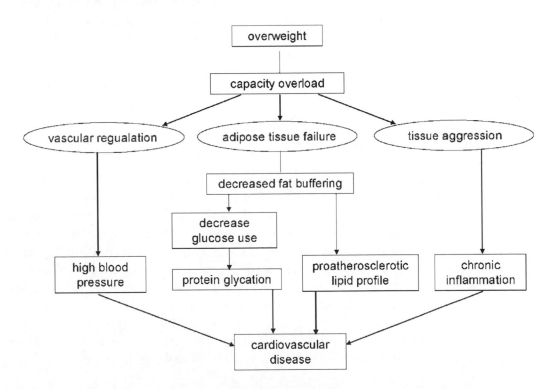

Figure 1. The mechanisms in the relationship between overweight and cardiovascular disease.

The National Cholesterol Education Program Adult Treatment Panel III (2002) published updated guidelines for the treatment of lipid disorders, greatly expanding the number of subjects eligible for therapy [47]. In the new recommendations, several important changes have been made in the way subjects at risk for CVD are identified and subsequently managed. Although the National Cholesterol Education Program Adult Treatment Panel III (2002) maintains that LDL cholesterol should be the primary target of any lipid-lowering therapy, it identifies non-HDL-cholesterol (HDL-C) as a secondary target in patients with elevated triacylglycerols. It is now recommended that subjects with two or more CVD risk factors be assessed for 10-year absolute CVD risk based on the Framingham Point Scale [48]. This methodology helps to identify those individuals who require more aggressive treatment. Lipoproteins are macromolecular complexes of lipids and proteins that originate mainly from the liver and intestine, and they are involved in the transport and redistribution of lipids within the body [49]. Lipid and lipoprotein metabolism can be viewed as a complex biological pathway containing multiple steps. Lipid homeostasis is achieved by the coordinated action of a large number of nuclear factors, binding proteins, apoenzymes and receptors [50]. Lipid metabolism is also closely linked with energy metabolism and is subjected to many hormonal controls that are essential for adjustment to environmental and internal conditions [51]. Genetic variability has been found for components regulating plasma lipid levels in men. The challenge has been to find not only which variants but also how many are required in order to be able to forecast CVD risk and be able to successfully recommend treatments. Judging from the current status of the field, this challenge will continue for years to come. Additionally, although the pathogenesis of the relationship between postprandial triacylglycerol rich lipoprotein (TRL) and CVD remains unclear, experimental evidence has been able to provide several plausible mechanisms. Atherogenic effects may be mediated directly by TRL particles or components of the particles. A variety of in vitro and clinical studies suggest that postprandial chylomicrons and VLDL are associated with adverse effects on the arterial endothelium [52,53]. Incubation with remnant lipoproteins has been shown to induce an elevation in the expression of intercellular adhesion molecule-1, vascular cell adhesion molecule-1 and tissue factor in a human umbilical vein endothelial cell model, in part through a redox-sensitive mechanism [54]. Furthermore, indirect mechanisms of TRL atherogenicity may be related to metabolic changes associated with the presence of postprandial TRL [55].

Numerous studies have demonstrated that excess adipose tissue is responsible for increasing cardiovascular deaths in adolescents and adults up to 75 years of age [56–59]. A number of more recent studies have specifically reported on the effect of excess adipose tissue on direct measures of macrovascular disease [60-62]. BMI was associated with both fatty streaks and raised lesions in the right coronary artery and stenosis in the left anterior descending artery. Systemic inflammation and the production of adipokines by adipose tissue have been considered to be important mechanisms involved in adverse effects of adiposity on the vessel wall. In addition, these same adipose tissue-derived factors have been shown to influence gene expression and cell function in endothelial cells, arterial smooth muscle cells, and monocytes/macrophages. These represent the major cell types of the artery wall and are key components involved in the defense of vessel wall homeostasis.

5.3. Roles of Genetic Factors in the Development of Overweight Related with CVD

The regulation of body weight and energy homeostasis is subject to complex regulatory mechanisms that maintain the balance between energy intake, energy expenditure and energy stores. As has been shown in animal models and in human studies, genetic factors play an important role in this regulation as well as in the development of overweight [63]. Based on current pathogenesis studies, it has been estimated that 30-70% of the development of overweight is related to the involvement of genetic factors [64,65].

The last edition of the Human Obesity Gene Map, which was published in October of 2005, reported that more than 600 loci from single-gene mutations in mouse models of obesity, non-syndromic human obesity cases due to single-gene mutations, obesity related Mendelian disorders, transgenic and knockout mice models, QTLs from cross-breeding experiments and genome-wide scans, and genes or markers are associated or linked with the obesity phenotype [66]. The number of studies that have reported associations between DNA sequence variation in specific genes and obesity phenotypes has also increased considerably, with 426 findings of positive associations with 127 candidate genes. Based on the current results of the last edition of the Human Obesity Gene Map, we calculated the numbers of candidate genes and studies related with the phenotype of overweight. As seen in Table 1, we found that most research determinations of overweight applied simple anthropometric measurements such as BMI, body weight, body fat, waist circumference, waist-to-hip ratio, and fat mass. These measurements reflect the visceral fat accumulation and can be used as an indicator of health risks associated with visceral obesity. Although rarely seen, there were some indices that measured the levels of serum hormone and the metabolic rate. Many studies have suggested that these measurements indicate a certain degree of relationship between overweight and CVD [67]. We believe that with continued development of new techniques for measuring overweight, the mechanism of the relationship between overweight and CVD will become much clearer.

Over the last few years, genetic methods based on chip technology have been exponentially developed. With a growing number of genes and loci indexed in the gene map, it has been possible to replicate several genes and QTLs that were identified from association and genome scan studies. The large number of genes and loci depicted in the overweight gene map provides a good indication of the complexity of the task that has to be undertaken in order to identify genes associated with an overweight susceptibility. Although false positive associations are abundant in the literature, 20% to 30% of these genetic associations have been shown to have modest but real effects on common disease risk [68]. This would suggest that perhaps as many as 20 to 30 of the overweight candidate genes that have been identified in this report could contribute to the risk of overweight in humans. There are increasing numbers of other loci that continue to be reported, but due to space limitation, it is not possible to provide a comprehensive description of all of these overweight candidate genes that might be related to CVD.

5.3.1. Leptin (LEP) Gene

Leptin is a recently discovered protein hormone that is the product of the obese gene. It is mainly produced in adipose tissues and plays a key role in the regulation of food intake, energy expenditure and body weight homeostasis [69]. Therefore, the amount of leptin is related to the amount and distribution of body fat. The increased plasma leptin levels that occur with overweight have been positively associated with cardiovascular complications in humans. In addition, this effect has been observed independent of BMI and traditional cardiac risk factors [70].

Similar to that described for resistin, leptin has also been found to have multiple effects on cells of the artery wall. Recent studies that measured coronary artery calcium have demonstrated that hyperleptinemia was associated with coronary atherosclerosis, with the association determined to be independent of insulin resistance [71,72]. Other studies have shown that leptin may have a role in neointimal formation in response to arterial injury [73]. In endothelial cells, leptin induces oxidative stress, increases production of MCP-1 and endothelin-1, and potentiates proliferation [74–77]. In smooth muscle cells, leptin promotes migration, proliferation and hypertrophy [56]. Leptin also contributes to increases in activation and cytokine production by macrophages, neutrophils, and T lymphocytes [78–80]. It also promotes calcification of cells of the vascular wall and facilitates thrombosis by increasing platelet aggregation [81,82]. All these effects of leptin point to a proatherogenic role.

Since the identification of the LEP gene at 7q31.3 as the human homolog to the mouse obesity (ob) gene [83], sequence variation in LEP has been studied extensively. Although mutations in the LEP gene are known to cause rare obesity syndromes [84,85] and be responsible for obesity in several animal models [86], LEP variations are exceedingly rare within the general population [87-89]. The interest in LEP as a susceptibility gene for human obesity has also led to the identification of several common polymorphisms in the 5' regulatory region, G2548A, A19G, and C1887T. These regions have been shown to have an association with lower LEP levels or obesity in several studies [90-93]. Although the results from these studies remain controversial, evidence does strongly support the relationship between the LEP sequence variation and CVD.

Furthermore, there are different functions of leptin that depend upon different genders. Estrogen appears to increase leptin production, while androgen appears to decrease its production. However, many discrepancies exist in the data for these previous studies. If sex steroid hormones are indeed directly regulating the production of leptin, then a sex steroid hormone response element should be present in the leptin gene. After reviewing the cDNA sequence of the leptin gene, we found there was a consensus sequence for the estrogen response element in its promoter region [94]. The transfection of a leptin-luciferase reported the construction into ER-positive MCF-7 breast cancer cells and in estrogen receptor (ER)-negative JEG-3 choriocarcinoma cells, which normally produce leptin [95]. Overall, these results suggest that 1) the leptin gene has an estrogen response element, 2) leptin promoter activation may depend upon coactivators present in the leptin-producing cells, and 3) different effects of estrogen may be due to the actual type of ER that is expressed in the target tissue.

5.3.2. Adiponectin Gene

SNPs of the adiponectin gene have been widely studied in relation with overweight. Adiponectin is a product of adipocytes, and its level in humans is decreased in overweight subjects [96]. There are 3 different oligomers for adiponectin, each of which may have a different biologic function [97,98]. Levels of adiponectin increase with weight loss or with pharmacological treatment of insulin resistance. Adiponectin has been shown to have a role in regulating systemic substrate metabolism, and as several recent publications have suggested, it may also have a role in modulating the cardiovascular system.

As might be expected based on the above observations, adiponectin promotes an antiatherogenic and antiinflammatory program of gene expression and function in the vessel wall cells. Adiponectin downregulates expression of adhesion molecules on the endothelial cells and thereby reverses the effects of resistin [99]. Adiponectin also reduces proliferation in a receptor-independent fashion in the vascular smooth muscle cells [100,101] and can reduce lipid accumulation along with downregulating the expression of scavenger receptors in macrophages [102]. Additionally, adiponectin also reduces endothelial oxidative stress and proliferation [103,104]. Studies have shown that adiponectin levels were inversely correlated to the progression of coronary artery calcium in both diabetic and nondiabetic subjects [105]. Adiponectin levels after treatment with insulin sensitizers have also been shown to be the best predictor of improvement in the carotid arterial wall stiffness and when there are mutations of the adiponectin gene, they are strongly associated with coronary artery disease in humans [106]. In an experiment using the homeostasis model assessment to determine insulin resistance, HDL cholesterol and high-molecular-weight adiponectin levels were found to be positively correlated, while both total serum adiponectin and high-molecular-weight adiponectin levels were negatively correlated with triglyceride and circulating inflammatory markers [97,98]" Serum high-molecular-weight adiponectin level is significantly lower in men with coronary artery disease, a finding that was independent of other cardiac risk factors [107].

The heritabilities for the genetic component of the adiponectin levels have been estimated to be in the range of 40-70% [108]. While several whole genome scans have been carried out in order to identify specific loci, the results have not been consistent [109-111]. More recent genome scans have indicated that the link can be explained by variations in the adiponectin gene (ADIPOQ) [112,113]. The associations between some of these ADIPOQ polymorphisms and overweight-related phenotypes have been the subject of several recent reviews [114,115].

Although the relationship between adiponectin plasma concentrations and the presence of overweight is well established, the evidence linking the ADIPOQ gene locus with adiponectin levels, overweight, and the prevalence of CVD has yet to be completely clarified [116,117]. For example the situation that has been described for the 276G>T (rs1501299) and 45T>G (rs2241766) SNPs exemplify the controversial status of the other polymorphisms in the ADIPOQ gene. While these two SNPs are the ones that have been studied the most, there are other population specific SNPs that have also been found to have interesting associations. The 276T minor allele was found to be significantly associated with lower fasting glucose and HOMA-IR in Korean subjects [118], with lesser T2DM risk in Japanese [119] and with a lower risk of coronary artery disease among Italian [120] and American [121] diabetic subjects. Other studies carried out by Lacquemant et al. [122] in France and by Ohashi et al. [123] in Japan did not find any significant association between the 276G>T polymorphism and the risk of CVD. Conversely, Filippi et al. [124] found in a large case-control study that the 276G>T polymorphism was associated with lower adiponectin levels, worse clinical profiles and increased coronary artery disease in Italian subjects. The controversy is even more marked for the 45T>G polymorphism, which consists of a synonymous mutation in exon 2 (Gly15Gly). Although there have been numerous studies no significant association between the 45T>G polymorphism and adiponectin concentrations was reported [125,126]. Overall, it appears that the locus is related to a cluster of phenotypes spanning plasma adiponectin levels, abdominal overweight and the risk of CVD. However, at the present time the support for these findings is not unanimous [113]. The final outcomes might depend on very distant mechanisms of the homeostatic system. In fact, it has proven really difficult to be able to capture differences in the highly regulated system that have been previously described, as there are many other relevant factors that could potentially modulate these associations.

5.3.3. Perilipin (PLIN A) Gene

The perilipin gene is emerging as a potential major player for overweight and other metabolic traits [127]. In the late 1980s, Londos' laboratory first identified a heavily PKA-phosphorylated protein that they named as perilipin (PLIN A). The name resulted from its physical location surrounding lipid droplets [128]. PLIN A was only found in adipocytes and in steroidogenic cells [129]. These cells possess intracellular neutral lipid storage deposits that are metabolized by hormone sensitive lipase (HSL) in adipocytes and by cholesterol esterase in steroidogenic cells, respectively [130,131].

Due to differential splicing, the PLIN A gene generates four different products (Perilipin A, B, C and D) that play a critical role in the hydrolysis of neutral lipids. In agreement with functional studies in cultured cells, perilipin knockout mice showed that an absence of perilipin resulted in leanness, increased basal lipolysis, enhanced leptin production, and resistance to diet-induced overweight. It also reversed overweight in a genetic model of overweight caused by leptin resistance [132] in addition to presenting an increased risk of glucose intolerance and peripheral IR [133]. These data suggest that the PLIN gene may have a role in modulating adipose tissue functions in humans. We have investigated the association of various PLIN polymorphisms with measures of overweight, lipid metabolism and insulin sensitivity in independent samples from Caucasian and Asian subjects [134–138]. In normal subjects from a Mediterranean Spanish population [134] we have reported that PLIN1:6209T>C (rs2289487) and PLIN4:11482G>A (rs894160) polymorphisms were significantly associated with lower body mass index in women. The same was true for the rare allele A carriers at PLIN4 (11482A). Moreover, the PLIN4 variant was associated with significantly lower waist-to-hip ratio, plasma glucose, and triglyceride concentrations in these normal weight subjects. In addition, PLIN1 and PLIN4 variants were associated with a lower overweight risk in women. It appears that when the variant allele is present, there is a higher resistance to both storing and/or mobilizing fat. Furthermore, PLIN variation is also responsible for a higher susceptibility to IR in Asian women who consume a high-saturated fat, low carbohydrate diet [127]. This finding confirms the observation that when under chronic dietary stress, subjects with the variant allele present a worse metabolic response. This genetic variability is also related to changes in the functional capacity of the adipose tissue that are only expressed when an excess of work stresses the system.

5.3.4. Peroxisome Proliferator-Activated Receptor-Gamma2 Isoform (PPAR-2) Gene

Gene–diet interactions play an important role on phenotypes related to overweight and metabolic syndrome [139,140]. In particular, peroxisome proliferator-activated receptor-gamma2 isoform (PPAR-2) has been shown to be one of the most promising candidate genes and is an excellent example of the relevance of the gene–nutrient interactions [141]. PPAR-2 regulates not only the adipocyte differentiation but also the metabolism of lipid and glucose.

Among several variants in the PPAR-2 gene that are related with overweight, the Pro12Ala polymorphism has been proven to be associated with increased insulin sensitivity and reduced risk for the development of diabetes [142,143]. Presumably, it may have a protective effect on myocardial infarction. The Quebec Family Study [144] found higher values for the BMI, visceral adipose tissue area, waist circumference and fasting glucose concentrations in the Pro12 homozygotes. These associations were not observed among the carriers of the Ala allele. In addition, unlike the subjects with the Pro12 allele, the carriers of the Ala allele did not respond to a higher fat diet. Another recent randomized controlled trial [145] enrolled 522 subjects with impaired glucose tolerance and then randomly assigned each to an intensive diet and exercise intervention group or to a control group. By year 3 of the intervention, the odds ratio for the development of type 2 diabetes in subjects with the Ala allele was found to be twofold higher as compared to those with the Pro12Pro genotype. However, none of the Ala12 homozygotes in the study developed diabetes during the trials that examined dietary and exercise intervention. The findings of this study provide strong support for a gene-diet weight-related interaction in subjects with the Pro12Ala polymorphism of PPAR-2.

5.3.5. The GR Gene (GRL)

Since 19 mutations in the GR gene (GRL) were first reported in 1991, a number of other mutations within the human GRL gene have been described [146]. Weaver and colleagues performed the first study to find a potential association between the GRL gene mutation and components associated with overweight [147]. In the Quebec Family Study, the 4.5 kb allele was found to be associated with a higher abdominal visceral fat (AVF) area in both men and women, which was independent of the total body fat mass [148]. Examination of the total variance in the AVF area in these subjects found that the polymorphism accounted for 41% and 35% of the variance in men and women, respectively. However, the association between the 1220A>G polymorphism in exon 2 and overweight has been further hampered by contradictory results in recent years, even though the vast majority of reports were negative [149,150]. In addition, the number of these negative findings continues to rise [151–156]. In spite of any functional effects for the 1220A>G receptor variant [157–161], there are only a few studies that have presented data indicating there is a marginal association between this polymorphism and overweight [162,163]. Unfortunately, these results are not really all that statistically robust. In a recent prospective study, female subjects with the GRL BclI polymorphism were found to have a substantial increase in body weight, subcutaneous adiposity, and fat mass [164]. A significantly higher BMI was seen in the polymorphism carriers when compared to the noncarriers [159]. In a further study that examined the mutated GRL gene in a group of white Australians who were of Anglo-Celtic extraction, the authors suggested that the gene conferred a nearly absolute likelihood of being overweight [165].

5.3.6. Lipoprotein Lipase (LPL) Gene

Lipoprotein lipase (LPL) is the key enzyme for the hydrolysis of circulating triglycerides into free fatty acids and glycerol [166]. LPL has the highest activity in adipose tissues, and in the heart and skeletal muscle. It plays an important role in adipocyte lipid storage and supplying muscle fuel and thereby, plays a role in the regulation of lean muscle mass and overweight.

The hormonal control of LPL in adipose tissues is very complex and involves regulation that occurs at the transcriptional and post-transcriptional levels [167]. In general, cortisol and insulin appear to promote lipid accumulation by increasing the activity of LPL, while growth hormone and estrogen appear to exert the opposite effect [168]. In human subjects, postheparin LPL activity has proven to be a convenient way to study LPL regulation by the sex steroid hormones. In obese women, fasting postheparin plasma LPL activity showed an inverse correlation with plasma estradiol levels and a positive correlation with plasma-free testosterone [169]. In addition, different sex steroid hormones exhibited different functions with regard to the regulation of LPL. Although it is well documented that sex steroid hormones regulate the activity of LPL, it is not clear whether the regulation is direct or indirect, and if direct, whether the regulation is genomic or nongenomic. Estrogen generally decreases the production of LPL in adipose tissues in both rats and humans. If sex steroid hormones are going to directly regulate LPL, a sex steroid hormone response element should be present in the LPL genome. Homma et al. [170] prepared a pLPL-CAT construct, along with an ER expression vector, and introduced this into differentiated fat cells. Estrogen markedly decreased the LPL mRNA in the genetically manipulated cells. A search of the LPL promoter for an estrogen response element did not find a classical ERE but did demonstrate the presence of an AP-1-like TGAATTC sequence that was responsible for the suppression of the LPL gene transcription by estrogen. The effects of androgens on LPL in adipose tissues are less clear because of the aromatization of androgen to estrogen. However, when an aromatase inhibitor was given to men along with testosterone, LPL activity was increased in postheparin plasma, suggesting that androgens may increase LPL production in adipose tissues.

Associations have been reported between LPL polymorphisms and lipid fractions and CVD risk in a population-based cohort, case-control, and cross-sectional studies [171–173]. These studies have shown that there are significant relationships between the T-93G (rs1800590), D9N (rs1801177), G188E, N291S (rs268), PvuII (rs285), HindIII (rs320), and S447X (rs328) polymorphisms and high-density lipoprotein cholesterol, triglycerides, myocardial infarction, and coronary stenosis. Carriers of 9N or 291S have modestly adverse lipid profiles, while carriers of the less common allele of HindIII or of 447X have modestly advantageous profiles. These LPL genotype studies confirm the existence of a close interrelationship between the high-density lipoprotein cholesterol and triglyceride pathways. Additionally, all of these results demonstrate that LPL is a key enzyme in lipoprotein metabolism and a major candidate gene for overweight related with CVD.

6. CONCLUSION

Despite remarkable progress in the diagnosis and treatment of overweight and CVD, they remain the most critical global health threats, as they contribute to more than one-third of the global morbidity. Thanks to the remarkable progress that has been made in gene studies, numerous possible susceptibility genes for overweight have been identified [174,175]. Genetic variants or single nucleotide polymorphisms in many candidate genes have also been found to be associated with increased or decreased risks for overweight related with CVD. This review summarizes the actual findings on the genetic background of overweight related with CVD. It has been demonstrated that polymorphisms of several candidate genes of overweight can affect weight loss and maintenance in response to weight reducing programs. Because of the differences of ethnicity, gender, age, levels of adiposity, absence or presence of concomitant disorders, there have been some discordant results reported in some previous studies. Although the results are not completely consistent, a meta-analysis on already published data could perhaps bring resolution of the contrary findings. By improving our knowledge on genetic determinants of the overweight related with CVD, we expect to be able to better assist in the development of more effective and individually tailored therapeutic strategies.

REFERENCES

[1]   Pi-Sunyer FX. Obesity: criteria and classification. *Proc Nutr Soc* 2000; 59:505–509.

[2]   WHO: Prevalence of excess body weight and obesity in children and adolescents. Fact Sheet No. 2.3, May 2007. *www.euro.who.int*

[3]   Wyatt HR. The prevalence of obesity. *Prim Care* 2003; 30:267–279.

[4]   Barsh GS; Farooqi IS; O'Rahilly S. Genetics of body-weight regulation. *Nature* 2000; 404:644–651.

[5]   Yanovski SZ; Yanovski JA. Obesity. *N Engl J Med* 2002; 346:591–602.

[6]   Ivković-Lazar T. Current diagnostic methods of the specific distribution of adipose tissue. *Med Pregl* 2000; 53:584–587.

[7]   *Heart Disease and Stroke Statistics – Update, American Heart Association*, Dallas, TX, 2004.

[8]   R Ross. Atherosclerosis – an inflammatory disease. *N Engl J Med* 1999; 340:115–126.

[9]   Bjorntorp P. The regulation of adipose tissue distribution in humans. *Int J Obes* 1996; 20:291–302.

[10]   Tchernof A; Poehlman ET; Despres JP. Body fat distribution, the menopause transition, and hormone replacement therapy. *Diabetes Metab* 2000; 26:12–20.

[11]   Wade GN; Gray JM. Cytoplasmic 17b-[3H] estradiol binding in rat adipose tissues. *Endocrinology* 1978; 103:1695–1701.

[12]   Watson GH; Manes JL; Mayes JS; McCann JP. Biochemical and immunological characterization of oestrogen receptor in the cytosolic fraction of gluteal, omental and perirenal adipose tissues from sheep. *J Endocrinol* 1993; 139:107–115.

[13]   Mayes JS; McCann JP; Ownbey TC; Watson GH. Regional differences and up-regulation of progesterone receptors in adipose tissues from oestrogen-treated sheep. *J Endocrinol* 1996; 148:19–25.

[14]   Pedersen SB; Fuglsig S; Sjogren P; Richelsen B. Identification of steroid receptors in human adipose tissue. *Eur J Clin Invest* 1996; 26:1051–1056.

[15]   McCann JP; Mayes JS; Hendricks GR; Harjo JB; Watson GH. Subcellular distribution and glycosylation pattern of androgen receptor from sheep omental adipose tissue. *J Endocrinol* 2001; 169:587–593.

[16]   Luconi M; Forti G; Baldi E. Genomic and nongenomic effects of estrogens: molecular mechanisms of action and clinical implications for male reproduction. *J Steroid Biochem Mol Biol* 2002; 80:369–381.

[17]   Pietras RJ; Nemere I; Szego CM. Steroid hormone receptors in target cell membranes. *Endocrine* 2001; 14:417–427.

[18]   Bouchard L; Tremblay A; Bouchard C; Perusse L. Contribution of several candidate polymorphisms in the determination of adiposity changes: results from the Quebec Family Study. *Int J Obes* 2007; 31:891–899.

[19] Joshipura KJ; Ascherio A; Manson JE; Stampfer MJ; Rimm EB; Speizer FE; Hennekens CH; Spiegelman D; Willett WC. Fruit and vegetable intake in relation to risk of ischemic stroke. *JAMA* 1999; 282:1233–1239.

[20] Bhatnagar A. Environmental cardiology: studying mechanistic links between pollution and heart disease, *Circ Res* 2006; 99:692–705.

[21] Ramos KS; Partridge CR; Teneng I. Genetic and molecular mechanisms of chemical atherogenesis. *Mutat Res* 2007; 621:18–30.

[22] Lee DH; Lee IK; Song K; Steffes M; Toscano W; Baker BA; Jacobs DR. A strong dose–response relation between serum concentrations of persistent organic pollutants and diabetes: results from the national health and examination survey 1999–2002. *Diabetes Care* 2006; 29:1638–1644.

[23] Lee DH; Lee IK; Jin SH; Steffes M; Jacobs DR Jr. Association between serum concentrations of persistent organic pollutants and insulin resistance among nondiabetic adults: results from the national health and nutrition examination survey. *Diabetes Care* 2007; 30:622–628.

[24] Lee DH; Lee IK; Porta M; Steffes M; Jacobs DR. Relationship between serum concentrations of persistent organic pollutants and the prevalence of metabolic syndrome among non-diabetic adults: results from the National Health and Nutrition Examination Survey 1999–2002. *Diabetologia* 2007; 50:1841–1851.

[25] Martinet W; Knaapen MW; De Meyer GR; Herman AG; Kockx MM. Elevated levels of oxidative DNA damage and DNA repair enzymes in human atherosclerotic plaques, *Circulation* 2002; 106:927–932.

[26] Mastin JP. Environmental cardiovascular disease, *Cardiovasc. Toxicol* 2005; 5:91–94.

[27] Jones OA; Maguire ML; Griffin JL. Environmental pollution and diabetes: a neglected association. *Lancet* 2008; 371:287–288.

[28] Franchini M; Mannucci PM. Short-term effects of air pollution on cardiovascular diseases: outcomes and mechanisms. *J Thromb Haemostasis* 2007; 5:2169–2174.

[29] Dockery DW; Pope CA; Xu X; Spengler JD; Ware JH; Fay ME; Ferris BJ; Speizer FE. An association between air pollution and mortality in six US cities. *N Engl J Med* 1993; 329:1753–1759.

[30] Peters A; Fröhlich M; Döring A; Immervoll T; Wichmann HE; Hutchinson WL; Pepys MB; Koenig W. Particulate air pollution is associated with an acute phase response in men; results from the MONICA-Augsburg Study. *Eur Heart J* 2001; 22:1198–1204.

[31] Zanobetti A; Schwartz AJ. The effect of particulate air pollution on emergency admissions formyocardial infarction: amulticity case-crossover analysis, *Environ. Health Perspect* 2005; 113:978–982.

[32] Parhofer KG; Barrett PH. Thematic review series: patient-oriented research. What we have learned about VLDL and LDL metabolism from human kinetics studies. *J Lipid Res* 2006; 47:1620–1630.

[33] Hutley L; Prins JB. Fat as an endocrine organ: relationship to the metabolic syndrome. *Am J Med Sci* 2005; 330:280–289.

[34] Trayhurn P. Endocrine and signalling role of adipose tissue: new perspectives on fat. *Acta Physiol Scand* 2005; 184:285–293.

[35] Ronti T; Lupattelli G; Mannarino E. The endocrine function of adipose tissue: an update. *Clin Endocrinol* (Oxf) 2006; 64:355–365.

[36] Hansen E; Hajri T; Abumrad NN. Is all fat the same? The role of fat in the pathogenesis of the metabolic syndrome and type 2 diabetes mellitus. *Surgery* 2006; 139:711–716.

[37] Regitz-Zagrosek V; Lehmkuhl E; Weickert MO. Gender differences in the metabolic syndrome and their role for cardiovascular disease. *Clin Res Cardiol* 2006; 95:136–147.

[38] Kabir M; Catalano KJ; Ananthnarayan S; Kim SP; Van Citters GW; Dea MK. Molecular evidence supporting the portal theory: a causative link between visceral adiposity and hepatic insulin resistance. *Am J Physiol Endocrinol Metab* 2005; 288:E454–461.

[39] Romanski SA; Nelson RM; Jensen MD. Meal fatty acid uptake in adipose tissue: gender effects in nonobese humans. *Am J Physiol Endocrinol Metab* 2000; 279:E455–462.

[40] Wells JC. The evolution of human fatness and susceptibility to obesity: an ethological approach. *Biol Rev Camb Philos Soc* 2006; 81:183–205.

[41] Jensen MD. Adipose tissue and fatty acid metabolism in humans. *J R Soc Med* 2002; 95:3–7.

[42] Seidell JC; Perusse L; Despres JP; Bouchard C. Waist and hip circumferences have independent and opposite effects on cardiovascular disease risk factors: the Quebec Family Study. *Am J Clin Nutr* 2001; 74:315–321.

[43] McCarty MF. A paradox resolved: the postprandial model of insulin resistance explains why gynoid adiposity appears to be protective. *Med Hypotheses* 2003; 61:173–176.

[44] Virtanen KA; Iozzo P; Hallsten K; Huupponen R; Parkkola R; Janatuinen T. Increased fat mass compensates for insulin resistance in abdominal obesity and type 2 diabetes: a positron-emitting tomography study. *Diabetes* 2005; 54:2720–2726.

[45] Poirier P; Giles TD; Bray GA; Hong Y; Stern JS; Pi-Sunyer FX; Eckel RH. Obesity and cardiovascular disease: pathophysiology, evaluation, and effect of weight loss. *Arterioscler Thromb Vasc Biol* 2006; 26: 968–976.

[46] Klein S; Burke LE; Bray GA; Blair S; Allison DB; Pi-Sunyer X; Hong Y; Eckel RH. Clinical implications of obesity with specific focus on cardiovascular disease: a statement for professionals from the American Heart Association Council on Nutrition, Physical Activity, and Metabolism. *Circulation* 2004; 110:2952–2967.

[47] National Cholesterol Education Program Adult Treatment Panel III. Third Report of the National Cholesterol Education Program (NCEP) Expert Panel on Detection, Evaluation, and Treatment of High Blood Cholesterol in Adults (Adult Treatment Panel III) final report. *Circulation* 2002; 106:3143–3421.

[48] Wilson PW; D'Agostino RB; Levy D; Belanger AM; Silbershatz H; Kannel WB. Prediction of coronary heart disease using risk factor categories. *Circulation* 1998; 97:1837–1847.

[49] Rainwater DL; Kammerer CM; Carey KD; Dyke B; VandeBerg JF; Shelledy WR; Moore PH Jr; Mahaney MC; McGill HC Jr; VandeBerg JL. Genetic determination of HDL variation and response to diet in baboons. *Atherosclerosis* 2002; 161:335–343.

[50] 50.Rainwater DL; Kammerer CM; VandeBerg JL. Evidence that multiple genes influence baseline concentrations and diet response of Lp(a) in baboons. *Arterioscler Thromb Vasc Biol* 1999; 19:2696–2700.

[51] Baroukh N; Ostos MA; Vergnes L; Recalde D; Staels B; Fruchart J; Ochoa A; Castro G; Zakin MM. Expression of human apolipoprotein A-I/C-III/A-IV gene cluster in mice

reduces atherogenesis in response to a high fat-high cholesterol diet. *FEBS Letters* 2001; 502:16–20.

[52] Speidel MT; Booyse FM; Abrams A; Moore MA; Chung BH. Lipolyzed hypertriglyceridemic serum and triglyceriderich lipoprotein cause lipid accumulation in and are cytotoxic to cultured human endothelial cells. High density lipoproteins inhibit this cytotoxicity. *Thromb Res* 1990; 58:251–264.

[53] Vogel RA; Corretti MC; Plotnick GD. Effect of a single high-fat meal on endothelial function in healthy subjects. *Am J Cardiol* 1997; 79:350–354.

[54] Doi H; Kugiyama K; Oka H; Sugiyama S; Ogata N; Koide SI; Nakamura SI; Yasue H. Remnant lipoproteins induce proatherothrombogenic molecules in endothelial cells through a redox-sensitive mechanism. *Circulation* 2000; 102:670–676.

[55] Griffin BA. Lipoprotein atherogenicity: an overview of current mechanisms. *Proc Nutr Soc* 1999; 58:163–169.

[56] Hu FB; Willett WC; Li T; Stampfer MJ; Colditz GA; Manson JE. Adiposity as compared with physical activity in predicting mortality among women. *N Engl J Med* 2004; 351:2694–2703.

[57] Calle EE; Thun MJ; Petrelli JM; Rodrigues C; Heath CDW. Body mass index and mortality in a prospective cohort of U.S. adults. *N Engl J Med.* 1999; 341:1097–1105.

[58] Stevens J; Cai J; Pamuk ER; Williamson DF; Thun MJ; Wood JL. The effect of age on the association between body mass index and mortality. *N Engl J Med* 1998; 338:1–7.

[59] van Dam RM; Willett WC; Manson JE; Hu FB. The relationship between overweight in adolescence and premature death in women. *Ann Intern Med* 2006; 145:91–97.

[60] Elkeles RS; Fehert MD; Flather MD; Godsland IF; Nugara F; Richmod W; Rubens MB; Wang D. The association of coronary calcium score and conventional cardiovascular risk factors in type 2 diabetic subjects asymptomatic for contrary heart disease (The PREDICT Study). *Diabet Med.* 2004; 21:1129–1134.

[61] Cassidy AE; Bielak LF; Zhou Y; Sheedy PF; Turner ST; Breen JF; Araoz PA; Kullo IJ; Lin X; Peyser PA. Progression of subclinical coronary atherosclerosis: does obesity make a difference? *Circulation* 2005; 111:1877–1882.

[62] McGill HC; McMahan CA; Hederick EE; Zieske AW; Malcom GT; Tracy RE. Strong JP. Obesity accelerates the progression of coronary atherosclerosis in young men. *Circulation* 2002; 105:2712–2718.

[63] Bell CG; Walley AJ; Froguel P. The genetics of human obesity. *Nat Rev Genet* 2005; 6:221–234.

[64] Loos RJ; Bouchard C. Obesity: is it a genetic disorder? *J Int Med* 2003; 254:401-425.

[65] Comuzzie AG; Allison DB. The search for human obesity genes. *Science* 1998; 280:1374–1377.

[66] Rankinen T; Zuberi A; Chagnon YC; Weisnagel SJ; Argyropoulos G; Walts B; Perusse L; Bouchard C. The human obesity gene map: the 2005 update. *Obesity* 2006; 14:529–644

[67] Dervaux N; Wubuli M; Megnien JL; Chironi G; Simon A. Comparative associations of adiposity measures with cardiometabolic risk burden in asymptomatic subjects. *Atherosclerosis* 2008; 201:413–417.

[68] Lohmueller KE; Pearce CL; Pike M; Lander ES; Hirschhorn JN. Meta-analysis of genetic association studies supports a contribution of common variants to susceptibility to common disease. *Nat Genet* 2003; 33:77–82.

[69]   Friedman JM; Halaas JL. Leptin and the regulation of body weight in mammals. *Nature* 1998; 395:763–770.

[70]   Berg AH; Scherer PE. Adipose tissue, inflammation, and cardiovascular disease. *Circ Res* 2005; 96:939–949.

[71]   Reilly MP; Igbal N; Schutta M; Wolfe ML; Scally M; Localio AR; Rader DJ; Kimmel SE. Plasma leptin levels are associated with coronary atherosclerosis in type 2 diabetes. *J Clin Endocrinol Metab* 2004; 89: 3872–3878.

[72]   Bodary PF; Gu S; Shen Y; Hasty AH; Buckler JM; Eitzman DT. Recombinant leptin promotes atherosclerosis and thrombosis in apolipoprotein E-deficient mice. *Arterioscler Thromb Vasc Biol* 2005; 25:119–122.

[73]   Stephenson K; Tunstead J; Tsai A; Gordon R; Henderson S; Dansky HM. Neointimal formation after endovascular arterial injury is markedly attenuated in db/db mice. *Arterioscler Thromb Vasc Biol* 2003; 23:2027–2033.

[74]   Bouloumie A; Marumo T; Lafontan M; Busse R. Leptin induces oxidative stress in human endothelial cells. *FASEB J* 1999; 13:1231–1238.

[75]   Yamagishi SI; Edelstein D; Du XL; Kaneda Y; Guzman M; Brownlee M. Leptin induces mitochondrial superoxide production and monocyte chemoattractant protein-1 expression in aortic endothelial cells by increasing fatty acid oxidation via protein kinase A. *J Biol Chem* 2001; 276:25096–25100.

[76]   Park HY; Kwon HM; Lim HJ; Hong BK; Lee JY; Park BE; Jang Y; Cho SY; Kim HS. Potential role of leptin in angiogenesis: leptin induces endothelial cell proliferation and expression of matrix metalloproteinases in vivo and in vitro. *Exp Mol Med* 2001; 33:95–102.

[77]   Quehenberger P; Exner M; Sunder-Plassmann R; Ruzicka K; Bieglmayer C; Endler G; Muellner C; Speiser W; Wagner O. Leptin induces endothelin-1 in endothelial cells in vitro. *Circ Res* 2002; 90:711–718.

[78]   Shin HJ; Oh J; Kang SM; Lee JH; Shin MJ; Hwang KC; Jang Y; Chung JH. Leptin induces hypertrophy via p38 mitogen-activated protein kinase in rat vascular smooth muscle cells. *Biochem Biophys Res Commun* 2005; 329:18–24.

[79]   Martin-Romero C; Santos-Alvarez J; Goberna R; Sanchez-Margalet V. Human leptin enhances activation and proliferation of human circulating T lymphocytes. *Cell Immunol* 2000; 199:15–24.

[80]   Caldefie-Chezet F; Poulin A; Tridon A; Sion B; Vasson MP. Leptin: a potential regulator of polymorphonuclear neutrophil bactericidal action? *Leukoc Biol* 2001; 69:414–418.

[81]   Parhami F; Tintut Y; Ballard A; Fogelman AM; Demer LL. Leptin enhances the calcification of vascular cells: artery wall as a target of leptin. *Circ Res* 2001; 88:954–960.

[82]   Nakata M; Yada T; Soejima N; Maruyama I. Leptin promotes aggregation of human platelets via the long form of its receptor. *Diabetes* 1999; 48:426–429.

[83]   Zhang Y; Proenca R; Maffei M; Barone M; Leopold L; Friedman JM. Positional cloning of the mouse obese gene and its human homologue. *Nature* 1994; 372:425–432.

[84]   Montague CT; Farooqi IS; Whitehead JP; Soos MA; Rau H; Wareham NJ; Sewter CP; Digby JE; Mohammed SN; Hurst JA; Cheetham CH; Earley AR; Barnett AH; Prins JB; O'Rahilly S. Congenital leptin deficiency is associated with severe early-onset obesity in humans. *Nature* 1997; 387:903–908.

[85]   Strobel A; Issad T; Camoin L; Ozata M; Strosberg AD. A leptin missense mutation associated with hypogonadism and morbid obesity. *Nat Genet* 1998; 18:213–215.

[86]   Friedman JM; Halaas JL. Leptin and the regulation of body weight in mammals. *Nature* 1998; 395:763–770.

[87]   Considine RV; Considine EL; Williams CJ; Nyce MR; Magosin SA; Bauer TL; Rosato EL; Colberg J; Caro JF. Evidence against either a premature stop codon or the absence of obese gene mRNA in human obesity. *J Clin Invest* 1995; 95:2986–2988.

[88]   Maffei M; Stoffel M; Barone M; Moon B; Dammerman M; Ravussin E; Bogardus C. Absence of mutations in the human OB gene in obese/diabetic subjects. *Diabetes* 1996; 45:679–682.

[89]   Carlsson B; Lindell K; Gabrielsson B; Karlsson C; Bjarnason R; Westphal O; Karlsson U; Sjostrom L; CarlssonLM. Obese (ob) gene defects are rare in human obesity. *Obes Res* 1997; 5:30–35.

[90]   Hager J; Clement K; Francke S. A polymorphism in the 5_ untranslated region of the human ob gene is associated with low leptin levels. *Int J Obes Relat Metab Disord* 1998; 22:200–205.

[91]   Mammes O; Betoulle D; Aubert R. Novel polymorphisms in the 5_ region of the LEP gene: association with leptin levels and response to low-calorie diet in human obesity. *Diabetes* 1998; 47:487–489.

[92]   Hoffstedt J; Eriksson P; Mottagui-Tabar S; Arner P. A polymorphism in the leptin promoter region (_2548 g/a) influences gene expression and adipose tissue secretion of leptin. *Horm Metab Res* 2002; 34:355–359.

[93]   Jiang Y; Wilk JB; Borecki I. Common variants in the 5_ region of the leptin gene are associated with body mass index in men from the National Heart, Lung, and Blood Institute Family Heart Study. *Am J Hum Genet* 2004; 75: 220–230.

[94]   Shimizu H; Shimomura Y; Nakanishi Y; Futawatari T; Ohtani K; Sato N; Mori M. Estrogen increases in vivo leptin production in rats and human subjects. *J Endocrinol* 1997; 154:285–292.

[95]   O'Neil JS; Burow ME; Green AE; McLachlan JA; Henson MC. Effects of estrogen on leptin gene promoter activation in MCF-7 breast cancer and JEG-3 choriocarcinoma cells: selective regulation via estrogen receptors alpha and beta. *Mol Cell Endocrinol* 2001; 176:67–75.

[96]   Matsuzawa Y; Funahashi T; Kihara S; Shimomura I. Adiponectin and metabolic syndrome. *Arterioscler Thromb Vasc Biol* 2004; 24:29–33.

[97]   Bobbcrt T; Rochlitz II; Wegewitz U; Akpulat S; Mai K; Weickcrt MO; Mohlig M; Pfeiffer AFH; Spranger J. Changes of adiponectin oligomer composition by moderate weight reduction. *Diabetes* 2005; 54:2712–2719.

[98]   Aso Y; Yamamoto R; Wakabayashi S; Uchida T; Takayanagi K; Takebaysahi K; Okuno T; Inoue T; Node K; Tobe T; Inukai T; Nakano Y. Comparison of serum high-molecular weight (HMW) adiponectin with total adiponectin concentrations in type 2 diabetic patients with coronary artery disease using a novel enzyme-linked immunosorbent assay to detect HMW adiponectin. *Diabetes* 2006; 55:1954–1960.

[99]   Kobashi C; Urakaze M; Kishida M; Kibayashi E; Kobayashi H; Kihara S; Funahashi T; Takata M; Temaru R; Sato A; Yamazaki K; Nakamura N; Kobayashi M. Adiponectin inhibits endothelial synthesis of interleukin-8. *Circ Res* 2005; 97:1245–1252.

[100] Arita Y; Kihara S; Ouchi N; Maeda K; Kuriyama H; Okamoto Y; Kumada M; Hotta K; Nishida M; Takahashi M; Nakamura T; Shimomura I; Muraguchi M; Ohmoto Y; Funahashi T; Matsuzawa Y. Adipocyte-derived plasma protein adiponectin acts as a platelet-derived growth factor-BB-binding protein and regulates growth factor-induced common postreceptor signal in vascular smooth muscle cell. *Circulation* 2002; 105:2893–2898.

[101] Wang Y; Lam KS; Xu JY; Lu G; Xu LY; Cooper GJ; Xu A. Adiponectin inhibits cell proliferation by interacting with several growth factors in an oligomerization-dependent manner. *J Biol Chem* 2005; 280:18341–18347.

[102] Ouchi N; Kihara S; Arita Y; Nishida M; Matsuyama A; Okamoto Y; Ishigami M; Kuriyama H; Kishida K; Nishizawa H; Hotta K; Muraguchi M; Ohmoto Y; Yamashita S; Funahashi T; Matsuzawa Y. Adipocytederived plasma protein, adiponectin, suppresses lipid accumulation and class A scavenger receptor expression in human monocyte-derived macrophages. *Circulation* 2001; 103:1057–1063.

[103] Chen H; Montagnani M; Funahashi T; Shimomura I; Quon MJ. Adiponectin stimulates production of nitric oxide in vascular endothelial cells. *J Biol Chem* 2003; 278:45021–45026.

[104] Motoshima H; Wu X, Mahadev K; Goldstein BJ. Adiponectin suppresses proliferation and superoxide generation and enhances eNOS activity in endothelial cells treated with oxidized LDL. *Biochem Biophys Res Commun* 2004; 315:264–271.

[105] Maahs DM; Ogden LG; Kinney GL; Wadwa P; Snell-Bergeon JK; Dabelea D; Hokanson JE; Ehrlich J; Eckel RH; Rewers M. Low plasma adiponectin levels predict progression of coronary artery calcification. *Circulation* 2005; 111:747–753.

[106] Araki T; Emoto M; Teramura M; Yokoyama H; Mori K; Hatsuda S; Maeno T; Shinohara K; Koyama H; Shoji T; Inaba M; Nishizawa Y. Effect of adiponectin on carotid arterial stiffness in type 2 diabetic patients treated with pioglitazone and metformin. *Metabolism* 2006; 55:996–1001.

[107] Kumada M; Kihara S; Sumitsuji S; Kawamoto T; Matsumoto S; Ouchi N; Arita Y; Okamoto Y; Shimomura I; Hiraoka H; Nakamura T; Funahashi T; Matsuzawa Y. Association of hypoadiponectinemia with coronary artery disease in men. *Arterioscler Thromb Vasc Biol* 2003; 23:85–89.

[108] Comuzzie AG; Funahashi T; Sonnenberg G; Martin LJ; Jacob HJ; Black AE. The genetic basis of plasma variation in adiponectin, a global endophenotype for obesity and the metabolic syndrome. *J Clin Endocrinol Metab* 2001; 86:4321–4325.

[109] Lindsay RS; Funahashi T; Krakoff J; Matsuzawa Y; Tanaka S; Kobes S. Genome-wide linkage analysis of serum adiponectin in the Pima Indian population. *Diabetes* 2003; 52:2419–2425.

[110] Chuang LM; Chiu YF; Sheu WH; Hung YJ; Ho LT; Grove J. Biethnic comparisons of autosomal genomic scan for loci linked to plasma adiponectin in populations of Chinese and Japanese origin. *J Clin Endocrinol Metab* 2004; 89:5772–5778.

[111] ejero ME; Cai G; Göring HH; Diego V; Cole SA; Bacino CA; Butte NF; Comuzzie AG. Linkage analysis of circulating levels of adiponectin in hispanic children. *Int J Obes* (Lond) 2007; 31:535–542.

[112] Pollin TI; Tanner K; O'Connell JR; Ott SH; Damcott CM; Shuldiner AR. Linkage of plasma adiponectin levels to 3q27 explained by association with variation in the APM1 gene. *Diabetes* 2005; 54:268–274.

[113] Guo X; Saad MF; Langefeld CD; Williams AH; Cui J; Taylor KD. Genome-wide linkage of plasma adiponectin reveals a major locus on chromosome 3q distinct from the adiponectin structural gene: the IRAS Family Study. *Diabetes* 2006; 55:1723–1730.

[114] Yang WS; Chuang LM. Human genetics of adiponectin in the metabolic syndrome. *J Mol Med* 2006; 84:112–121.

[115] Gable DR; Hurel SJ; Humphries SE. Adiponectin and its gene variants as risk factors for insulin resistance, the metabolic syndrome and cardiovascular disease. *Atherosclerosis* 2006; 188:231–244.

[116] Heid IM; Wagner SA; Gohlke H; Iglseder B; Mueller JC; Cip P. Genetic architecture of the APM1 gene and its influence on adiponectin plasma levels and parameters of the metabolic syndrome in 1,727 healthy Caucasians. *Diabetes* 2006; 55:375–384.

[117] Fumeron F; Aubert R; Siddiq A; Betoulle D; Pean F; Hadjadj S. Adiponectin gene polymorphisms and adiponectin levels are independently associated with the development of hyperglycemia during a 3-year period: the epidemiologic data on the insulin resistance syndrome prospective study. *Diabetes* 2004; 53:1150–1157.

[118] Jang Y; Lee JH; Kim OY; Koh SJ; Chae JS; Woo JH. The SNP276G>T polymorphism in the adiponectin (ACDC) gene is more strongly associated with insulin resistance and cardiovascular disease risk than SNP45T>G in nonobese/nondiabetic Korean men independent of abdominal adiposity and circulating plasma adiponectin. *Metabolism* 2006; 55:59–66.

[119] Hara K; Boutin P; Mori Y; Tobe K; Dina C; Yasuda K. Genetic variation in the gene encoding adiponectin is associated with an increased risk of type 2 diabetes in the Japanese population. *Diabetes* 2002; 51:536–540.

[120] Bacci S; Menzaghi C; Ercolino T; Ma X; Rauseo A; Salvemini L. The t276 G/T single nucleotide polymorphism of the adiponectin gene is associated with coronary artery disease in type 2 diabetic patients. *Diabetes Care* 2004; 27:2015–2020.

[121] Qi L, Doria A; Manson JE; Meigs JB; Hunter D; Mantzoros CS. Adiponectin genetic variability, plasma adiponectin, and cardiovascular risk in patients with type 2 diabetes. *Diabetes* 2006; 55:1512–1516.

[122] Lacquemant C; Froguel P; Lobbens S; Izzo P; Dina C; Ruiz J. The adiponectin gene SNPt45 is associated with coronary artery disease in Type 2 (non-insulin-dependent) diabetes mellitus. *Diabet Med* 2004; 21:776–781.

[123] Ohashi K; Ouchi N; Kihara S; Funahashi T; Nakamura T; Sumitsuji S. Adiponectin I164T mutation is associated with the metabolic syndrome and coronary artery disease. *J Am Coll Cardiol* 2004; 43:1195–1200.

[124] Filippi E; Sentinelli F; Romeo S; Arca M; Berni A; Tiberti C. The adiponectin gene SNPt276G>T associates with early-onset coronary artery disease and with lower levels of adiponectin in younger coronary artery disease patients. *J Mol Med* 2005; 83:711–719.

[125] Berthier MT; Houde A; Cote M; Paradis AM; Mauriege P; Bergeron J. Impact of adiponectin gene polymorphisms on plasma lipoprotein and adiponectin concentrations of viscerally obese men. *J Lipid Res* 2005; 46:237–244.

[126] Vasseur F; Helbecque N; Lobbens S; Vasseur-Delannoy V; Dina C; Clement K. Hypoadiponectinaemia and high risk of type 2 diabetes are associated with adiponectin-encoding (ACDC) gene promoter variants in morbid obesity: evidence for a role of ACDC in diabesity. *Diabetologia* 2005; 48:892–899.

[127] Corella D; Qi L; Tai ES; Deurenberg-Yap M; Tan CE; Chew SK. Perilipin gene variation determines higher susceptibility to insulin resistance in Asian women when consuming a high-saturated fat, lowcarbohydrate diet. *Diabetes Care* 2006; 29:1313–1319.

[128] Londos C; Gruia-Gray J; Brasaemle DL; Rondinone CM; Takeda T; Dwyer NK. Perilipin: possible roles in structure and metabolism of intracellular neutral lipids in adipocytes and steroidogenic cells. *Int J Obes Relat Metab Disord* 1996; 20:S97–S101.

[129] Blanchette-Mackie EJ; Dwyer NK; Barber T; Coxey RA; Takeda T; Rondinone CM. Perilipin is located on the surface layer of intracellular lipid droplets in adipocytes. *J Lipid Res* 1995; 36:1211–1226.

[130] Greenberg AS; Egan JJ; Wek SA; Garty NB; Blanchette-Mackie EJ; Londos C. Perilipin, a major hormonally regulated adipocyte-specific phosphoprotein associated with the periphery of lipid storage droplets. *J Biol Chem* 1991; 266:11341–11346.

[131] Moore HP; Silver RB; Mottillo EP; Bernlohr DA; Granneman JG. Perilipin targets a novel pool of lipid droplets for lipolytic attack by hormone-sensitive lipase. *J Biol Chem* 2005; 280:43109–43120.

[132] Martinez-Botas J; Anderson JB; Tessier D; Lapillonne A; Chang BH; Quast MJ. Absence of perilipin results in leanness and reverses obesity in Lepr(db/db) mice. *Nat Genet* 2000; 26:474–479.

[133] Tansey JT; Sztalryd C; Gruia-Gray J; Roush DL; Zee JV; Gavrilova O. Perilipin ablation results in a lean mouse with aberrant adipocyte lipolysis, enhanced leptin production, and resistance to diet-induced obesity. *Proc Natl Acad Sci USA* 2001; 98:6494–6499.

[134] Qi L; Corella D; Sorli JV; Portoles O; Shen H; Coltell O. Genetic variation at the perilipin (PLIN) locus is associated with obesity-related phenotypes in White women. *Clin Genet* 2004; 66:299–310.

[135] Corella D; Qi L, Sorli JV; Godoy D; Portoles O; Coltell O. Obese subjects carrying the 11482G>A polymorphism at the perilipin locus are resistant to weight loss after dietary energy restriction. *J Clin Endocrinol Metab* 2005; 90:5121–5126.

[136] Jang Y; Kim OY; Lee JH; Koh SJ; Chae JS; Kim JY. Genetic variation at the perilipin locus is associated with changes in serum free fatty acids and abdominal fat following mild weight loss. *Int J Obes* (Lond) 2006; 30:1601–1608.

[137] Qi L; Tai ES; Tan CE; Shen H; Chew SK; Greenberg AS. Intragenic linkage disequilibrium structure of the human perilipin gene (PLIN) and haplotype association with increased obesity risk in a multiethnic Asian population. *J Mol Med* 2005; 83:448–456.

[138] Qi L; Shen H; Larson I; Schaefer EJ; Greenberg AS; Tregouet DA. Gender-specific association of a perilipin gene haplotype with obesity risk in a white population. *Obes Res* 2004; 12:1758–1765.

[139] Ginsberg HN; Kris-Etherton P; Dennis B; Elmer PJ; Ershow A; Lefevre M; Pearson T; Roheim P; Ramakrishnan R; Reed R; Stewart K; Stewart P; Phillips K; Anderson N. Effects of reducing dietary saturated fatty acids on plasma lipids and lipoproteins in healthy subjects: the DELTA Study, protocol 1. *Arterioscler Thromb Vasc Biol* 1998; 18:441–449.

[140] Yang W; Kelly T; He J. Genetic epidemiology of obesity. *Epidemiol Rev* 2007; 29:49–61.

[141] Lindi VI; Uusitupa MI; Lindstrom J; Louheranta A; Eriksson JG; Valle TT; Hamalainen H; Ilanne-Parikka P; Keinanen-Kiukaanniemi S; Laakso M; Tuomilehto J. Finnish Diabetes Prevention Study, Finnish Diabetes Prevention Study. Association of the Pro12Ala polymorphism in the PPAR-gamma2 gene with 3-year incidence of type2diabetes and bodyweight change inthe Finnish Diabetes Prevention Study. *Diabetes* 2002; 51:2581–2586.

[142] Talmud P. Gene–environment interaction and its impact on coronary heart disease risk. *Nutr Metab Cardiovasc Dis* 2007; 17:148–152.

[143] Altshuler D; Hirschhorn JN; Klannemark M; Lindgren CM; Vohl MC; Nemesh J; Lane CR; Schaffner SF; Bolk S; Brewer C; Tuomi T; Gaudet D; Hundson TJ; Daly M; Gropp L; Lander ES. The common PPAR-gamma Pro12Ala polymorphism is associated with decreased risk of type 2 diabetes. *Nat. Genet* 2000; 26:76–80.

[144] Knouff C; Auwerx J. Peroxisome proliferator-activated receptor-gamma calls for activation inmoderation: lessons from genetics and pharmacology. *Endocr Rev* 2004; 25:899–918.

[145] Robitaille J; Despres JP; Perusse L; Vohl MC. The PPARgammaP12A polymorphism modulates the relationship between dietary fat intake and components of themetabolic syndrome: results from the Quebec Family Study. *Clin Genet* 2003; 63:109–116.

[146] Hurley DM; Accili D; Stratakis CA. Point mutation causing a single amino acid substitution in the hormone binding domain of the glucocorticoid receptor in familial glucocorticoid resistance. *J. Clin. Invest.* 1991; 87:680–686.

[147] Weaver JU; Hitman GA; Kopelman PG. An association between a BclI restriction fragment length polymorphism of the glucocorticoid receptor locus and hyperinsulinaemia in obese women. *J. Mol. Endocrinol* 1992; 9:295–300.

[148] Buemann B; Vohl MC; Chagnon M. Abdominal visceral fat is associated with a BclI restriction fragment length polymorphism at the glucocorticoid receptor gene locus. *Obes Res* 1997; 5:186–192.

[149] Rosmond R. The glucocorticoid receptor gene and its association to metabolic syndrome. *Obes Res* 2002; 10:1078–1086.

[150] Rosmond R. Association studies of genetic polymorphisms in central obesity: a critical review. *Int J Obes Relat Metab Disord* 2003; 27:1141–1151.

[151] Dobson MG; Redfern CP; Unwin N; Weaver JU. The N363S polymorphism of the glucocorticoid receptor: potential contribution to central obesity in men and lack of association with other risk factors for coronary heart disease and diabetes mellitus. *J Clin Endocrinol Metab* 2001; 86:2270–2274.

[152] Ikeda Y; Dalziel B; Heilbronn L. Polymorphisms in the glucocorticoid receptor gene in Japanese population. *In The Endocrine Society, 83rd Annual Meeting*; 2001 June 20–23; Denver, Colorado.

[153] Van Rossum EF; Koper JW; Huizenga NA. A polymorphism in the glucocorticoid receptor gene, which decreases sensitivity to glucocorticoids in vivo, is associated with low insulin and cholesterol levels. *Diabetes* 2002; 51:3128–3134.

[154] Cercato C; Frazzatto EST; Halpern A; Villares SMF. The N363S polymorphism of the glucocorticoid receptor: lack of association with visceral obesity. Int J Obes Relat Metab Disord 2003; 27:S70.

[155] Verdich C; Holst C; Echwald SM. Genes associated with body coposition for given BMI in men. *Int J Obes Relat Metab Disord* 2003; 27:S75.

[156] Syed AA; Irving JAE; Redfern CPF. Low prevalence of the N363S polymorphism of the glucocorticoid receptor in South Asians living in the United Kingdom. *J Clin Endocrinol Metab* 2004; 89:232–235.

[157] DE Lange P; Koper JW; Huizenga NA. Differential hormonedependent transcriptional activation and -repression by naturally occurring human glucocorticoid receptor variants. *Mol Endocrinol* 1997; 11:1156–1164.

[158] Karl M; Lamberts SW; Detera-Wadleigh SD. Familial glucocorticoid resistance caused by a splice site deletion in the human glucocorticoid receptor gene. *J Clin Endocrinol Metab* 1993; 76:683–689.

[159] Huizenga NA; Koper JW; De Lange P. A polymorphism in the glucocorticoid receptor gene may be associated with and increased sensitivity to glucocorticoids in vivo. *J Clin Endocrinol Metab* 1998; 83:144–151.

[160] Ray DW; Littlewood AC; Clark AJ. Human small cell lung cancer cell lines expressing the proopiomelanocortin gene have aberrant glucocorticoid receptor function. *J Clin Invest* 1994; 93:1625–1630.

[161] Gaitan D; Debold CR; Turney MK. Glucocorticoid receptor structure and function in an adrenocorticotropin-secreting small cell lung cancer. *Mol Endocrinol* 1995; 9:1193–1201.

[162] Diblasio AM; Vanrossum EF; Maestrini S. The relation between two polymorphisms in the glucocorticoid receptor gene and body mass index, blood pressure and cholesterol in obese patients. *Clin Endocrinol* (Oxf.) 2003; 59:68–74.

[163] Roussel R; Reis AF; Dubois-Laforgue D. The N363S polymorphism in the glucocorticoid receptor gene is associated with overweight in subjects with type 2 diabetes mellitus. *Clin Endocrinol* (Oxf.) 2003; 59:237–241.

[164] Tremblay A; Bouchard L; Bouchard C. Long-term adiposity changes are related to a glucocorticoid receptor polymorphism in young females. *J Clin Endocrinol Metab* 2003; 88:3141–3145.

[165] Lin RC; Wang WY; Morris BJ. High penetrance, overweight, and glucocorticoid receptor variant: case-control study. *Br Med J* 1999; 319:1337–1338.

[166] Goldberg IJ; Merkel M. Lipoprotein lipase: physiology, biochemistry, and molecular biology. *Front Biosci* 2001; 6:D388–D405.

[167] Enerback S, Gimble JM. Lipoprotein lipase gene expression: physiological regulators at the transcriptional and posttranscriptional level. *Biochim Biophys Acta* 1993; 1169:107–125.

[168] Bjorntorp P. The regulation of adipose tissue distribution in humans. *Int J Obes* 1996; 20:291–302.

[169] Iverius PH, Brunzell JD. Relationship between lipoprotein lipase activity and plasma sex steroid level in obese women. *J Clin Invest* 1988; 82:1106–1112.

[170] Homma H, Kurachi H, Nishio Y, Takeda T, Yamamoto T, Adachi K, Morishige K, Ohmichi M, Matsuzawa Y, Murata Y. Estrogen suppresses transcription of lipoprotein lipase gene. Existence of a unique estrogen response element on the lipoprotein lipase promoter. *J Biol Chem* 2000; 275:11404–11411.

[171] Corella D; Guillen M; Portoles O. Gender specific associations of the Trp64Arg mutation in the beta3-adrenergic receptor gene with obesity-related phenotypes in a Mediterranean population: interaction with a common lipoprotein lipase gene variation. *J Intern Med* 2001; 250:348–360.

[172] Garenc C; Perusse L; Bergeron J. Evidence of LPL gene-exercise interaction for body fat and LPL activity: the HERITAGE Family Study. *J Appl Physiol* 2001; 91:1334–1340.

[173] Jemaa R; Tuzet S; Portos C; Betoulle D; Apfelbaum M; Fumeron F. Lipoprotein lipase gene polymorphisms: associations with hypertriglyceridemia and body mass index in obese people. *Int J Obes Relat Metab Disord* 1995; 19:270–274.

[174] Aoi N; Soma M; Nakayama T; Rahmutula D; Kosuge K; Izumi Y; Matsumoto K. Variable number of tandem repeat of the 5'-flanking region of type-C human natriuretic peptide receptor gene influences blood pressure levels in obesity-associated hypertension. *Hypertension Research* 2004; 27:711–716.

[175] Kosuge K; Soma M; Nakayama T; Aoi N; Sato M; Haketa A; Uwabo J; Izumi Y; Matsumoto K. Human Uncoupling Protein 2 and 3 Genes Are Associated with Obesity in Japanese. *Endocrine* 2008; 34:87–95.

In: Overweightness and Walking
Editor: Caleb I. Black, pp. 177-191

ISBN: 978-1-60741-298-4
© 2010 Nova Science Publishers, Inc.

Chapter 8

OBESITY AS A COMPLICATION OF CANCER IN CHILDREN

Josephine Ho, Alexander K.C. Leung[*] and Aru Narendran

The University of Calgary, Alberta Children's Hospital, Calgary, Alberta, Canada

ABSTRACT

It is well known that the prevalence of obesity in the general population of children is increasing and that this is likely related to sedentary lifestyles and poor eating habits. Obesity is also being seen as a complication of treatments being used for cancer therapy in children as well as cancer itself. This can have a significant impact on a child's future health, especially since survival rates are being improved for many childhood cancers. When obesity results as a complication of a cancer or as a side effect of a treatment for cancer, children will be at risk for problems such as dyslipidemia, impaired glucose tolerance, hypertension, and cardiovascular disease.

Obesity as a complication of cancer in children can be either short-term or long-term. Treatment for cancer such as high dose steroids can result in transiently increased appetite, Cushing's syndrome and obesity during the treatment course. However, other forms of therapy such as radiation to the hypothalamus or surgical manipulation near the hypothalamic/pituitary region can result in permanent damage and cause hypothalamic obesity. In addition, tumors that invade or disrupt the hypothalamic/pituitary region can result in permanent hypothalamic dysregulation and cause obesity.

Trends in the prevalence of childhood cancer related obesity will be examined and a review of the etiology and pathogenesis behind these causes of obesity will be discussed. Current pharmacologic and surgical treatment options will also be reviewed.

Key words: obesity, childhood cancer, complications

[*] Corresponding author: Telefax: (403) 230-3322, e-mail: aleung@ucalgary.ca

INTRODUCTION

It is well known that childhood obesity is increasing in the general population [1, 2]. Obesity has become an epidemic illness in most developed countries. Between 1960 and 2000, the prevalence of obesity amongst American adults increased from 13.4% to 30.9% [3, 4]. In children in the United States the prevalence of obesity was estimated at 17% in the years 2003 to 2004 [5]. In parallel to this, childhood survival from cancer has been improving due to improved treatments available. The 5-year survival rates of childhood cancers combined improved from 56% in 1974 to 1976, up to 77% in 1992 to 1998 [6]. With this improvement in survival, long-term health consequences related to the cancer itself (for example, brain tumors in the hypothalamic region), or to treatments for cancer (for example, corticosteroid therapy, cranial irradiation) can have a significant impact on long-term health in childhood cancer survivors [7].

The World Health Organization has established the diagnosis of obesity based on the Body Mass Index (BMI), which is calculated as the patient's weight in kilograms divided by the square of the height in meters. In children, appropriate BMI measurements can vary depending on age and gender. Obesity in children has been defined as a BMI greater than or equal to the 95th percentile and overweight as a BMI from the 85th to 94th percentile [5]. It is important to note that in a child, BMI can improve if their weight remains stable over a period of time when their height is increasing.

Prevention of obesity remains an important issue for childhood survivors from cancer due to the fact that it is a potentially modifiable risk factor for other diseases. Childhood obesity is an important predictor of future development of obesity as an adult [8] as well as its associated complications both in childhood and adulthood [9]. Obesity can lead to cardiovascular disease, type 2 diabetes mellitus, hypertension and dyslipidemia [10]. Cardiovascular disease is particularly concerning in childhood survivors of cancer because they may have already received potentially cardiotoxic chemotherapy and radiation [7]. In addition to cardiovascular disease, obesity is a risk factor for certain forms of cancer, gastroesophageal reflux, obstructive sleep apnea, degenerative joint disease, gout, back pain, and polycystic ovary syndrome [11].

EPIDEMIOLOGY

Most of the data on obesity following childhood cancer are from populations of children who have been treated for acute lymphoblastic leukemia with or without cranial irradiation. This is likely because childhood acute lymphoblastic leukemia is the most common pediatric cancer [12]. The other largely studied population is children who have been treated for central nervous system tumors, with craniopharyngiomas being the most common. In both of these populations, the development of obesity has been shown to be increased compared to the normal population [7, 13-15].

In a large study of 1,765 adult survivors of childhood acute lymphoblastic leukemia, the odds of developing obesity defined as a body mass index greater than or equal to 30 kg/m^2, was 2.59 for females and 1.86 for males compared to healthy adult siblings [14]. Female survivors were more likely to be overweight than their siblings and obesity was not associated with chemotherapy or radiation doses less than 20 Gy [14].

In a study of 921 adults who had been treated for central nervous system malignancies as children, females who had brain tumors treated at a young age with high doses of cranial radiation had the greatest risk of developing obesity [13]. Interestingly, approximately 40% of these adults were below the 10th percentile for height [13].

Obesity is a recognized risk factor for cardiovascular disease and is part of the metabolic syndrome. The metabolic syndrome can include features such as altered lipid profile, hypertension, impaired fasting glucose, obesity, and increased waist circumference [16]. In a study of fifty survivors of non-brain tumor malignancies, 16% were found to have features of the metabolic syndrome compared to none of the age matched controls [17]. In this same study, childhood cancer survivors had higher glucose and insulin levels and increased weight compared with their age matched controls [17]. An increase in the risk of age and sex adjusted cardiovascular mortality ratio has been reported as 3.8 for survivors of childhood leukemia [18] which suggests that early intervention is necessary in order to alter any potential modifiable risk factors for cardiovascular disease.

ETIOLOGY AND PATHOGENESIS

A complex neuroendocrine feedback loop exists that regulates energy balance in individuals. This feedback loop is comprised of the afferent system, central nervous system processing unit, and the efferent system. In the afferent system, neural signals from the vagus nerve as well as hormonal signals such as ghrelin (increases with fasting), leptin (information about the size of peripheral adipocyte energy stores) and insulin (mediates a satiety signal) are generated [19]. Other peripheral afferent signals also include low blood glucose and macronutrients such as protein. Within the brain, various neurotransmitters such as dopamine from the dorsomedial and arcuate nuclei, norepinephrine from the locu coeruleus, and serotonin from the median raphe have been shown to have effects on appetite and satiety [19]. The central nervous system processing unit consists of the ventromedial hypothalamus (ventromedial and arcuate nuclei), paraventricular nuclei, and lateral hypothalamus. Disruptions in any of these regions can lead to obesity. The efferent system coordinates energy storage and expenditure by sending signals that control appetite, modulating the sympathetic and parasympathetic nervous system and affecting the daily energy expenditure [19]. Energy balance is extremely complex and multiple genetic, hormonal and behavioral factors can affect it. Some specific mechanisms for obesity in children who have had childhood cancer will be discussed.

Energy Balance

As in other healthy children, disruption in the balance between energy intake and energy expenditure can result in obesity. Studies have shown that compared to healthy controls, there is a decreased physical activity level in people who have been diagnosed with acute lymphoblastic leukemia or craniopharyngioma as children. However, energy intake was not significantly increased [20, 21]. Harz et al evaluated the food intake in 27 patients with childhood onset of craniopharyngioma and 1027 healthy children aged 7 years to 16 years as controls [20]. No significant difference in caloric intake was noted between the two groups. Movement counts measured by accelerometry were also compared in 19 patients with history of craniopharyngioma and 26 controls matched for BMI and age. Patients with craniopharyngioma showed significantly less physical activity compared to controls [20].

In patients treated for acute lymphoblastic leukemia as children, physical activity was found to be less common in cancer survivors than controls [22]. These individuals also had a higher median percentage of body fat compared to controls but the BMI was only slightly increased [22]. In another study, cardiopulmonary fitness was assessed by measuring peak oxygen consumption in children that had been treated for acute lymphoblastic leukemia using cranial irradiation compared to survivors of other childhood malignancies who did not require cranial irradiation and controls [23]. The children with acute lymphoblastic leukemia were found to have reduced energy expenditure compared to both controls and children who had been diagnosed with other malignancies [23].

Exogenous Corticosteroid-Induced Obesity

Treatment for childhood cancer often includes supraphysiologic doses of glucocorticosteroids which can result in increased appetite and Cushing syndrome. Clinical features of Cushing syndrome include moon-face, posterior cervical fat pad, truncal obesity, thin skin, easy bruising, hypertension, and striae.

Food intake has been shown to increase during corticosteroid treatment [24]. Exogenous corticosteroid-induced obesity during treatment for childhood cancer is usually self-limited and will resolve after discontinuation of the supra-physiologic doses of corticosteroid. In a retrospective analysis of 60 children with childhood craniopharyngioma, the dose and duration of perioperative dexamethasone therapy was found to have short-term effects on the weight gain but did not appear to have effects on the development of long-term severe obesity [25]. Of the 60 children studied, 40% developed severe obesity with a BMI greater than three standard deviations. Cumulative doses and duration of dexamethasone given perioperatively were similar for patients who developed severe obesity compared to those who maintained normal weight. In addition, cumulative dose of dexamethasone correlated positively with weight gain during the first year after surgery but did not correlate with long-term severe obesity. The only significant difference between the children who developed severe obesity in the long-term compared with those who did not was a higher BMI at the time of diagnosis of craniopharyngioma [25].

Endogenous Corticosteroid-Induced Obesity

Up-regulated 11β-hydroxysteroid dehydrogenase activity has been implicated as a cause of Cushing-like obesity following suprasellar operations for tumors in the hypothalamic region when receiving only replacement doses of glucocorticoids [26]. In a study of patients aged 9 to 22 years with hypothalamic obesity who were also ACTH deficient and receiving only replacement doses of glucocorticoids, cortisone conversion to the more active cortisol appeared to be increased. The authors hypothesized that this could be the potential mechanism for increased Cushing-like obesity in children who are only receiving physiologic doses of corticosteroid hormone replacement [26].

Hypothalamic Obesity

Obesity resulting from injury to the hypothalamic region of the brain is seen in children with acute lymphoblastic leukemia requiring cranial irradiation or brain tumors. Intractable weight gain can be present at diagnosis of a brain tumor or develop following neurosurgical interventions or cranial irradiation [27-30]. This intractable weight gain is felt to be the result of damage to the ventromedial hypothalamus which promotes excessive energy intake and decreased energy expenditure.

The ventromedial hypothalamus usually receives information from the hormones insulin, leptin and grehlin which are related to energy intake and adipocyte stores. The action of these hormones on the ventromedial hypothalamus then result in the release of various other signals that have affects on the feeding behavior. Neurons that release neuropeptide Y and agouti-related peptide stimulate feeding while neurons that release α- melanocyte-stimulating hormone and cocaine-amphetamine regulate transcript signal satiety [19, 31].

In patients with hypothalamic obesity, excessive insulin secretion has been found. One hypothesis is that hyperphagia results from ventromedial hypothalamus lesions resulting in damage to the satiety center. Increases in insulin levels are secondary to the obesity that develops [32]. In another hypothesis, ventromedial hypothalamus damage results in the loss of inhibition to the vagus nerve. The vagus nerve stimulates the pancreatic beta-cell to secrete excessive amounts of insulin. With the increased insulin secretion, food that is ingested is stored in adipose tissue resulting in obesity [32, 33].

Leptin Resistance

Leptin is a 167 amino acid peptide hormone that is secreted by adipose tissue and signals the hypothalamus to suppress appetite [34,35]. Leptin inhibits hypothalamic neuropeptide Y which results in a decrease in appetite [34-36]. Abnormalities in leptin signaling can be due to leptin deficiency or leptin resistance [37].

In a study by Roth et al, 14 patients aged 7 to 21 years old were evaluated for serum leptin levels following neurosurgical treatment for their craniopharyngioma [34]. Leptin levels were found to be significantly elevated compared to controls in patients who were had suprasellar tumours. In contrast, those with intrasellar tumors had almost normal leptin levels. The authors hypothesized that hypothalamic obesity developed in patients with suprasellar craniopharyngiomas due to hypothalamic insensitivity to endogenous leptin [34].

Cranial irradiation appears to be a risk factor for elevated leptin levels [38, 39], although this finding has not been consistently shown in other studies. In a cross-sectional study of 26 patients assessing the relationship of leptin levels with BMI in childhood survivors of acute lymphocytic leukemia, cranial irradiation was not found to play a role in the relationship of leptin and BMI [40]. Children who developed growth hormone deficiency following treatment for childhood cancer and were untreated for the growth hormone deficiency have been reported to have increased levels of leptin [41].

Patel et al examined 37 patients aged 3.5 years to 21 years with a history of craniopharyngioma, germinoma, optic nerve glioma, astrocytoma or head trauma and compared them to 138 healthy children aged 5 years to 18.2 years [42]. Of the 37 patients, all had cranial surgery and 24 had additional cranial radiation. Any pituitary hormone deficits were appropriately replaced. Higher mean serum leptin levels were found compared to healthy children with simple obesity and similar age and pubertal status [42]. Serum leptin binding activity was significantly lower in patients with a past history of hypothalamic damage compared to healthy children. The authors hypothesized that the low leptin binding activity which indicates higher free leptin levels together with the elevated leptin levels compared to controls could be consistent with central leptin insensitivity due to hypothalamic damage [42].

Genetic Factors

Obesity is a polygenic trait and several candidate genes have been investigated in the general population including those involved in energy intake (leptin receptor [LEPR], leptin [LEP] , agouti-related protein [AGRP], adiponectin [APJ]), energy expenditure (G-protein β3 subunit [GNβ3] , uncoupling protein 2 [UCP2], UCP3, insulin-induced gene 2 [INSIG2]), lipolysis and lipogenesis (tumor necrosis factor-α, interleukin-6, peroxisome proliferator activated receptor [PPAR-γ2], Ghrelin) [43].

Genetic variation in the leptin receptor gene (LEPR) has been hypothesized to be a risk factor for obesity. One of these polymorphisms, Gln223Arg has been studied and found to have various effects. These include lower leptin binding affinity, higher serum levels of leptin, and higher BMIs [44-47]. In a study using a cohort of childhood cancer survivors (The Childhood Cancer Survivor Study [48]), genotyping of the leptin receptor gene polymorphism Gln223Arg of 600 non-hispanic, causcasian adult survivors of childhood acute lymphoblastic leukemia was performed [49]. Female survivors who were overweight were more likely to be homozygous for the Arg allele than those with a Gln allele. In particular, female patients who had received cranial radiation and were homozygous for the Arg allele had a six times higher odds of being overweight. Interestingly, male survivors of childhood acute lymphoblastic leukemia in this cohort had a similar distribution of genotype regardless of weight. The authors concluded that leptin receptor gene polymorphism Gln223Arg could influence the future development of obesity in female survivors of childhood acute lymphoblastic leukemia who were exposed to cranial radiation [49].

Growth Hormone Deficiency

Growth hormone deficiency can cause increased fat mass and a decrease in lean body mass with a resultant increase in obesity [50]. This could suggest that children who are growth hormone deficient resulting from the childhood cancer or following treatment of the cancer could be at an increased risk for obesity. Neurosurgical procedures or cranial irradiation can result in damage to the hypothalamic-pituitary axis and cause growth hormone deficiency in childhood cancer survivors. The prevalence of growth hormone deficiency in adult survivors of acute lymphoblastic leukemia has been estimated at 58% in those treated with cranial irradiation at a mean of approximately 25 years following the diagnosis [51]. In addition, body mass index and waist to hip ratio has been found to be higher in patients with lower growth hormone levels [51]. Percentage of abdominal fat in patients with growth hormone deficiency following treatment of craniopharyngioma has been shown to be higher than healthy controls without growth hormone deficiency that were matched for BMI [52].

Interestingly, some studies have noted that even patients who receive no cranial irradiation or neurosurgical procedures for treatment of their acute lymphoblastic leukemia are at an increased risk for growth hormone deficiency [39, 51]. The mechanism of developing growth hormone deficiency in the absence of iatrogenic procedures or radiotherapy is unclear.

There has been a postulated relationship between growth hormone deficiency and leptin levels. Brennan et al compared 32 patients who had received cranial radiation as children for acute lymphoblastic leukemia with 35 age and BMI matched young adults [41]. Dual x-ray absorptiometry was used to assess fat mass and lean body mass and serum leptin levels were measured. Lean body mass was decreased and serum leptin levels were significantly increased in patients treated with cranial radiation compared to controls. When the patient group was sub-divided by growth hormone status, those with severe growth hormone deficiency had the highest leptin concentration per unit fat mass [41].

Hypogonadism

Untreated hypogonadism in childhood cancer survivors has been noted to be a risk factor for developing hyperinsulinemia, impaired glucose tolerance, and diabetes [53]. In addition, patients who have hypogonadism following treatment for testicular cancer have been shown to have a higher waist to hip ratio than those that do not have hypogonadism [54]. Further studies are necessary to delineate the relationship between obesity and hypogonadism following treatment for childhood cancer.

TREATMENT

For patients with hypopituitarism, appropriate replacement of the deficient hormones is important in normalizing the balance of energy expenditure and energy intake. This may include appropriate thyroid hormone replacement, sex steroid hormone replacement, and growth hormone replacement when applicable. In addition, lifestyle modification including appropriate nutritional counseling and physical activity guidelines should always be initiated prior to undertaking more aggressive pharmacologic or surgical intervention. Unfortunately, lifestyle modification alone is often not sufficient in treating obesity that results from treatments for childhood cancer. A review of interventions that have been investigated in childhood survivors of cancer will be presented.

Pharmacotherapy

Somatostatin agonist

Ventromedial hypothalamus damage results in the loss of inhibition to the vagus nerve. The resulting over-stimulation of the vagus nerve leads to excessive secretion of insulin from the pancreatic beta-cells [32]. With the increased insulin secretion, food that is ingested is stored in adipose tissue resulting in obesity [32,33]. Somatostatin analogs bind to receptors on the pancreatic beta-cell membrane which causes a suppression of insulin release. Therefore, somatostatin analogs have the potential to decrease the weight gain seen in hypothalamic obesity.

Octreotide, a somatostatin agonist, has been investigated as a treatment for severe obesity following therapy for leukemia or brain tumours [32,55]. In a study by Lustig et al, nine children aged 10 years to 18 years with childhood cancer and hypothalamic obesity caused by cranial insult were recruited [55]. Seven had a past history of a brain tumour while the other two had received cranial radiation as part of their therapy for acute lymphocytic leukemia. Octreotide given subcutaneously was found to promote weight loss. In addition, this treatment demonstrated a reduction in insulin secretion and leptin levels [55].

Lustig et al conducted a further randomized, double-blind, placebo-controlled trial using octreotide in 18 subjects (mean age of 14.2 years) with hypothalamic obesity [32]. Underlying diagnoses included craniopharyngioma, hypothalamic astrocytoma, pineal germinoma and acute lymphoblastic leukemia requiring cranial irradiation. Octreotide was found to suppress insulin and stabilize weight and BMI. In addition, improved quality of life was found to correlate with the amount of insulin suppression.

Dextroamphetamine

The role of dextroamphetamine, a central nervous system stimulant, has been studied in a small series of children who had been treated for a craniopharyngioma. Dextroamphetamine is a sympathomimetic amine that has been used to treat children with attention deficit hyperactivity disorder. In children who have had a surgical resection for craniopharyngioma, obesity can result from decreased physical activity and impulsive eating due to hypothalamic insult. Mason et al found that treatment with dextroamphetamine for 24 months led to weight stabilization in five patients aged 6 years to 9.8 years who had craniopharyngioma and obesity and hyperphagia following treatment of the craniopharyngioma [56]. Children were more willing to participate in physical activity and their hyperactivity was improved. Although poor appetite can be a side effect of dextroamphetamine, caloric intake was not affected in this group of children [56]. Further long-term studies are necessary to assess if the weight stabilization persists long term.

Triiodothyronine

Triiodothyronine supplementation has been reported in 3 patients who were treated for brain tumors and developed hypothalamic obesity [57]. Fernandes et al described a 24-year-old woman with a pineal tumor and astrocytoma, 10-year-old boy with optic glioma, and a 12-year-old girl with a mixed germ cell tumor who all suffered from hypothalamic obesity [57]. Conservative management with nutritional counseling was unsuccessful and all patients were being appropriately treated for other pituitary hormonal deficits. In particular, all three patients had normal serum free thyroxine levels. Triiodothyronine supplementation resulted in weight loss for all patients ranging from 4.3 kg to 14 kg. The triiodothyronine level was supraphysiological in all patients but no symptoms of hyperthyroidism were noted. Hyperthyroidism can be associated with the side effect of osteoporosis, but in this small case series one patient had an improvement of bone mineral density while on the supraphysiologic triiodothyronine for her hypothalamic obesity [57]. The authors hypothesized that triiodothyronine supplementation might act by altering hypothalamic homeostasis although the exact mechanism is unclear [57]. Further investigation into the effectiveness of this treatment and potential long-term side effects are necessary before this therapy can be routinely recommended.

Surgical Management

Bariatric surgery

In morbidly obese patients, bariatric surgery can result in substantial weight loss [58]. Bariatric surgical approaches include procedures to reduce food absorption such as a jejunal bypass or a biliary diversion; or procedures that reduce food ingestion such as a gastroplasty [59]. In procedures that induce malabsorption, weight loss occurs from a negative energy balance. However, side effects such as malnutrition, vitamin deficiencies, electrolyte imbalances and liver failure can occur [60]. Procedures that restrict the storage capacity of the stomach can lead to decreased caloric intake by creating early satiety. Usually restrictive procedures are easier to perform and have less side effects than malabsorptive procedures [60].

General guidelines exist for the selection of children for bariatric surgery [61], but there is limited literature on bariatric surgery in survivors of childhood cancer. In general, these surgical procedures should not be undertaken unless all other measures have failed since this is a major and non-reversible surgery.

Inge et al reported a 14-year-old boy who developed severe obesity with a BMI greater than 60 mg/m^2 following hypothalamic injury after sub-total resection and cranial irradiation for a craniopharyngioma [62]. This patient was initially treated with caloric restriction, appropriate pituitary hormone replacement, and a trial of octreotide. All of these measures were not successful at weight loss. Laparoscopic Roux-en-Y gastric bypass surgery together with a truncal anterior vagotomy was performed which resulted in 49 kg of weight loss over two and a half years. Food cravings were reduced and levels of fasting insulin, ghrelin and leptin were decreased.

Laparoscopic adjustable gastric banding

Laparoscopic adjustable gastric banding is much less invasive than bariatric surgery and consists of placing a silicone band around the gastric body to reduce the volume of the stomach and decrease the sensation of hunger. This procedure still requires general anesthesia, but in contrast to bariatric surgery the laparoscopic adjustable gastric banding is reversible [59]. This procedure has been shown to induce significant weight loss. It is also associated with beneficial metabolic effects such as decrease in blood pressure, improved glucose and lipid metabolism, and a greater reduction of visceral fat compared to subcutaneous fat [59].

Laparoscopic adjustable gastric banding has been reported in a case series of four patients diagnosed with childhood craniopharyngiomas [63]. In this series, patients ranged from age 2 years to 21 years at the time of diagnosis of their craniopharyngioma. Following their treatments for craniopharyngioma, all patients developed morbid obesity which was refractory to conventional therapy including dietary restriction, behavioral therapy, and increased physical activity. In addition, treatment with silbutramine in one case and orlistat in another case failed to result in improvement of the morbid obesity. Laparoscopic adjustable gastric banding resulted in persistent weight loss and a change in food eating behavior with a specific reduction in the amount of sweets. The authors hypothesized that laparoscopic adjustable gastric banding may cause altered regulation of gastrointestinal satiety factors [63].

Truncal vagotomy

Ventromedialhypothalamus injury, which can occur as a result of tumor invasion, surgical injury or radiotherapy, might result in hypothalamic obesity. This is associated with hyperinsulinemia and hyperphagia. Truncal vagotomy is hypothesized to decrease hunger sensations and decrease food intake through various gastric and extra-gastric factors. Delayed gastric emptying, decreased gastric motility, lower gastric acid secretion, and increased gastric tone can all lead to prolonged satiety [64]. Decreasing vagally mediated insulin secretion may also have effects on food intake [65]. Truncal vagotomy has been reported to result in a significant weight reduction, decreased hunger sensation and a decrease in cravings for sweets and food with high fat content [64]. In addition, an improvement of basal and maximal plasma glucose and insulin levels during an oral glucose tolerance test following truncal vagaotomy has been shown [64].

There is very little evidence of the efficacy of truncal vagotomy in childhood survivors of cancer. Smith et al reported a girl who was diagnosed with a craniopharyngioma at the age of 12 years [65]. Following resection and radiotherapy, she developed hypothalamic obesity. Conservative management was not successful and she was felt to be a poor candidate for bariatric surgery. A truncal vagotomy was performed and she lost approximately 15 kg. In addition, her post-vagotomy insulin levels decreased [65]. Further investigation needs to be done regarding this therapy in obesity associated with childhood cancer.

CONCLUSION

Childhood cancer can cause obesity directly through hypothalamic lesions or invasion. More commonly, childhood cancer treatments can result in obesity following surgery or radiotherapy. Obesity is a significant concern in survivors of childhood cancer, since it is a risk factor for many diseases including hypertension, type 2 diabetes, cardiovascular disease, dyslipidemia, and many others. With the increasing survival of children from childhood cancers, awareness of obesity as a complication is important so that early conservative interventions can be initiated.

Unfortunately, many children who develop hypothalamic obesity as a result of their cancer or their cancer treatment will be very difficult to manage with nutrition, exercise, and behavioral therapy. More aggressive pharmacologic and surgical treatment options have been explored for children, but to date there are few trials and further research needs to be pursued to find effective and safe treatment options.

REFERENCES

[1] Ogden, CL; Flegal, KM; Carroll, MD; Johnson, CL. Prevalence and trends in overweight among US children and adolescents, 1999-2000. *JAMA.*, 2002, 288, 1728-1732.

[2] Ogden, CL; Carroll, MD; Curtin, LR; McDowell, MA; Tabak, CJ; Flegal, KM. Prevalence of overweight and obesity in the United States, 1999-2004. *JAMA.* 2006, 295, 1549-1555.

[3] Flegal, KM; Carroll, MD; Ogden, CL; Johnson, CL. Prevalence and trends in obesity among US adults, 1999-2000. *JAMA.*, 2002, 288, 1723-1727.

[4] Flegal, KM; Carroll, MD; Kuczmarski, RJ; Johnson, CL. Overweight and obesity in the United States: prevalence and trends, 1960-1994. *Int. J. Obes. Relat. Metab. Disord.*, 1998, 22, 39-47.

[5] Barlow, SE. Expert committee recommendations regarding the prevention, assessment, and treatment of child and adolescent overweight and obesity: summary report. *Pediatrics.*, 2007, 120 (Suppl 4), S164-S192.

[6] Jemal, A; Murray, T; Samuels, A; Ghafoor, A; Ward, E; Thun, MJ. Cancer statistics, 2003. *CA: Cancer J. Clin.*, 2003, 53, 5-26.

[7] Brouwer, CA; Gietema, JA; Kamps, WA; de Vries, EG; Postma, A. Changes in body composition after childhood cancer treatment: impact on future health status - a review. *Crit. Rev. Oncol. Hematol.*, 2007, 63, 32-46.

[8] Janssen, I; Katzmarzyk, PT; Srinivasan, SR; Chen, W; Malina, RM; Bouchard, C; et al. Utility of childhood BMI in the prediction of adulthood disease: comparison of national and international references. *Obes. Res.*, 2005, 13, 1106-1115.

[9] Cheung, YB; Machin, D; Karlberg, J; Khoo, KS. A longitudinal study of pediatric body mass index values predicted health in middle age. *J. Clin. Epidemiol.*, 2004, 57, 1316-1322.

[10] Yan, LL; Daviglus, ML; Liu, K; Stamler, J; Wang, R; Pirzada, A; et al. Midlife body mass index and hospitalization and mortality in older age. *JAMA.*, 2006, 295, 190-198.

[11] Haslam, DW; James, WP. Obesity. *Lancet.*, 2005, 366, 1197-1209.

[12] Oeffinger, KC. Are survivors of acute lymphoblastic leukemia (ALL) at increased risk of cardiovascular disease? *Pediatr. Blood Cancer.*, 2008, 50(Suppl 2), 462-467; discussion 468.

[13] Gurney, JG, Ness, KK; Stovall, M; Wolden, S; Punyko, JA; Neglia, JP; et al. Final height and body mass index among adult survivors of childhood brain cancer: childhood cancer survivor study. *J. Clin. Endocrinol. Metab.*, 2003, 88, 4731-4739.

[14] Oeffinger, KC; Mertens, AC; Sklar, CA; Yasui, Y; Fears, T; Stovall, M; et al. Obesity in adult survivors of childhood acute lymphoblastic leukemia: a report from the Childhood Cancer Survivor Study. *J. Clin. Oncol.*, 2003, 21, 1359-1365.

[15] Rogers, PC; Meacham, LR; Oeffinger, KC; Henry, DW; Lange, BJ. Obesity in pediatric oncology. *Pediatr. Blood Cancer.*, 2005, 45, 881-891.

[16] Third Report of the National Cholesterol Education Program (NCEP) Expert Panel on Detection, Evaluation, and Treatment of High Blood Cholesterol in Adults (Adult Treatment Panel III) final report. *Circulation.*, 2002, 106, 3143-3421.

[17] Talvensaari, KK; Lanning, M; Tapanainen, P; Knip, M. Long-term survivors of childhood cancer have an increased risk of manifesting the metabolic syndrome. *J. Clin. Endocrinol. Metab.*, 1996, 81, 3051-3055.

[18] Mertens, AC; Yasui, Y; Neglia, JP; Potter, JD; Nesbit, ME, Jr.; Ruccione, K; et al. Late mortality experience in five-year survivors of childhood and adolescent cancer: the Childhood Cancer Survivor Study. *J. Clin. Oncol.*, 2001, 19, 3163-3172.

[19] Lustig, RH. The neuroendocrinology of childhood obesity. *Pediatr. Clin. North Am.*, 2001, 48, 909-930.

[20] Harz, KJ; Muller, HL; Waldeck, E; Pudel, V; Roth, C. Obesity in patients with craniopharyngioma: assessment of food intake and movement counts indicating physical activity. *J. Clin. Endocrinol. Metab.*, 2003, 88, 5227-5231.

[21] Mayer, EI; Reuter, M; Dopfer, RE; Ranke, MB. Energy expenditure, energy intake and prevalence of obesity after therapy for acute lymphoblastic leukemia during childhood. *Horm. Res.*, 2000, 53, 193-199.

[22] Marinovic, D; Dorgeret, S; Lescoeur, B; Alberti, C; Noel, M; Czernichow, P; et al. Improvement in bone mineral density and body composition in survivors of childhood acute lymphoblastic leukemia: a 1-year prospective study. *Pediatrics.*, 2005, 116, e102-e108.

[23] Warner, JT; Bell, W; Webb, DK; Gregory, JW. Relationship between cardiopulmonary response to exercise and adiposity in survivors of childhood malignancy. *Arch. Dis. Child.*, 1997, 76, 298-303.

[24] Reilly, JJ; Brougham, M; Montgomery, C; Richardson, F; Kelly, A; Gibson, BE. Effect of glucocorticoid therapy on energy intake in children treated for acute lymphoblastic leukemia. *J. Clin. Endocrinol. Metab.*, 2001, 86, 3742-3745.

[25] Muller, HL; Heinrich, M; Bueb, K; Etavard-Gorris, N; Gebhardt, U; Kolb, R; et al. Perioperative dexamethasone treatment in childhood craniopharyngioma - influence on short-term and long-term weight gain. *Exp. Clin. Endocrinol Diabetes.*, 2003, 111, 330-334.

[26] Tiosano, D; Eisentein, I; Militianu, D; Chrousos, GP; Hochberg, Z. 11 beta-hydroxysteroid dehydrogenasc activity in hypothalamic obcsity. *J. Clin. Endocrinol. Metab.*, 2003, 88, 379-384.

[27] Didi, M; Didcock, E; Davies, HA; Ogilvy-Stuart, AL; Wales, JK; Shalet, SM. High incidence of obesity in young adults after treatment of acute lymphoblastic leukemia in childhood. *J. Pediatr.*, 1995, 127, 63-67.

[28] Sklar, CA; Mertens, AC; Walter, A; Mitchell, D; Nesbit, ME; O'Leary, M; et al. Changes in body mass index and prevalence of overweight in survivors of childhood acute lymphoblastic leukemia: role of cranial irradiation. *Med. Pediatr. Oncol.*, 2000, 35, 91-95.

[29] Craig, F; Leiper, AD; Stanhope, R; Brain, C; Meller, ST; Nussey, SS. Sexually dimorphic and radiation dose dependent effect of cranial irradiation on body mass index. *Arch. Dis. Child.*, 1999, 81, 500-504.

[30] Nysom, K; Holm, K; Michaelsen, KF; Hertz, H; Muller, J; Molgaard, C. Degree of fatness after treatment for acute lymphoblastic leukemia in childhood. *J. Clin. Endocrinol. Metab.*, 1999, 84, 4591-4596.

[31] Schwartz, MW; Woods, SC; Porte, D, Jr.; Seeley, RJ; Baskin, DG. Central nervous system control of food intake. *Nature.*, 2000, 404, 661-671.

[32] Lustig, RH; Hinds, PS; Ringwald-Smith, K; Christensen, RK; Kaste, SC; Schreiber, RE; et al. Octreotide therapy of pediatric hypothalamic obesity: a double-blind, placebo-controlled trial. *J. Clin. Endocrinol. Metabol.*, 2003, 88, 2586-2592.

[33] Jeanrenaud, B. An hypothesis on the aetiology of obesity: dysfunction of the central nervous system as a primary cause. *Diabetologia.*, 1985, 28, 502-513.

[34] Roth, C; Wilken, B; Hanefeld, F; Schroter, W; Leonhardt, U. Hyperphagia in children with craniopharyngioma is associated with hyperleptinaemia and a failure in the downregulation of appetite. *Eur. J. Endocrinol.*, 1998, 138, 89-91.

[35] Mantzoros, CS. The role of leptin in human obesity and disease: a review of current evidence. *Ann. Int. Med.*, 1999, 130, 671-680.

[36] Stephens, TW; Basinski, M; Bristow, PK; Bue-Valleskey, JM; Burgett, SG; Craft, L; et al. The role of neuropeptide Y in the antiobesity action of the obese gene product. *Nature.*, 1995, 377, 530-532.

[37] Strosberg, AD; Issad, T. The involvement of leptin in humans revealed by mutations in leptin and leptin receptor genes. *Trends Pharmacol. Sci.*, 1999, 20, 227-230.

[38] Link, K; Moell, C; Garwicz, S; Cavallin-Stahl, E; Bjork, J; Thilen, U; et al. Growth hormone deficiency predicts cardiovascular risk in young adults treated for acute lymphoblastic leukemia in childhood. *J. Clin. Endocrinol. Metab.*, 2004, 89, 5003-5012.

[39] Birkebaek, NH; Fisker, S; Clausen, N; Tuovinen, V; Sindet-Pedersen, S; Christiansen, JS. Growth and endocrinological disorders up to 21 years after treatment for acute lymphoblastic leukemia in childhood. *Med. Pediatr. Oncol.*, 1998, 30, 351-356.

[40] Siviero-Miachon, AA; Spinola-Castro, AM; Tosta-Hernandez, PD; de Martino Lee, ML; Petrilli, AS. Leptin assessment in acute lymphocytic leukemia survivors: role of cranial radiotherapy? *J. Pediatr. Hematol. Oncol.*, 2007, 29, 776-782.

[41] Brennan, BM; Rahim, A; Blum, WF; Adams, JA; Eden, OB; Shalet, SM. Hyperleptinaemia in young adults following cranial irradiation in childhood: growth hormone deficiency or leptin insensitivity? *Clin. Endocrinol.*, 1999, 50, 163-169.

[42] Patel, L; Cooper, CD; Quinton, ND; Butler, GE; Gill, MS; Jefferson, IG; et al. Serum leptin and leptin binding activity in children and adolescents with hypothalamic dysfunction. *J. Pediatr. Endocrinol. Metab.*, 2002, 15, 963-971.

[43] Ross, JA. Genetic susceptibility and body mass in childhood cancer survivors. *Pediatr. Blood Cancer.*, 2007, 48, 731-735.

[44] Mattevi, VS; Zembrzuski, VM; Hutz, MH. Association analysis of genes involved in the leptin-signaling pathway with obesity in Brazil. *Int. J. Obes. Relat. Metab. Disord.*, 2002, 26, 1179-1185.

[45] Quinton, ND; Lee, AJ; Ross, RJ; Eastell, R; Blakemore, AI. A single nucleotide polymorphism (SNP) in the leptin receptor is associated with BMI, fat mass and leptin levels in postmenopausal Caucasian women. *Hum. Genet.*, 2001, 108, 233-236.

[46] van Rossum, CT; Hoebee, B; van Baak, MA; Mars, M; Saris, WH; Seidell, JC. Genetic variation in the leptin receptor gene, leptin, and weight gain in young Dutch adults. *Obes. Res.*, 2003, 11, 377-386.

[47] Yiannakouris, N; Yannakoulia, M; Melistas, L; Chan, JL; Klimis-Zacas, D; Mantzoros, CS. The Q223R polymorphism of the leptin receptor gene is significantly associated with obesity and predicts a small percentage of body weight and body composition variability. *J. Clin. Endocrinol. Metab.*, 2001, 86, 4434-4439.

[48] Robison, LL; Mertens, AC; Boice, JD; Breslow, NE; Donaldson, SS; Green, DM; et al. Study design and cohort characteristics of the Childhood Cancer Survivor Study: a multi-institutional collaborative project. *Med. Pediatr. Oncol.*, 2002, 38, 229-239.

[49] Ross, JA; Oeffinger, KC; Davies, SM; Mertens, AC; Langer, EK; Kiffmeyer, WR; et al. Genetic variation in the leptin receptor gene and obesity in survivors of childhood acute lymphoblastic leukemia: a report from the Childhood Cancer Survivor Study. *J. Clin. Oncol.*, 2004, 22, 3558-3562.

[50] Rosen, T; Bosaeus, I; Tolli, J; Lindstedt, G; Bengtsson, BA. Increased body fat mass and decreased extracellular fluid volume in adults with growth hormone deficiency. *Clin. Endocrinol.*, 1993, 38, 63-71.

[51] Gurney, JG; Ness, KK; Sibley, SD; O'Leary, M; Dengel, DR; Lee, JM; et al. Metabolic syndrome and growth hormone deficiency in adult survivors of childhood acute lymphoblastic leukemia. *Cancer.*, 2006, 107, 1303-1312.

[52] Srinivasan, S; Ogle, GD; Garnett, SP; Briody, JN; Lee, JW; Cowell, CT. Features of the metabolic syndrome after childhood craniopharyngioma. *J. Clin. Endocrinol. Metab.*, 2004, 89, 81-86.

[53] Neville, KA; Cohn, RJ; Steinbeck, KS; Johnston, K; Walker, JL. Hyperinsulinemia, impaired glucose tolerance, and diabetes mellitus in survivors of childhood cancer: prevalence and risk factors. *J. Clin. Endocrinol. Metab.*, 2006, 91, 4401-4407.

[54] Nuver, J; Smit, AJ; Wolffenbuttel, BH; Sluiter, WJ; Hoekstra, HJ; Sleijfer, DT; et al. The metabolic syndrome and disturbances in hormone levels in long-term survivors of disseminated testicular cancer. *J. Clin. Oncol.*, 2005, 23, 3718-3725.

[55] Lustig, RH; Rose, SR; Burghen, GA; Velasquez-Mieyer, P; Broome, DC; Smith, K; et al. Hypothalamic obesity caused by cranial insult in children: altered glucose and insulin dynamics and reversal by a somatostatin agonist. *J. Pediatr.*, 1999, 135, 162-168.

[56] Mason, PW; Krawiecki, N; Meacham, LR. The use of dextroamphetamine to treat obesity and hyperphagia in children treated for craniopharyngioma. *Arch. Pediatr. Adolesc. Med.*, 2002, 156, 887-892.

[57] Fernandes, JK; Klein, MJ; Ater, JL; Kuttesch, JF; Vassilopoulou-Sellin, R. Triiodothyronine supplementation for hypothalamic obesity. *Metabolism.*, 2002, 51, 1381-1383.

[58] Fisberg, M; Baur, L; Chen, W; Hoppin, A; Koletzko, B; Lau, D; et al. Obesity in children and adolescents: Working Group report of the second World Congress of Pediatric Gastroenterology, Hepatology, and Nutrition. *J. Pediatr. Gastroenterol. Nutr.*, 2004, 39(Suppl 2), S678-S687.

[59] Pontiroli, AE; Pizzocri, P; Librenti, MC; Vedani, P; Marchi, M; Cucchi, E; et al. Laparoscopic adjustable gastric banding for the treatment of morbid (grade 3) obesity

and its metabolic complications: a three-year study. *J. Clin. Endocrinol. Metab.*, 2002, 87, 3555-3561.

[60] Bult, MJ; van Dalen, T; Muller, AF. Surgical treatment of obesity. *Eur. J. Endocrinol.*, 2008, 158, 135-145.

[61] Inge, TH; Krebs, NF; Garcia, VF; Skelton, JA; Guice, KS; Strauss, RS; et al. Bariatric surgery for severely overweight adolescents: concerns and recommendations. *Pediatrics.*, 2004, 114, 217-223.

[62] Inge, TH; Pfluger, P; Zeller, M; Rose, SR; Burget, L; Sundararajan, S; et al. Gastric bypass surgery for treatment of hypothalamic obesity after craniopharyngioma therapy. *Nat. Clin. Pract. Endocrinol. Metab.*, 2007, 3, 606-609.

[63] Muller, HL; Gebhardt, U; Wessel, V; Schroder, S; Kolb, R; Sorensen, N; et al. First experiences with laparoscopic adjustable gastric banding (LAGB) in the treatment of patients with childhood craniopharyngioma and morbid obesity. *Klin. Padiatr.*, 2007, 219, 323-325.

[64] Kral, JG. Effects of truncal vagotomy on body weight and hyperinsulinemia in morbid obesity. *Am. J. Clin. Nutr.*, 1980, 33(Suppl 2), 416-419.

[65] Smith, DK; Sarfeh, J; Howard, L. Truncal vagotomy in hypothalamic obesity. *Lancet.*, 1983, 1, 1330-1331.

In: Overweightness and Walking
Editor: Caleb I. Black, pp. 193-209

ISBN: 978-1-60741-298-4
© 2010 Nova Science Publishers, Inc.

Chapter 9

EFFECTIVENESS OF SCHOOL-BASED POLICIES TO REDUCE CHILDHOOD OBESITY

Ming-Chin Yeh[1], Nisha Beharie[2] and Janel Obenchain[1]*

[1]Nutrition and Food Science Track, Urban Public Health Program, Hunter College, City University of New York, New York, New York
[2]Department of Psychiatry and Community Medicine, Mount Sinai School of Medicine, New York, New York

ABSTRACT

The prevalence of childhood obesity has increased significantly over the past three decades. It is estimated that approximately 17% of all school-aged children are overweight or obese. Childhood obesity has a huge impact on the health of children as it is associated with an increased risk of hypertension, hypercholesterolemia, diabetes, and a wide range of additional physiological and psychosocial consequences.

Because school settings offer continuous, intensive contact with children during children's formative years, they have several advantages for implementation of interventions. For example, school educational programs can develop student attitudes, knowledge, and skills for a healthy lifestyle. In addition to education, schools can promote healthy dietary practices and regular physical activity by modifying school environments through offering healthier choices in cafeterias and vending machines and by providing physical activity curriculum. Overall, school infrastructure and physical environment, policies, curricula, and personnel have great potential to positively influence children's weight and health.

Based on prior review articles examining interventions implemented at school settings, strategies involving a combination of nutrition and physical activity interventions seem to be effective at achieving weight reduction in school settings. However, less attention has been paid to developing, implementing and evaluating school-based policy on childhood obesity prevention and management. This chapter intends to summarize evidence regarding the effectiveness of school-based policy

* Corresponding author: Email: myeh@hunter.cuny.edu

interventions and to provide possible policy recommendations for researchers, practitioners and policy makers.

We first provide the definition of overweight and obesity and describe the obesity trends in the US and the world. Physiological, psychosocial and economic consequences related to obesity are also presented. We then discuss school-based policies and programs. Finally, policy recommendations for preventing obesity are provided.

INTRODUCTION

This chapter attempts to address the childhood obesity epidemic by describing and analyzing school-based policies that work to both prevent and treat obesity and by offering suggestions for future policy and programming. Schools are chosen as the focal point as much national, state, and local policy can be effectively implemented in schools to ensure that children eat less energy dense food, consume less food and drinks high in sugar, and be more physically active.

Definition and Measures of Being Overweight and Obesity

Body Mass Index (BMI) is a common measure of weight status. Body mass index is defined as an individual's body weight in kilograms divided by the square of their height in meters (kg/m^2). For adults, a BMI below 18.5 is considered underweight and a BMI between 18.5 and 24.9 is normal weight. Being overweight is defined as having a BMI between 25 and 29.9, and being obese is defined as having a BMI equal to or higher than 30.

For children and teens, BMI is age and sex-specific and is often referred to as BMI-for-age. This measurement is obtained after BMI is calculated by plotting the BMI number on the Centers for Disease Control and Prevention (CDC) BMI-for-age growth charts (for either girls or boys) to obtain a percentile ranking. The percentile indicates the relative position of the child's BMI number among children of the same sex and age and is the most commonly used indicator to assess the size and growth patterns of individual children in the United States. The growth charts show the weight status categories used with children and teens (i.e. underweight, healthy weight, overweight, and obese). BMI-for-age weight status categories and the corresponding percentiles are shown in the following table. [1]

Weight Status Category	Percentile Range
Underweight	Less than the 5th percentile
Healthy weight	5th percentile to less than the 85th percentile
Overweight	85th to less than the 95th percentile
Obese	Equal to or greater than the 95th percentile

Global Obesity Trends

There is much discussion and awareness of the obesity epidemic in the United States. However, there is data to suggest that the rates of obesity are also rising globally. Most of these data come from industrialized or developed nations. According to a recent World Health Organization (WHO) report, the levels of obesity have risen dramatically from 1977 to 2004 among Organization for Economic Cooperation and Development (OECD) countries. The 2004 Health Statistics Data of the OECD reported that the rates of people who were overweight and obese rose from less than 20% in 1976 to more than 50% by 2001. [2] Obesity has, therefore, become an issue of increasing concern in recent years among developed or industrialized nations.

The WHO figures indicated that obesity is spreading around the world as a "global epidemic". According to the WHO, as of 2004, there were more people suffering from illnesses related to being overweight than from illnesses caused by malnutrition. Globally there were more than 1 billion overweight adults, of which at least 300 million were clinically obese, while 800 million suffered from malnutrition. [3] Consequently, many of the OECD countries began contemplating various measures to reverse the trend of rising obesity rates. For example, as of 2005 the European Union Parliament planned to introduce a directory on mandatory nutritional labeling of processed food products sold in supermarkets to help consumers make informed purchase and consumption decisions, [4] and rules were announced in January of 2008 requiring all prepackaged food to clearly display amounts of sugar, salt, fat, saturated fat, carbohydrates, and energy on the front of packaging. [5]

The rates of obesity among developing countries could also be of great concern as many of these countries become increasingly industrialized and adopt many of the same food production and eating patterns which have led to the epidemic seen in OECD countries and other developed nations. [6] This could lead to a period of time where obesity and malnutrition exist in juxtaposition to one another in developing countries (as is the case in some regions of the developed world as well). Many developing countries are in fact in a time of nutritional transition. The "nutrition transition" proposes that, if the trends continue, obesity rates among developing countries could parallel those of the developed countries. [7] Developing countries therefore have the opportunity to study and learn from the obesity epidemic that is currently affecting developed nations to prevent the same trajectory in their own countries.

Obesity Trends in the United States

A startling trend in obesity has emerged among the US population during the past several decades. The CDC's Behavioral Risk Factor Surveillance System (BRFSS) measured levels of obesity among adults nationwide and found that in 1991 only four states had obesity prevalence rates of 15 - 19 % and no states had rates above or above 20%. By 2008, however, only Colorado had a prevalence of obesity less than 20%. Of the forty nine states with prevalence greater than 20%, thirty-two states had prevalence equal to or greater than 25%. Six states, Alabama, Mississippi, Oklahoma, South Carolina, Tennessee, and West Virginia had a prevalence of obesity equal to or greater than 30%. [8]

Obesity trends among children

Obesity is also affecting children at an alarming rate. Data from the National Health and Nutrition Examination Survey (NHANES) reveal that the prevalence of obesity in children has increased dramatically over the past several decades. Between the study periods of 1976-1980 and 2003 - 2006, the prevalence of obesity increased from 5.0% to 12.4% for children between the ages of 2 - 5 years and from 6.5% to 17% for those aged 6 - 11. [9] Other studies have also illustrated this increase. For example, Hedley et al. found that the prevalence rate of obesity tripled in the past twenty to thirty years to 16.5% among U.S. children and teenagers aged 6 - 19 years, and doubled to 10.3% among preschool children aged 2 - 5 years. [10] This marked increase in childhood obesity deserves researchers' as well as policy makers' special attention.

CONSEQUENCES OF OBESITY

The rise in childhood obesity has coincided with the rise of obesity related co-morbidities among children. The consequences of childhood obesity can be broadly classified into physiological and psychosocial consequences.

Physiological Consequences

There are many physiological/medical consequences that can occur due to obesity. Some major conditions include: hypertension, diabetes, dyslipidemia and non-alcoholic fatty liver disease. [11] Obstructive sleep apnea syndrome [12] and orthopedic disorders [13] are also common. Conditions such as gastroesophageal reflux, [14] constipation, [15] and asthma [16] have also been reported.

While many of these diseases tend to occur later in life, it is concerning that these diseases are becoming more commonly seen in children, such as type 2 diabetes. [17 - 18] This form of diabetes has historically only affected an older population. However, type 2 diabetes and other conditions associated with more elderly populations, such as hypertension, [19] orthopedic complications, [13] and fatty liver stenosis, [20 - 21] are now commonly found among obese children and adolescents.

Psychosocial Consequences

There are a host of contextual factors that cause obese children and youth to be at risk for poor psychosocial outcomes. Overweight and obese children are commonly victimized and teased by their peers because their peers view them as different and undesirable. Although such victimization occurs commonly among adolescents, obese adolescents are more susceptible than their average-weight peers. [22] This behavior is often referred to as "weight-based peer victimization" and is defined as unsolicited bullying and teasing as a result of being overweight or obese. This peer victimization of obese adolescents has been associated with low self-esteem, body dissatisfaction, social isolation, marginalization, poor psychosocial adjustment, depression, eating disorders, and suicidal ideation and attempts, as well as poor academic performance. [22]

In addition to weight-based peer victimization, Falkner et al. found an association between obesity and academic performance (i.e. being held back in school and quitting school). The researchers found that obese girls were less likely to have associated with peers, reported more emotional problems, felt more hopeless, and reported more suicidal ideation when compared with their average weight peers. Similarly, obese boys reported that their "friends didn't care about them" more so than their average weight peers. [23]

There are also numerous studies that point to the deleterious effect of obesity on mental health during adolescence. For example, the results of a study conducted by Al Mamun et al. suggest that the perception of being overweight during adolescence is a significant risk factor for depression in young adult men and women. [24] Furthermore, while overweight children have been shown to maintain a positive self image, [25] overweight adolescents (particularly females) tend to develop negative self images that may carry on through adulthood. [26 - 27]

Economic Consequences

Given the significant health consequences of obesity, it stands to reason that there would also be greater associated economic costs. According to an article published in 2003, the costs of healthcare for overweight and obese individuals is estimated on average 37% more than the costs for normal weight individuals, adding an average of $732 to average medical bill to each American. The study also shows that obesity related medical costs account for almost 10% of all health expenditures in the US. [28]

In addition, childhood obesity alone has been shown to be associated with a near doubling of cost of hospitalizations during the time period of 1999 – 2005 due to a diagnosis of obesity from $125.9 to $237.6 million (accounting for inflation). Similarly, the burden on Medicaid has increased as obesity related hospitalizations cost Medicaid $188 million in 2005 as compared with $53.6 million in 2001. [29]

SCHOOL-BASED INTERVENTION

There have been extensive reviews examining interventions implemented at school settings. [30 – 33] For example, Katz et al. conducted a systematic review and meta-analysis of peer-review studies published between 1966 and 2004 to determine the effectiveness of school-based strategies for obesity. [34] Similarly to the results from many other review papers, Katz et al. concluded that a combination of nutrition and physical activity interventions seems to be effective at achieving weight reduction in school settings. However, less attention has been paid to developing, implementing and evaluating school-based policy on childhood obesity prevention and management. The following intends to shed some light on school-based policy interventions on childhood obesity prevention and management.

The Importance of School-Based Obesity Prevention Policies

Children spend more time in schools than in any other environment away from home. More than 48 million students attend 94,000 public, elementary, and secondary schools each day. [35] Many of these children are also eating a significant portion of their daily meals at school. The National School Lunch Program provided nutritionally balanced low-cost or free lunches for more than 30.5 million children each school day in 2008. [36] "School Lunch", however, is no longer just a lunch program. The program also provides cash reimbursements for school breakfast and afterschool snacks. Many children eat breakfast and lunch at school every day, and those children obtain an average of 47% of their total daily calories at school. [37] In addition, there are 7 states (Delaware, Illinois, Michigan, Missouri, New York, Oregon, and Pennsylvania) that require schools to provide snacks and dinner in areas where more than 50% of the children qualify for free or reduced price school meals. [38]

Given that children and adolescents are eating so many of their meals in the schools, the food offered there should be of high quality. However, the recent Third School Nutrition and Dietary Assessment study (SNDA III) has shown that although the majority of US schools offer breakfast and lunches that meet the U.S. Department of Agriculture (USDA) standards for key nutrients, such as protein, vitamins A and C, calcium and iron, less than one-third of public schools meet these standards for total fat and saturated fat. [39]

Furthermore, during the past few decades, there has been an increase in the number of food options available throughout the school day including "competitive foods" sold as a la carte options at meals, and items available to purchase from snack bars and vending machines. [40] These foods "compete" with the federally subsidized nutritionally balanced school meals for the student's lunch or pocket money. Unlike the National School Lunch Program meals, competitive foods are not required by the USDA to comply with the Dietary Guidelines for Americans. [41] The Dietary Guidelines for Americans are jointly published every five years by the Department of Health and Human Services (DHHS) and the USDA, most recently in 2005. [42] In contrast to the evolving Dietary Guidelines, the federal requirements for competitive foods were established in 1979 and have not been similarly updated. These 1979 requirements provide minimal standards that seem nutritionally arbitrary (e.g. candy bars are ok but jelly beans are not). Furthermore, these guidelines apply only to foods sold in the cafeteria. [41] Those "banned" jelly beans might still be available in the vending machine just outside in the hallway, along with the most common competitive foods sold: sodas, sports drinks, and higher-fat salty snacks. [43]

The trend of increasing availability of unhealthy foods, compounded by the lack of access to nutritious foods in schools as well as in communities, allows for both obesity and hunger to coexist in low-income communities. [39] Minority and low-income communities in particular are at increased risk for obesity, [44 - 45] presenting a challenge for school nutrition programs in balancing the need to prevent hunger as well as obesity. The aim of ensuring enough key nutrients and calories for the nation's hungry children may now be at odds with concerns of over consumption of poorer quality calories that may lead to obesity. For example, SNDA III data found that elementary school children in schools offering fried potatoes or dessert in school lunches more than once per week were much more likely to be obese than children in schools that served fried potatoes and desserts only once per week or less often. [46]

Significantly, considering the rapidly increasing cost of food, transportation, labor and benefits and indirect expense, federal policies do not provide adequate funding to government-sponsored school meal programs. [43] For example the Omnibus Budget Reconciliation Acts of 1980 and 1981 cut federal reimbursement levels for school meals, and when adjusted for inflation the original funding cut has never been restored. [47]

Lack of physical activity of our children has also contributed to the pediatric obesity epidemic. Policies (or lack of) have directly impacted the level at which students are active in schools and in their neighborhoods. For example, there is no federal law requiring physical education to be provided to students in the education system. There is also no incentive for offering physical education programs. The physical education curriculums are largely left up to states and school districts. As such, only 12% of states require elementary schools to provide recess that could potentially be used for physical activity. [48]

Large Scale School Programs and Policies Implemented to Combat Obesity

Despite some of the potential negative impacts that prior policies have had on the health outcomes related to childhood obesity, policies and programming have been implemented in response to the obesity epidemic at local, state, and federal levels.

Local schools and districts are striving to improve healthy food offerings through programs such as farm-to-school programs which link schools with local farms to provide locally grown fresh fruits and vegetables. [49] Similarly, some schools have created school gardening programs that the students participate in and benefit from by consuming the fresh produce that the gardens provide. [50]

At the state level there have been efforts to alter the competitive foods that are offered to students in schools to include more fresh fruits, vegetables, whole grain, and less sugary drinks. For example, between 2000 and 2006, the percentage of school districts prohibiting vending machines offering high-calorie, low nutrition foods and beverages rose from 4 to 30 percent; schools selling water in vending machines or school stores increased from 30 to 46 percent; and schools selling cookies, cake, or other high-fat baked goods in vending machines or school stores fell from 38 to 25 percent. [50]

Finally, national policies have been enacted to support the increase in the nutritional values of school meals. The Child Nutrition and WIC legislation covers all Federal child nutrition programs, including the School Breakfast, National School Lunch Programs, and the Special Supplement Nutrition Program for Women, Infants and Children (WIC). Along with other important provisions, the Child Nutrition and WIC Reauthorization Act of 2004 required all school districts participating in the National School Lunch Program to develop a wellness policy including goals for nutrition education and nutrition guidelines. Specifically, school wellness policies must include the following components to encourage student wellbeing: 1) standards and goals for nutrition education, physical activity, and other school-based activities; 2) nutrition guidelines for all foods available on each school campus during the school day; 3) assurance that guidelines for reimbursable school meals will not be less restrictive than federal regulations and guidelines; 4) a plan for measuring and implementing local wellness policy; and 5) involve parents, students, school food authority representatives, school board members, school administrators, and the public in developing the school wellness policy. [41] The Child Nutrition and WIC Reauthorization Act of 2004 is set to expire on September 30, 2009. By reauthorizing this act, Congress will have the opportunity to affect the nutrition of numerous children in many differing settings.

The legislation commonly known as "the Farm Bill" is another example of evolving federal policy promoting nutrition among children. Agricultural policies and funding allocations for nutritional programs promulgated by the "Farm Bill" can directly impact the nature and distribution of the nation's food supply. In addition to other important programs, such as emergency food assistance, the "Farm Bill" can impact children's access to fresh fruit and vegetables. The 2002 Farm Bill, the Farm Security and Rural Investment Act of 2002, created a pilot program to provide free fresh fruit and vegetable snacks to students in twenty-five schools in six states. Acting in synergy, the 2004 Child Nutrition and WIC Reauthorization Act slightly expanded the program and gave it permanent status. In turn, the 2008 Farm Bill, the Food, Energy and Conservation Act of 2008, expanded this Fresh Fruit and Vegetable Snack Program nationwide. [51]

Increased attention is also being paid to physical activity. At the local level, some school districts are providing policy leadership encouraging children to walk and bicycle to school. States are also promulgating policies, such as increasing the qualifications of physical education instructors. The number of states that have policies requiring certain standards of new hires of physical education instructors for high schools, middle schools and elementary schools are 48, 43 and 28 respectively. [52]

Individually Focused Programs in Schools

Although school-based intervention programs often focus on working with students, very few obesity prevention policies enacted by states have focused on students in the school individually or with their families. However, one common policy is individualized BMI tracking. Arkansas was the first state to mandate that all public schools perform BMI assessments and has had 94 to 99 percent participation rates by schools. It has been shown that obesity rates have not increased since 2003 in that state. [53] Currently, California, Delaware, Florida, Illinois, Kansas, Maine, Missouri, New York, Pennsylvania, Tennessee, and West Virginia have incorporated measurement of student BMI levels as part of either health examinations or physical education activities. [54] Despite high participation rates, few studies, with the exception of Arkansas noted above, have examined the effectiveness or impact of school based BMI measurement. Additionally, parents have reported concerns about maintaining their child's privacy, conducting respectful measurements, and reporting results in a neutral manner that avoid weight labeling. [55] BMI tracking among school children deserves further investigation.

Community-Based or Large Scale Programs and Policies Outside of the School

Despite the fact that the schools are an opportune location for programs and policies targeted at obesity prevention and reduction, these efforts must be augmented with national policies and programming targeted to obesity prevention and reduction outside of schools.

The childhood obesity epidemic must be looked at from an ecological model that includes a variety of domains as a means of intervention including the homes, communities, childcare facilities, and after school programs. [56] To combat the so-called "obesogenic" environment, a term referring to those environments that promote weight gain primarily by either encouraging overconsumption or deterring physical activity, multi-level approaches are needed. [57]

A review of health promotion and disease prevention efforts reveal that increasing physical activity in adults can be cost effective. [58] This would also be true for those efforts that increase physical activity for children and adolescents. Walk to School programs are one example of community-based programs aimed at increasing activity. [59] The Wonders of Walking program in Colorado is another success story. [60] This program consisted of one session (45 – 60 min) featuring education on the benefits of exercise, activity, goal-setting, social support, and problem-solving to reduce sedentary time and maximize walking. In addition, an "open-loop feedback system" was employed to encourage youth to set specific walking goals and to frequently review goal attainment. This is an approach that has shown to increase activity in obese and normal weight children. [61 – 62]

Large scale polices that impact children and adolescents may also affect people of all ages. Legislation requiring chain restaurants and fast-food outlets to list calories and other nutrition information is a policy that can affect people of all ages in many different settings. New York City passed a regulation requiring large chain restaurants to post nutrition information on menus or menu boards [63] and several states have also adopted similar policies. [64] Policies regarding restaurant and fast-food meals are of particular importance as it was estimated in 2007 that nearly half (47.9%) of all food expenditures are spent eating outside the home. This has increased from 34% in 1974, and nearly doubled what it was in 1955. [65] In addition, studies have linked frequent eating out to higher caloric intake, weight gain, and obesity. [66 – 68] Survey results conducted by Burton et al. also showed that consumers significantly underestimated the levels of calories, fat, and saturated fat in less-healthful restaurant items. Actual fat and saturated fat levels were twice consumers' estimates, and calories approached twice more than what consumers expected. In the subsequent experiment, for items for which levels of calories, fat, and saturated fat substantially exceeded consumers' expectations, the provision of nutrition information had a significant influence on consumer's product attitude, purchase intention, and choice. [69] Thus, policies such as providing calorie labeling information could potentially reduce the amount of calories consumed.

In addition to providing more information on making healthier choices, policies can also induce changes in the physical environment that increase the ability to make healthier choices. For example, polices reducing disparities in lack of access to healthy foods are a promising means towards encouraging healthier eating. A report issued by the Institute for Agriculture and Trade Policy cited several successful examples of farmers markets in low-income neighborhoods around the country, as well as cooperative grocery stores and community gardens in impoverished neighborhoods of the Minneapolis/St. Paul metropolitan area. [70] Another solution is to improve offerings in the small convenience stores that many urban neighborhoods rely on. The District of Columbia, Philadelphia, Los Angeles, New York, and many other cities are working on policies to encourage healthier options in these neighborhood corner stores. [71]

CONCLUSION

Recommendations Provided by the Centers for Disease Control and Prevention

The CDC recently published a report outlining twenty-four recommended community strategies and measurements to prevent obesity in the United States. [72] A large majority of these recommendations are aimed at reducing obesogenic environments for adults and children alike. These are as follows:

Strategies to promote the availability of affordable healthy food and beverages:
1. Communities should increase availability of healthier food and beverage choices in public service venues.
2. Communities should improve availability of affordable healthier food and beverage choices in public service venues.
3. Communities should improve geographic availability of supermarkets in underserved areas.
4. Communities should provide incentives to food retailers to locate in and/or offer healthier food and beverage choices in underserved areas.
5. Communities should improve availability of mechanisms for purchasing foods from farms.
6. Communities should provide incentives for the production, distribution and procurement of foods from local farms.

Strategies to support healthy food and beverages choices:
1. Communities should restrict availability of less healthy foods and beverages in public service venues.
2. Communities should institute smaller portion size options in public service venues.
3. Communities should limit advertisements of less healthy foods and beverages.
4. Communities should discourage consumption of sugar-sweetened beverages.

Strategies to create safe communities that support physical activity:
1. Communities should improve access to outdoor recreational facilities.
2. Communities should enhance infrastructure supporting bicycling.
3. Communities should enhance infrastructure supporting walking.
4. Communities should support locating schools within easy walking distance of residential areas.
5. Communities should improve access to public transportation.
6. Communities should zone for mixed use development.
7. Communities should enhance personal safety in areas where persons are or could be physically active.
8. Communities should enhance traffic safety in areas where persons are or could be physically active.

Strategies to encourage communities to organize for change:
1.   Communities should participate in community coalitions or partnerships to address obesity.

More importantly, for the purposes of this chapter, some proposed *strategies directly address the childhood obesity epidemic*. These recommendations are:

1.   Communities should require physical education in schools.
2.   Communities should increase the amount of physical activity in PE programs in schools.
3.   Communities should increase opportunities for extracurricular physical activity.
4.   Communities should reduce screen time in public service venues (such as day care settings and schools).
5.   Communities should encourage the support of breastfeeding.

Implications and Policy Recommendations

While all of these community-based recommendations are excellent suggestions, many of the suggested community level changes would be easier to implement and enforce if federal and state policies in the area of food distribution and physical activity were strengthened. For example, simply recommending that communities require physical education in schools will not result in improved physical education programs if economic support and an enforceable policy is lacking. A community-only approach will only continue to favor those more affluent communities with the resources and support to implement such recommendations.

Policies should be strengthened to bring accountability and not just recommendations to provide healthy food and encourage physical activity. Schools must be accountable to provide healthy food instead of competitive food. Despite improvements in the quality of competitive foods available in schools, much more progress is needed. For example, as of 2006, more than three-fourths of high schools sold sodas or high-sugar fruit drinks, and almost half of high schools allow students to buy food and beverages from vending machines or school stores. [50] From a health perspective, competitive foods should be restricted in schools as they have been found to directly affect health outcomes of the students. However, many schools may rely on the extra revenue provided by the easily sold high-fat, high-sugar foods and beverages often found in vending machines. [43] In order to hold the school accountable for improving the competitive food options, the community may also need to consider ensuring the school does not suffer from the loss of revenue. The good news is that the cities of New York, Los Angeles and Chicago have already made steps to improve the food being sold in vending machines and many schools have been able to maintain revenue following these changes. [73]

Accountability extends beyond the school doors, however. Communities also have accountability in encouraging the availability of healthy food options. This is particularly important for schools that have "open campuses" allowing the children to leave the school grounds during the lunch period. For example, there is data to suggest that the proximity of fast food restaurants to schools affects adolescent obesity. These establishments should therefore be regulated either by requiring that the food served be less calorie-dense and include more fruits and vegetables or by limiting the proximity and/or density of these establishments to the schools. [74]

Finally, the federal policies that govern the nation's food supply and the food industry must be evaluated as a complex whole. Although the federal government is taking policy action to combat childhood obesity, federal policy may have in fact inadvertently contributed to the childhood obesity epidemic through food-assistance and agricultural programs that failed to promote healthful fruit and vegetable consumption. For example, the 2007 WIC food assistance package revision, implemented in 2009, includes fruits and vegetables for the first time as part of aligning the package with the 2005 Dietary Guidelines for Americans. [75] Likewise, the subsidization of commodity corn by our agricultural policy has consequentially encouraged the production of high-fructose corn syrup, a plentiful, inexpensive sweetener with characteristics promoting the shelf-life, desirability, and cheapness of calorie-dense packaged foods and beverages. [76]

All of our federal food and nutrition policy, including our agricultural policy, should reflect the goals of the Dietary Guidelines. These Guidelines recommend that Americans consume 2 to 6 ½ cups of fruit and vegetables combined daily depending on age, gender, and activity level. [77] However, the most recent per capita food availability data (adjusted for loss) show that in 2006 there was only enough fruit available in any form (including juice) to provide less than one cup per person per day, and only enough vegetables in any form (including beans, lentils, legumes, and dehydrated vegetables) to provide less than two cups per person per day. [78] In sum, federal policies must be accountable and coherent as a whole in striving to combat childhood obesity by reflecting the goals promulgated in the Dietary Guidelines for Americans, particularly in the important school setting.

REFERENCES

[1] Centers for Disease Control and Prevention (CDC). *About BMI for Children and Teens: Healthy Weight – It's not a diet, it's a lifestyle!* http://www.cdc.gov/healthy weight/assessing/bmi/ childrens_BMI/about_childrens_BMI.html.

[2] Organization for Economic Cooperation and Development (OECD), *Health Data*, 2004, www.oecd.org.

[3] World Health Organization (WHO). *"Obesity and Overweight"*. Geneva 2004, http://www.who.int/dietphysicalactivity/publications/facts/obesity/en/.

[4] Laureiro, M. L., Nayga, R. M. (2005). *Obesity rates in OECD countries: An international perspective.* http://ageconsearch.umn.edu/bitstream/24454/1/ pp05lo01.pdf. Accessed 9/18/2009.

[5] Traynor, I. & Boseley, S. EU brings in compulsory food labelling to curb obesity. *The Guardian.* January 31, 2008. http://www.guardian. foodanddrink. Accessed 9/25/2009.

[6] Wang, Y., Monteiro, C. & Popkin, B. M. (2002). Trends of obesity and underweight in older children and adolescents in the United States, Brazil, China, and Russia. *Am J Clin Nutr.*, 75(6), 971-7.

[7] Popkin, B. M. & Gordon-Larsen, P. (2004). The nutrition transition: worldwide obesity dynamics and their determinants. *Int J Obes Relat Metab Disord, 28* Suppl 3, S2-9.

[8]   Centers for Disease Control and Prevention (CDC). "*US Obesity Trends*". Available at: http://www.cdc.gov/obesity/data/trends.html. Accessed 9/26/2009.

[9]   Centers for Disease Control and Prevention (CDC). NHANES Surveys (1976–1980 and 2003–2006). Available at http://www.cdc.gov/obesity.

[10] Hedley, A. A., Ogden, C. L., Johnson, C. L., Carroll, M. D., Curtin, L. R. & Flegal, K. M. (2004). Prevalence of overweight and obesity among US children, adolescents, and adults, 1999-2002. *JAMA, 291(23)*, 2847-50.

[11] Lee, Y. S. (2009). Consequences of Childhood Obesity. *Ann Acad Med Singapore*, 38, 75-81.

[12] American Sleep Apnea Association. "*Sleep Apnea Information*". Available at: http://www.sleepapnea.org/info/index.html. Accessed 9/18/ 2009.

[13] Wills, M. (2004). Orthopedic Complications of Childhood Obesity. *Pediatric Physical Therapy, 16(4)*, 230-235.

[14] Hampel, H., Abraham, N. S. & El-Serag, H. B. (2005). Meta-analysis: obesity and the risk for gastroesophageal reflux disease and its complactions, *Ann Intern Med, 143(3)*, 199-211.

[15] Fishman, L., Lenders, C., Fortunato, C., Noonan, C. & Nurko, S. (2004). Increased prevalence of constipation and fecal soiling in a population of obese children. *J Pediatr., 145(2)*, 253-254.

[16] Gennuso, J., Epstein, L. H., Paluc, R. A. & Cerny, F., (1998). The relationship between asthma and overweight in urban minority children and adolescents. *Arch Pediatr Adolesc Med, 152*, 1197-1200.

[17] McCall, A. & Raj, R. (2009). Exercise for the prevention of obesity and diabetes in children. *Clin Sports Med, 28*, 393–421.

[18] Weigensberg, M. & Goran, M. (2009). Type 2 diabetes in children and adolescents. *Lancet, 373*, 1743-1744.

[19] Liao, C., Su, T., Chien, K., Wang, J., Chiang, C., Lin, C., Lin, R.S., Lee, Y. & Sung, F. (2009). Elevated blood pressure, obesity, and hyperlipidemia. *J Pediatr, 155(1)*, 79-83.

[20] Loomba, R., Sirlin, C. B., Schwimmer, J. B. & Lavine, J. E. (2009) Advances in pediatric nonalcoholic fatty liver disease. *Hepatology, 50(8)*, 1–12.

[21] Feldstein, A. E., Charatcharoenwitthaya, P., Treeprasertsuk, S., Benson, J. T., Enders, F. B. & Angulo, P., (2009) The natural history of nonalcoholic fatty liver disease in children: A follow-up study for up to 20-years. doi:10.1136/gut.2008.171280 *Gut* published online 21 Jul 2009.

[22] Robinson S. (2006) Victimization of obese adolescents. *J Sch Nurs, 22(4)*, 201-206.

[23] Falkner, N. H., Neumark-Sztainer, D., Story, M., Jeffery, R. W., Beuhring, T. & Resnick, M. D. (2001) Social, educational, and psychological correlates of weight status in adolescents. *Obes Res, 9(1)*, 32-42.

[24] Al Mamun, A., Cramb, S. & McDermott, B. M., O'Callaghan, M., Najman, J.M., Williams, G.M. (2007) Adolescents' perceived weight associated with depression *Obesity, 15(12)*, 3097-3105.

[25] French, S. A., Story, M. & Perry, C. L. (1995). Self-esteem and obesity in children and adolescents: a literature review. *Obes Res, 3*, 479-90.

[26] Davison K. K., Schmalz, D. L., Young, L. M. & Birch L. L. (2008). Overweight girls who internalize fat stereotypes report low psychosocial well-being. *Obesity, 16 Suppl 2*, S30-8.

[27] Borzekowski, D. L., Bayer, A. M. (2005). Body image and media use among adolescents. *Adolesc Med Clin.*, *16(2)*, 289-313.

[28] Finkelstein, E. A., Fiebelkorn, I. C. & Wang, G. (2003). National medical spending attributable to overweight and obesity: how much, and who's paying? *Health Aff.* Suppl Web Exclusives:W3-219-26.

[29] Trasande, L., Liu, Y., Fryer, G. & Weitzman, M. (2009). Effects of childhood obesity on hospital care and costs, 1999–2005. *Health Affairs, 28(4)*, w751–w760.

[30] Katz, D. L., O'Connell, M., Yeh, M. C., Nawaz, H., Njike, V., Anderson, L. M., Cory, S. & Dietz, W. (2005). Public health strategies for preventing and controlling overweight and obesity in school and worksite settings: a report on recommendations of the Task Force on Community Preventive Services. *MMWR Recomm Rep, 54*(RR-10), 1-12.

[31] Kropski, J. A., Keckley, P. H,, Jensen, G. L. (2008). School-based obesity prevention programs: an evidence-based review. *Obesity.* May; *16(5)*, 1009-18.

[32] Brown, T. & Summerbell, C. (2009). Systematic review of school-based interventions that focus on changing dietary intake and physical activity levels to prevent childhood obesity: an update to the obesity guidance produced by the National Institute for Health and Clinical Excellence. *Obes Rev, 10(1)*, 110-41.

[33] Katz, D. L. (2009). School-based interventions for health promotion and weight control: not just waiting on the world to change. *Annu Rev Public Health, 30*, 253-72.

[34] Katz, D. L., O'Connell, M., Njike, V. Y., Yeh, M. C. & Nawaz, H. (2008). Strategies for the prevention and control of obesity in the school setting: systematic review and meta-analysis. *Int J Obes*, *32(12)*, 1780-9.

[35] Frumkin, H. (2006). Introduction: Safe and healthy school environments. In *Safe and Healthy School Environments*, edited by H. Frumkin, R.J. Geller, I.L. Rubin, and J. Nodvin, 3–10. New York: Oxford University Press.

[36] United States Department of Agriculture. (USDA). National School Lunch Program Fact Sheet. Available at: http://www.fns.usda.gov/cnd/Lunch/. Accessed 9/27/09.

[37] Briefel, R. R., Wilson, A., Gleason, P. M. Consumption of low-nutrient dense foods and beverages at school, home and other locations among school lunch participants and nonparticipants. *J Am Diet Assoc.*, 2009, *109* (suppl 1), S79-S90.

[38] Fox, M. K., Hamilton, W., Lin, B. H. (2004). Effects of food assistance and nutrition programs on health and nutrition. *Vol. 3. Literature Review. Food Assist. Nutr. Res. Rep.* 19–3.

[39] Gordon, A., and M.K. Fox. (2007). School Nutrition Dietary Assessment Study-III: Summary of Findings. http://www.fns.usda.gov/oane/menu/Published/CNP/FILES/SNDAIII-SummaryofFindings.pdf. Accessed 10/27/2008.

[40] Institute of Medicine (IOM). (2007). *Nutrition Standards for Foods in Schools: Leading the way toward healthier youth.* Washington, D.C.: National Academies Press.

[41] Story, M., Nanney, M. S. & Schwartz, M. B. (2009). Schools and obesity prevention: Creating school environments and policies to promote healthy eating and physical activity. *The Milbank Quarterly*, *87(1)*, 71–100.

[42] U. S. Department of Health and Human Services and U.S. Department of Agriculture. (2005). "Dietary Guidelines for Americans, 2005," 6th ed. U.S. Government Printing Office, Washington, DC.

[43] School Nutrition Association (SNA). *A Matter of Standards: 2008 Legislative Issue Paper*.http://www.schoolnutrition.org/uploadedFiles/School_Nutrition/106_Legislative Action/SNAPositionStatements/IndividualPositionStatements/SNA.Final.IP.2008.pdf. Accessed 8/15/ 2009.

[44] Black, J. & Macinko, J. Neighborhoods and obesity. *Nutr Rev.*, 2008, *66*, 2-20.

[45] Drewnowski, A. Obesity, diets, and social inequalities. *Nutr Rev.*, 2009, *67*(Suppl 1), S36-S39.

[46] Fox, M., Dod, A.H., Wilson, A., Gleason, P.M. (2009) Association between school food environment and practices and body mass index of US public school children. *J Am Diet Assoc.*, *109*, S108-S117.

[47] Martin, J. (2008). Overview of Federal Child Nutrition Legislation. In *Managing Child Nutrition Programs: Leadership for Excellence*, 2nd ed., edited by J. Martin and C.B. Oakley, 145–99. Sudbury, Mass.: Jones and Bartlett.

[48] National Association for Sport and Physical Education (NASPE) and American Heart Association (AHA). (2006). *Shape of the Nation Report: Status of Physical Education in the USA*. Reston, Va.

[49] Story, M., Kaphingst, K., Robinson-O'Brian, R. & Glanz, K. (2008) Creating healthy food and eating environments: Policy and environmental approaches. *Annu. Rev. Public Health*, *29*, 253-72.

[50] O'Toole, T. P., Anderson, S., Miller, C. & Guthrie, J. (2007). Nutrition services and foods and beverages available at school: Results from the School Health Policies and Programs Study 2006. *J Sch Health, 77(8)*, 500–521.

[51] Economic Research Service. United States Department of Agriculture. 2008 Farm Bill Side by Side. Availalbe at: http://www.ers.usda.gov/FarmBill/2008/titles/ titleIVNutrition.htm. Accessed 9/27/09.

[52] Lee, S. M., Burgeson, C. R., Fulton, J. E. & Spain, C. G. (2007) Physical education and physical activity: Results from the School Health Policies and Programs Study 2006. *J Sch Health, 77(8)*, 435–63.

[53] Justus, M. B., Ryan, K.W., Rockenbach, J., Katterapalli, C. & Card-Higginson, P. (2007). Lessons learned while implementing a legislated school policy: body mass index assessments among Arkansas's public school students. *J Sch Health, 77(10)*, 706–13.

[54] Trust for America's Health. 2007. *F as in Fat: How Obesity Policies Are Failing in America, 2007*. Available at http://healthyamericans.org/reports/obesity2007/Obesity 2007Report.pdf. Accessed 6/20/ 2008.

[55] Kubik, M. Y., Story, M. & Rieland, G. (2007). Developing school-based BMI screening and parent notification programs: Findings from focus groups with parents of elementary school students. *Health Education & Behavior*, *34(4)*, 622–33.

[56] Davison, K. K. & Birch, L. L. (2001). Childhood overweight: a contextual model and recommendations for future research. *Obes Rev*, *2(3)*, 159-71.

[57] Yeh, M. C. & Katz, D. L. (2006). Food, nutrition and the health of urban populations. In Freudenberg N, Galea S, Vlahov D (eds.). *Cities and the Health of the Public.* Nashville: Vanderbilt University Press. 106-125.

[58] Kahn, E. B., Ramsey, L. T., Brownson, R. C., et al. (2002). The effectiveness of interventions to increase physical activity: a systematic review. *Am J Prev Med*, *22(4S)*, 73–107.

[59] Vaughn, A. E., Ball, S. C., Linnan, L. A., Marchetti, L. M., Hall, W. L. & Ward, D. S. (2009). Promotion of walking for transportation: a report from the Walk to School day registry. *J Phys Act Health.*, *6(3)*, 281-8.

[60] Walders-Abramson, N., Wamboldt, F. S., Curran-Everett, D. & Zhang, L. (2009). Encouraging physical activity in pediatric asthma: A Case–Control Study of the Wonders of Walking (WOW) Program. *Pediatric Pulmonology.* *44*, 909–916.

[61] Goldfield, G. S., Kalakanis, L. E., Ernst, M. M., Epstein, L. H. (2000). Open-loop feedback to increase physical activity in obese children. *Int J Obes Relat Metab Disord.* *24,* 888–892.

[62] Roemmich, J. N., Gurgol, C. M. & Epstein, L. H.. (2004). Open-loop feedback increases physical activity of youth. *Med Sci Sports Exerc*, *36*, 668–673.

[63] Bassett, M. T., Dumanovsky, T., Huang, C., Silver, L. D., Young, C., Nonas, C., Matte, T. D., Chideya, S. & Frieden, T. R. (2008). Purchasing behavior and calorie information at fast-food chains in New York City, 2007. *Am J Public Health*, *98(8),* 1457-1459.

[64] Kuo, T., Jarosz, C. J., Simon, P. & Fielding, J. E. (2009). Menu labeling as a potential strategy for combating the obesity epidemic: a health impact assessment. *Am J Public Health, 99(9)*, 1680-1686.

[65] National Restaurant Association. 2007. *Industry research.* http://www.restaurant.

[66] Bowman, S. A., Gortmaker, S. L., Ebbeling, C. B., Pereira, M. A. & Ludwig, D. S. (2004). Effects of fast-food consumption on energy intake and diet quality among children in a national household survey. *Pediatrics, 113*, 112–18.

[67] McCrory, M. A., Fuss, P. J., Hays, N. P., Vinken, A. G., Greenberg, A. S. & Roberts, S. B. (1999). Overeating in America: association between restaurant food consumption and body fatness in healthy adult men and women ages 19 to 80. *Obes. Res., 7*, 564–71.

[68] Pereira, M. A., Kartashov, A. I., Ebbeling, C. B., Van Horn, L., Slattery, M. L., et al. (2005) Fastfood habits, weight gain, and insulin resistance (the CARDIA study): 15-year prospective analysis. *Lancet, 365, 36*–42.

[69] Burton, S., Creyer, E. H., Kees, J. & Huggins, K. (2006). Attacking the obesity epidemic: the potential health benefits of providing nutrition information in restaurants. *Am. J. Public Health, 96*, 1669–75.

[70] Levy, J. (2007). *10 Ways to get healthy, local foods into low-income neighborhoods: A Minneapolis resource guide.* http://www.iatp.org/iatp/publications.cfm?accountID=258&refID=97319.

[71] Healthy Corner Stores Network. Participant Profiles by State. Available at http://healthycornerstores.org/profiles/?order=location. Accessed 9/29/2009.

[72] Center for Disease Control and Prevention. (2009). Recommended Community Strategies and Measurements to Prevent Obesity in the United States. MMWR; 58 (No. RR-7).

[73] Story, M., Kaphingst, K. M., French, S. The role of schools in obesity prevention. *Future Child.* 2006, *16*, 109-142.

[74] Davis, B. & Carpenter, C. (2009). Proximity of fast-food restaurants to schools and adolescent obesity. *Am J Public Health*, *99*, 505–510.

[75] Food and Nutrition Service. United States Department of Agriculture. *WIC Food Packages.* Available at: http://www.fns.usda.gov/wic/benefitsandservices/foodpkg.htm. Accessed 9/29/ 2009.

[76] Global Development and Environment Institute, Tufts University. *Sweetening the Pot*. http://www.ase.tufts.edu/gdae/Pubs/rp/PB09-01SweeteningPotFeb09.pdf.   Accessed 9/1/09.

[77] United States Department of Agriculture. *Food Guide Pyramid*. Available at: www.mypyramid.gov. Accessed 12/20/2008.

[78] Economic Research Service. United States Department of Agriculture, *Food Consumption Data*. Available at: http://www.ers.usda.gov/Data/FoodConsumption/ FoodGuideIndex.htm. Accessed 1/10/2009.

In: Overweightness and Walking
Editor: Caleb I. Black, pp. 211-222

ISBN: 978-1-60741-298-4
© 2010 Nova Science Publishers, Inc.

Chapter 10

OVERWEIGHT AND OBESITY AMONG COMMUNITY-DWELLING OLDER ADULTS: HEALTH-RELATED ISSUES AND TREATMENT

M. Y. Mimi Tse*, W. Y. Peony Lai, S. M. Rose Heung and F. F. Iris Benzie

The Hong Kong Polytechnic University, Kowloon, Hong Kong

ABSTRACT

Background

Good dietary habits are important for health enhancement, while inadequate nutrition may increase susceptibility to and delay recovery from illness. To meet the needs of frail older persons and to promote functional longevity, health education on proper nutrition and exercise is important. Obesity is a relatively serious problem in Hong Kong Chinese, as elsewhere in the developed world, owing to the associated increased risks for Type 2 diabetes mellitus, cardiovascular disease and cancer.

Project Aims & Preliminary Findings

In this study, the prevalence of overweight and obesity among community-dwelling older persons was explored, and health-related issues regarding obesity were discussed. The study also examined the effects of a nutrition education program.

A total of 61 older persons (12 males and 49 females, ages ranging from 60 to 89 years, with mean age 73 years) from two elderly community centers took part in the study. Education level, self-reported health status, body mass index, dietary habits and physical exercise pattern were recorded.

Over 50% reported receiving no formal education. The majority were suffering from at least one chronic illness (hypertension, diabetes, hyperlipidemia or osteoporosis). None

---

* Corresponding author: Tel: 852 2766 6541; Fax: 852 2364 9663; Email: hsmtse@inet.polyu.edu.hk

knew their BMI. The prevalence of overweight and obesity were very high, with 70% (n=38) overweight or obese.

Consumption of 'desirable' foods (fruits, vegetables, dairy and bean curd products) was low. Participants' intake of fruits and vegetables was inadequate, with 65% of the participants consuming ≤ 1 serving of fruit/day and 33% consuming < 3 servings of vegetables/day. The majority (80%) did not consume any dairy products.

Intervention: Nutrition Education Programme

A nutrition and lifestyle program (NLP) was provided to these elderly in the community centers, and a learning contract approach was used to encourage older people to adhere to the programe.

The NLP lasted for 8 weeks, and covered nutritional labeling, identifying healthy and unhealthy snacks and food (e.g. those high in cholesterol, saturated fat, salt), meal planning, and encouraging physical activity.

Evaluation & Conclusion

Participating elderly were followed up weekly regarding their learning contract on dietary modification and physical activity. Participation in the nutrition education program was high (nearly 95%); participants demonstrated increased knowledge and awareness of their health and nutritional status and were willing to follow the advice on dietary modification and lead a more active lifestyle.

Nutrition behavior is a complex process; a holistic health promotion approach seems to be essential for implementing healthy nutrition behavior.

INTRODUCTION

Obesity is a global epidemic. More than one billion adults are overweight and over 300 million have a BMI of $\geq 30 kgm^2$ (WHO, 1998; WHO, 2000). It has been suggested that obesity will become the leading cause of death among the various 'lifestyle-related diseases' in the USA (Mokdad et al., 2000). Non-communicable diseases, namely type 2 diabetes, cardiovascular diseases, hypertension, stroke and certain cancers, are chronic and disabling, and are largely preventable. As such, obesity and overweight are major contributing factors for the development of non-communicable diseases. In Hong Kong, 63% of all deaths are related to non-communicable diseases including cancer, heart diseases, stroke and external causes of morbidity and mortality. To promote the health of our population, the problem of obesity and overweight is a key issue to tackle.

In Hong Kong, the prevalence of obesity is similar to that of Japan but less severe as compared with European populations (Janus et al., 1997; Yoshiike, 1998; Seidell & Flegal, 1997). Nearly half of women aged 45 or over were overweight (BMI $\geq 25 kgm^2$), and nearly 10% of these were obese (BMI $\geq 30 kgm^2$), though no significant differences were found among different age groups for men. Prevalence was highest (over 53%) among the 55-64 age group for both genders (Department of Health, 2005).

Measurement of Obesity

Obesity is defined as a condition in which there is an excess of body fat (Western Pacific Regional Office of WHO, 2000). Among all screening tests for obesity, the most common involve measuring waist-hip ratio and waist circumference, in which waist cut-off points differ significantly with different studies (Li, 2002). Some techniques to measure body fat are also expensive, complicated and not readily available, including, for example, computerized tomography, densitometry, dual-energy X-ray absorptiometry and magnetic resonance imaging (Department of Health, 2005; Heymsfield, 2005). Body mass index (BMI) is calculated as weight in kilograms divided by height in meters squared, and individuals are classified as underweight, normal, overweight or obese according to pre-defined BMI cut-off points. BMI is regarded as the most commonly used tool, and is easy to measure, highly reliable and best correlated to body fat content (Bray, 2004). BMI is commonly used as a marker for obesity in epidemiological studies.

For classification of adult body weight, the World Health Organization (WHO) defines a BMI of 18.5-24.9kgm² as the optimal or normal range, and BMIs of ≥25 and ≥30kgm² as overweight and obese respectively (WHO, 1998). As increasing evidence has shown that the risk of co-morbidities in relation to BMI differs among different races, the WHO has issued guidelines with different cut-off values to classify overweight and obesity for Asian populations (Table 1).

Impact of Overweight and Obesity on Older Persons' Health

Obesity poses a significant issue to the health of older persons; it was suggested that increasing age would also result in increases in body mass index as well as cardiovascular risk, including glucose intolerance, hypertension, dyslipidemia and obesity (Ko et al., 1997).

It is well known that obesity is related to negative physical and psychological health consequences. There is increased risk of various kinds of diseases. In terms of physical health consequences, disorders include cardiovascular disease such as hypertension and coronary heart disease, stroke, pulmonary disease such as obstructive sleep apnea, musculoskeletal diseases such as osteoarthritis, gastrointestinal disease such as nonalcoholic fatty liver disease, infertility, metabolic syndrome including type II diabetes mellitus, and even cancer. As for psychological consequences, lowered self-esteem, anxiety and mood disorders such as depression are also reported (Becker et al., 2001; Istfan & Anderson, 2007; WHO, 1998).

Table 1. Classification of BMI for Adult Asians by WHO

Classification	BMI (kg/m2)
Underweight	<18.5
Normal range	18.5-22.9
Overweight:	≥23
Pre-obese	23-24.9
Obese I	25-29.9
Obese II	≥30

Prevalence of Overweight and Obesity among Community-Dwelling Older Persons

The prevalence of overweight and obesity among community-dwelling older persons was explored. A total of 61 older persons (12 males and 49 females; ages ranging from 60 to 89 years, with mean age 73 years) from two elderly community centers took part in the study. Education level, self-reported health status, body mass index, dietary habits and physical exercise pattern were recorded. The demographic data are shown in table 2.

Over 50% reported receiving neither formal education nor any nutrition education. The majority suffered from at least one chronic illness (hypertension, diabetes, hyperlipidemia or osteoporosis). None knew their Body Mass Index (BMI). The prevalence of overweight and obesity were very high, with 70% (n=38) overweight or obese.

Table 2. Demographic data (N=61)

All participants (N=61)	
Age	
Mean±SD	73.62 ± 7.870
Range	60-89
Gender	**Number (Percent)**
Female	49 (80.3%)
Male	12 (19.7%)
Presence of Chronic Diseases	**Number (Percent)**
No chronic diseases	8 (13.1%)
One or more chronic diseases	53 (86.9%)
Health Conditions	**Number (Percent)**
Hypertension	33 (54.1%)
Non-insulin dependent diabetes	17 (27.9%)
Hyperlipidemia	8 (13.1%)
Osteoporosis	10 (16.4%)
Arthritis	4 (6.6%)
Other diseases such as respiratory diseases, cardiovascular diseases, gout, thyroid disease	11 (18%)
Religion	**Number (Percent)**
No religion	26 (42.6%)
Buddist	30 (49.2%)
Christian	3 (4.9%)
Catholic	1 (1.6%)
Others: Japanese religion	1 (1.6%)
Living Condition	**Number (Percent)**
Living alone	16 (26.2%)
Living with wife/husband	10 (16.4%)
Living with children	16 (26.2%)
Living with wife/husband and children	17 (27.9%)
Living with other people	2 (3.3%)

Table 2. (Continued)

All participants (N=61)	
Marital Status	**Number (Percent)**
Single	1 (1.6%)
Married	31 (50.8%)
Divorced/Separated	3 (4.9%)
Widowed	26 (42.6%)
Education Level	**Number (Percent)**
No formal education	30 (49.2%)
Primary education	24 (39.3%)
Junior secondary education	4 (6.6%)
Secondary education	0 (0%)
Tertiary education	3 (4.9%)
Received Nutrition Education	**Number (Percent)**
No nutrition education received	30 (49.2%)
Had received nutrition education (group or individual consultation)	31 (50.8%)

Intervention: Nutrition and Lifestyle Program

A nutrition and lifestyle program (NLP) was provided to these elderly in the community centers, and a learning contract approach was used to encourage them to adhere to the program. The nutrition and lifestyle program lasted for 8 weeks, and covered nutritional labeling, identifying healthy and unhealthy snacks and food (e.g. those high in cholesterol, saturated fat, salt), meal planning, and encouraging physical activity.

There were two practical sessions: visiting the virtual supermarket and healthy Chinese tea. The virtual supermarket visit tapped into the knowledge acquired in the previous class and required the participants to choose snacks of their own by reading food labels, and hopefully to make a healthy choice. For the Chinese tea session, participants were treated to 'dim sum', which reinforced the knowledge acquired by encouraging them to take an 'appropriate' amount of healthy 'dim sum', but to avoid over eating.

Dietary and Lifestyle Pattern: Before and after the Nutrition and Lifestyle Program

Before attending the nutrition and lifestyle program, consumption of 'desirable' foods (fruits & vegetables) was low. Participants' intake of fruits and vegetables was inadequate, with 65% of the participants consuming ≤ 2 servings of fruit per day, which means that only 35% consumed an adequate amount of > 2 servings of fruit per day. Also, 33% of the participants were consuming < 3 servings of vegetables per day, which means that 67% of them consumed > 3 servings of vegetables per day. In terms of physical activity and exercise, it was good to find that 77% of the participants exercised for 30 to 60 minutes per day, which is considered to be adequate.

58 older adults completed the NLP. Upon completion of the NLP, 26% of the participants understood their BMI and its interpretation as a health marker. Also, there were significant increases in both the consumption of 'desirable' foods and exercise (p <0.05). Participants' intake of fruits and vegetables was adequate, with 87% of the participants consuming 3 servings of fruit per day and 92% consuming more than 3 servings of vegetables per day. All participants (100%) exercised for more than 60 minutes per day.

The NLP was effective in terms of achieving desirable food consumption and improving understanding of BMI and the risk factors associated with obesity and overweight.

Table 3. Dietary and lifestyle pattern: pre- (n=61) and post-NLP (n=58)

	Pre-NLP (N=61)	Post-NLP (N=58)	
Knowledge of the BMI	**Number (Percent)**	**Number (Percent)**	**p-value**
Don't know what BMI is	61 (100%)	43 (74.1%)	**0.000#**
Know what BMI is	0 (0%)	15 (25.9%)	
BMI	**Number (Percent)**	**Number (Percent)**	**p-value**
Underweight (<18.5)	4 (6.6%)	2 (3.4%)	0.915
Normal weight (18.5-22.9)	19 (31.1%)	21 (36.2%)	
Overweight (23-24.9)	16 (26.2%)	16 (27.6%)	
Severely overweight (25-30)	18 (29.5%)	15 (25.9%)	
Obese (>30)	4 (6.6%)	4 (6.9%)	
Grocery shopping	**Number (Percent)**	**Number (Percent)**	**p-value**
Done by themselves	44 (72.1%)	41 (70.7%)	0.999
Done by their wives/husbands	5 (8.2%)	5 (8.6%)	
Done by their children	11 (18%)	11 (19%)	
Done by a maid or someone else	1 (1.6%)	1 (1.7%)	
Meal preparation	**Number (Percent)**	**Number (Percent)**	**p-value**
By themselves	42 (68.9%)	39 (67.2%)	0.998
By their wives/husbands	7 (11.5%)	7 (12.1%)	
By their children	11 (18%)	11 (19%)	
By a maid or someone else	1 (1.6%)	1 (1.7%)	
Habit of eating breakfast	**Number (Percent)**	**Number (Percent)**	**p-value**
Have breakfast every day	58 (95.1%)	57 (98.3%)	0.334
Do not have breakfast every day	3 (4.9%)	1 (1.7%)	
The number of main meals per day	**Number (Percent)**	**Number (Percent)**	**p-value**
Two main meals per day	5 (8.2%)	2 (3.4%)	0.271
Three or more main meals per day	56 (91.8%)	56 (96.6%)	
Snack-eating habit	**Number (Percent)**	**Number (Percent)**	**p-value**
No snacks	30 (49.2%)	28 (48.3%)	0.988
Frequent snacks	14 (23%)	14 (24.1%)	
Occasional snacks or when hungry between main meals	17 (27.9%)	16 (27.6%)	
Consumption of bread & cereals per day	**Number (Percent)**	**Number (Percent)**	**p-value**
<3 servings	0 (0%)	0 (0%)	**0.002#**
3 - 4 servings	9 (14.8%)	0 (0%)	
≥5 servings	52 (85.2%)	58 (100%)	

Table 3. (Continued)

	Pre-NLP (N=61)	Post-NLP (N=58)	
Consumption of meat group per day	Number (Percent)	Number (Percent)	p-value
<1 servings	5 (8.2%)	0 (0%)	0.000#
1-2 servings	21 (34.4%)	2 (3.4%)	
≥2 servings	35 (57.4%)	56 (96.6%)	
Consumption of milk group per day	Number (Percent)	Number (Percent)	p-value
<0.5 servings	45 (73.8%)	5 (8.6%)	0.000#
0.5-1 servings	7 (11.5%)	3 (5.2%)	
≥1 servings	9 (14.8%)	50 (86.2%)	
Consumption of fluid per day	Number (Percent)	Number (Percent)	p-value
<3 cups	1 (1.6%)	1 (1.7%)	0.002#
3-5 cups	14 (23%)	1 (1.7%)	
≥5 cups	46 (75.4%)	56 (96.6%)	
Consumption of vegetables per day	Number (Percent)	Number (Percent)	p-value
<2 servings	9 (14.8%)	0 (0%)	0.002#
≥2 servings and <3 servings	11 (18%)	5 (8.6%)	
≥3 servings	41 (67.2%)	53 (91.4%)	
Consumption of fruits per day	Number (Percent)	Number (Percent)	p-value
<2 servings	40 (65.6%)	8 (13.8%)	0.000#
2-3 servings	21 (34.4%)	50 (86.2%)	
Risk of under-nourishment	Number (Percent)	Number (Percent)	p-value
At risk of under-nourishment	5 (8.2%)	4 (6.9%)	0.789
Not at risk of under-nourishment	56 (91.8%)	54 (93.1%)	
Drinking alcohol	Number (Percent)	Number (Percent)	p-value
Every day	1 (1.6%)	1 (1.7%)	0.931
Sometimes	6 (9.8%)	4 (6.9%)	
Never	48 (78.7%)	46 (79.3%)	
Quit two or more years ago	6 (9.8%)	7 (12.1%)	
Smoking	Number (Percent)	Number (Percent)	p-value
Every day	2 (3.3%)	2 (3.4%)	0.809
Sometimes	1 (1.6%)	0 (0%)	
Never	46 (75.4%)	44 (75.9%)	
Quit two or more years ago	12 (19.7%)	12 (20.7%)	
Physical exercise	Number (Percent)	Number (Percent)	p-value
Do physical exercise every day	58 (95.1%)	58 (100%)	0.232
Physical exercise two days per week	1 (1.6%)	0 (0%)	
Physical exercise three days per week	2 (3.3%)	0 (0%)	
Duration of daily physical exercise	Number (Percent)	Number (Percent)	p-value
<30 minutes	1 (1.6%)	0 (0%)	0.000#
30-60 minutes	47 (77%)	18 (31%)	
>60 minutes	13 (21.3%)	40 (69%)	

* Chi-squared test was used.

\# A p value of < 0.05 was considered statistically significant.

Recommendations: Management of Overweight and Obesity for Older Adults

The World Health Organization (2003) suggests that healthy diets and regular physical activities are essential components of an effective weight management strategy.

1. Energy balance

The balance between energy intake and energy expenditure determines body weight and body fat. A negative energy balance can be induced by a reduction in energy consumed and an increase in energy expended. It will result in a decrease in body fat stores and weight loss (Department of Health, 1991).

2. Calculating total energy requirement

The basal metabolic rate (BMR) for elderly people can be determined by using the Schofield equations (Table 1.1). Determination of total energy requirements is done by multiplying the BMR value with a physical activity (PA) factor of 1.4 for a non-active lifestyle. The PA for a moderately active lifestyle is 1.5, while it is 1.6 for a very active lifestyle (Todorovic & Micklewright, 2007).

For an adult to lose 1 to 2 pounds per week (equivalent to 3500kcal or 500kcal/day x 7days), s/he would have to remove 500 to 600 kcal from the total daily energy requirements.

For elderly people, the energy needed for weight reduction is controversial. According to one theory, elderly people can lose 1 to 2 pounds per 2 weeks by removing 250 to 300 kcal from total daily energy requirements (Example 1).

Example 1:
A 65-year old lady, sedentary lifestyle, weight 65 kg, height 1.64 m (BMI 24.2)

$$BMR = 9.2 \times 65 + 687$$

$$= 1285 \text{ kcal} \times 1.4$$

$$= 1799 \text{ kcal}$$

Subtract 300 kcal for weight loss
Gives a daily calorie allowance of 1499 kcal per day

Table 4. Equations for estimating basal metabolic rate (Schofield equations)

Females over 60 yrs (kcal/day)		Males over 60 yrs (kcal/day)	
60 – 74 years	9.2W + 687	60 – 74 yrs	11.9W + 700
75 years +	9.8W + 624	75 years +	8.3W + 820

W = weight in kg

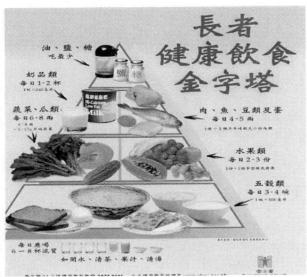

Grains & cereals 3-4 bowls
Vegetables 6-8 portions
Fruits 2-3 portions
Meat, poultry, fish, dry beans & eggs 4-5 portions
Dairy products 1-2 glasses
Eat less fat, oil, salts & sweets
Drink 6-8 glasses of fluid every day, including water, tea, fruit juice, soup

Figure 1. Healthy Eating Pyramid for the Elderly

3. Regular Meals

To increase satiety and prevent snacking on high-fat, energy-dense foods, elderly people's diet should include three main meals and two to three healthy snacks between meals (Holt et al., 1992). To get a wide range of essential nutrients, a well-balanced diet based on the Healthy Eating Pyramid should be planned, and the number of servings suggested for the daily diet in the Healthy Eating Pyramid should be followed (Figure 1) (SH Ho Centre for Gerontology and Geriatrics, 2006). Controlling portion size can help in achieving appropriate calorie intake and enhancing weight loss (Marchessault et al., 2007).

4. Diet Modification

In order to reduce energy intake and enhance satiety, the following strategies should be applied in choosing low-energy dense foods (Example 2):

emphasizing high-fiber food such as whole grains and cereals, vegetables and fruits (Marchessault et al., 2007; Grace, 2001)
choosing lean cuts of meat and trimming off the skin or fat of poultry (Grace, 2001)

choosing low-fat cooking methods such as boiling, steaming, stewing or simmering instead of frying or deep-frying

avoiding food with high fat content, including sausages, canned food such as spam and corned beef, and pastry items such as egg tarts and baked barbecued pork puffs

choosing skim or low-fat milk, low-fat yogurt or cheese

substituting lower-fat foods for high-fat foods

minimizing the consumption of sugary foods such as honey, candy, condensed milk, and dessert or sweetened beverages.

avoiding alcoholic beverages

5. Physical Activity

To promote health, psychological wellbeing, and a healthy body weight, the elderly should engage in regular physical activities which they can tolerate and enjoy, e.g. a 15-minute brisk walk after each meal (WHO, 2003).

Example 2: 24-hour Diet Recall for Tom

Wake up (6:30am)	
Breakfast (8:00am)	Wheat bread 1 slice
	Oatmeal (dry) 4 tablespoons
	Whole egg 1
	Cucumber 1 piece
Lunch (12:30pm)	Rice 2 bowls
	Meat 3 teals
	Boiled vegetables 1 bowl
Dinner (7:30pm)	Rice 2 bowls
	Meat 3 teals
	Boiled vegetables 1 bowl
Bedtime (10:30pm)	
Recommendation:	
Regular meals	
• having breakfast at 7:00am • adding healthy snacks at 3:00pm, e.g. 1 medium fruit, 1 glass of skim milk or a packet of soda crackers	
Portion control	
• learning the appropriate portion sizes, such as sandwiches for breakfast, 1 to 1 1/2 bowls of rice for lunch and dinner	
Physical activity	
• 15 minutes' brisk walking after breakfast, lunch and dinner	

REFERENCES

Becker, E. S., Margraf, J., Turke, V., Soeder, U. & Neumer, S. (2001). Obesity and mental illness in a representative sample of young women. *International Journal of Obesity and Related Metabolic Disorders*, *25*(Suppl 1), S5-9.

Bray, G. A. (2004). *Classification and evaluation of the overweight patient. In G.A. Bray & C. Bouchard (Eds.),* Handbook of obesity: Clinical applications (2nd ed., p.1-32). New York: Dekker.

Department of Health (1991). *Healthy dietary reference values for food energy and nutrients for United Kingdom.* HMSO: London.

Department of Health (2005). *Population Health Survey* 2003/2004. Hong Kong: Department of Health.

Department of Health (2005). *Tackling Obesity: Its Causes, the Plight and Preventive Actions.* Hong Kong: Department of Health.

Grace, C. M. (2001). *Dietary management of obesity. In P. G. Kopelman (Eds.),* Management of Obesity and Related Disorders (129-158). United Kingdom: Martin Duntiz

Heymsfield, S. B., Lohman, T. G., Wang, Z. & Going, S. (2005). *Human Body Composition* (2nd ed.). Champaign: Human Kinetics.

Holt, S., Brand, J., Soveny, C. & Hansky, J. (1992). Relationship of satiety to postprandial glycaemic, insulin, and cholecystokinin responses. *Appetite, 18,* 129-41.

Istfan, N. W. & Anderson, W. A. (2007). Steps for the medical evaluation of the obese patient. In Apovian, C.M. & Lenders, C. M. (2007), *A Clinical Guide for Management of Overweight and Obese Children and Adults* (15-28). New York: CRC Press.

Janus, E. D., Cockram, C., Fielding R., Hedley, A., Ho, P., Lam, K. (1997). *Hong Kong cardiovascular risk factor prevalence study* 1995-1996. Hong Kong: University of Hong Kong.

Ko, G. T. C., Chan, J. C. N., Woo, J., Lau, E. M. C., Yeung, V. T. F., Chow, C. C., Wai, H. P. S., Li, J. K. Y., So, W. Y. & Cockram, C. S. (1997). The effect of age on cardiovascular risk factors in Chinese women. *International Journal of Cardiology*, *61*, 221-227.

Kwok, P. & Tse, L. Y. (2004). Overweight and obesity in Hong Kong – What do we know? *Public Health & Epidemiology Bulletin*, *13(4)*, 53-60.

Li G., Chen X., Jang, Y., Wang J., Xing, X., Yang, W., Hu, Y. (2002). Obesity, coronary heart disease risk factors and diabetes in Chinese: an approach to the criteria of obesity in the Chinese population. *Obesity Reviews*, 3(3), 167-172.

Marchessault, G., Thiele, K., Armit, E., Chapman, G. E., Levy-Milne, R. & Barr, S. I. (2007). Canadian dietitians' understanding of non-dieting approaches in weight management. *Canadian Journal of Dietetic Practice and Research, 68,* 67-72.

Mokdad, A. H., Serdula, M. K., Dietz, W. H., Bowman, B. A., Marks, J. S. & Jeffery, P. (2000). The continuing epidemic of obesity in the United States. *JAMA, 284*(13), 1650-1651.

Seidell, J. C. & Flegal, K. M. (1997). Assessing obesity: classification and epidemiology. *British Medical Bulletin*, *53*, 238-252.

SH Ho Centre for Gerontology and Geriatrics (2006). *Principles of Healthy Eating for the Elderly.* June 9 2009, retrieved from website: http://healthyageing.sph.cuhk.edu.hk/healthy%20diet_en.htm

Todorovic, V. E. & Micklewright, A. (2007). *A pocket guide to clinical nutrition* (3rd ed.). The Parental and Enteral Nutrition Group of the British Dietetic Association: Britain.

Western Pacific Regional Office of World Health Organization (2000). *The Asia Pacific perspective: Redefining obesity and its treatment.* WPRO: Australia.

World Health Organization (1998). *Prevention and Management of the Global Epidemic of Obesity. Report of the WHO Consultation on Obesity.* WHO: Geneva.

World Health Organization (2000). *Obesity: Preventing and Managing the Global Epidemic. WHO Obesity Technical Report Series no.894.* WHO: Geneva.

World Health Organization (2003). *Global strategy on diet, physical activity and health: Fact sheet – Obesity and overweight.*

World Health Organization (2003). *Factsheet: Obesity and overweight – global strategy on diet, physical activity and health.*

Yoshiike, N., Matsumura, Y., Zaman, M. M. & Yamaguchi, M. (1998). Descriptive epidemiology of body mass index in Japanese adults in a representative sample from the National Nutrition survey 1990-94. *International Journal of Obesity and Related Metabolic Disorders*, 22, 684-687.

INDEX

D

E

H

M

N

O

P

Q

R

T

U

V

X

W

Y